ANATOMICAL CHART COMPANY

DISEASES
&DISORDERS
FOURTH EDITION

The World's Best Anatomical Charts

ANATOMICAL CHART COMPANY

DISEASES & DISORDERS

FOURTH EDITION

The World's Best Anatomical Charts

CLINICAL EDITOR

ADELE WEBB, PHD, RN, FNAP, FAAN

Senior Academic Director of Workforce Solutions
Capella University
Minneapolis, Minnesota

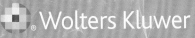

Philadelphia • Baltimore • New York • Londo
Buenos Aires • Hong Kong • Sydney • Tokyo

Acquisitions Editor: Crystal Taylor
Development Editor: Amy Millholen
Editorial Coordinator: Jeremiah Kiely
Editorial Assistant: Parisa Saranj
Marketing Manager: Tyrone Williams
Senior Production Project Manager: Alicia Jackson
Design Coordinator: Holly McLaughlin
Artist/Illustrator: Jen Clements
Manufacturing Coordinator: Margie Orzech-Zeranko
Prepress Vendor: SPi Global

Fourth Edition

Library of Congress Cataloging-in-Publication Data
Names: Webb, Adele A., author. | Anatomical Chart Co.
Title: Diseases & disorders : the world's best anatomical charts / Adele Webb.
Other titles: Diseases and disorders | Preceded by (work): Diseases & disorders.
Description: Fourth edition. | Philadelphia : Wolters Kluwer, [2020] | At head of title: Anatomical Chart Company. | Preceded by Diseases & disorders : world's best anatomical charts / Anatomical Chart Company. 3rd ed. c2008.
Identifiers: LCCN 2019003914 | ISBN 9781975110239
Subjects: | MESH: Disease | Pathology | Anatomy | Atlas
Classification: LCC QM25 | NLM QZ 17 | DDC 611.0022/3—dc23 LC record available at https://lccn.loc.gov/2019003914

CCS1020

CONTENTS

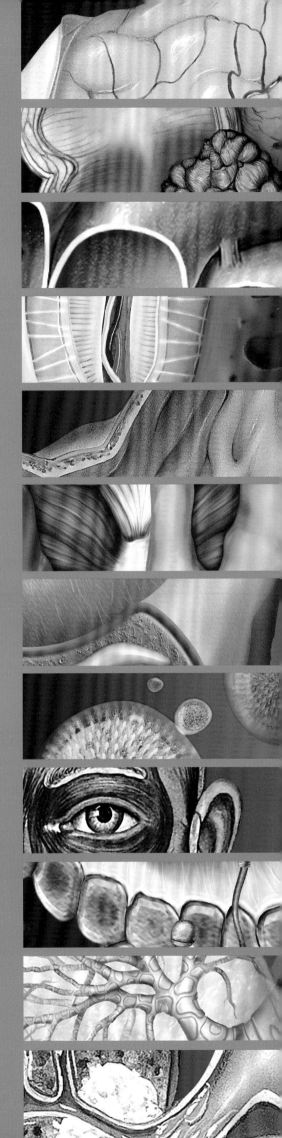

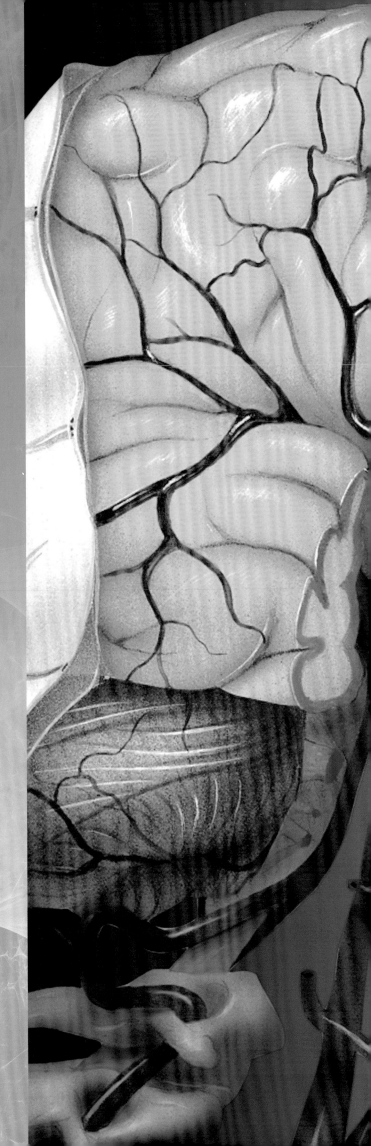

BRAIN DISEASES & DISORDERS

Understanding
Alzheimer's Disease

The most common form of dementia is Alzheimer's disease (AD), a slowly progressive disorder that destroys the neurons and communication pathways of the brain. It is the seventh leading cause of death in adults in the United States, and it is perhaps the most devastating chronic disease for patients and their families.

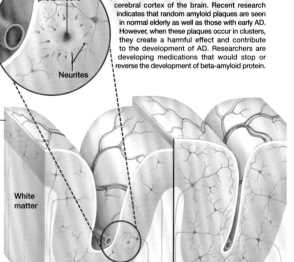

Hippocampus: memory and learning

Nucleus basalis of Meynert: relay center of neurons requiring acetylcholine

Amygdala: emotions

Hippocampus: memory and learning

Parietal lobe: language, sense of temperature, touch, pain, and space

Frontal lobe: reasoning, personality, movement, speech

Occipital lobe: vision

Temporal lobe: hearing, memory, language

The Aging Brain and Dementia

At birth, the brain contains as many nerve cells called neurons as it will ever have—many billions of neurons! Unlike other cells of our body, such as skin or bone, neurons cannot reproduce themselves. Therefore, as we age, neurons that die from normal wear and tear and injury are not replaced. The normal effects of aging can cause mild forgetfulness and reduced reflexes. However, there are diseases known as dementias that mimic these age-related changes in their early stages. Dementia is characterized by the progressive, yet dramatic, decline of cognitive function.

Diagnosing Alzheimer's Disease

Unfortunately, certain diagnosis of AD is done only by examining the brain at the time of death when an autopsy can supply an adequate sample of brain tissue. However, a thorough workup can help identify some of the hallmark features of AD and guide doctors toward this diagnosis. For example, blood tests to eliminate the possibility of infectious or metabolic disturbances; an MRI scan to reveal structural problems or history of strokes; and finally, neuropsychological tests to evaluate memory, spatial tasks, reaction time, and executive functioning. All of these tests help identify the areas of cognition that are impaired and distinguish one type of dementia from another.

Risk Factors

- Age. AD affects 1%-2% of seniors aged 65, and quickly rises to 35%-50% by age 85.
- On average, people with AD live 8-10 years after they are diagnosed.
- Genetics. Although the causes of AD are largely unknown, in some cases genetic factors are responsible. About 20% of patients with AD will have one or more siblings or parents affected.
- Gender. Women are at a slightly greater risk of developing AD than men; the reason for this still remains unknown.
- Education. An educated, or a higher functioning brain, appears to have an "extra reserve" that can delay the onset or decrease the risk of AD. However, crossword puzzles and other mental exercises have not been shown to protect against AD.
- Exercise. Some studies have suggested that ongoing physical exercise may be helpful in slowing the development or progression of AD.

Stages of Alzheimer's Disease

Managing AD involves two important considerations:

1. Enabling patients to be as independent as possible while maintaining their quality of life.
2. Providing support for the families. By understanding the general stages of AD, patients and their families can plan for the future.

Stage I:
Early or Mild Phase
Some early symptoms of AD go unnoticed because the patient's social skills cover up these difficulties:
- Continual forgetfulness
- Difficulty recalling new names and recent conversations
- Personality changes, such as decreased motivation and drive, or becoming easily upset or anxious
- Disorientation or becoming lost in familiar surroundings

Stage II:
Middle or Moderate Phase
- Worsening of memory, especially with current events
- Depression, withdrawal, or agitation
- Requiring help in decision making and managing personal finances
- Increasing dependence on others for daily care

Stage III:
Late or Severe Phase
- Unawareness of time and place
- Inability to identify close family members at times
- Increasing insecurity, suspicion, and agitation
- Disturbed sleep
- Slower and more difficult movement and coordination
- Constant dependence on others for daily care; this may require families to seek nursing home care for their loved one

Management of Alzheimer's Disease

Currently there is no cure for AD. However, there are several aspects of care that can help the patients and families manage the disease.

For the patients:
- Provide a calm and stable home environment.
- Minimize situations that may lead to agitation and anxiety.
- Provide as many structured activities throughout the day as possible, keeping the interests of the patient in mind.
- Medications may be prescribed by the doctor to treat the emotional and cognitive symptoms of AD.
- Work to avoid common complications of advanced-stage AD:
  Pneumonia and other infections
  Falls and fractures
  Wandering

For the families and caregivers:
- Ask for help from others when you need it.
- Maintain your own health.
- Ask questions about the patient's medical needs.
- Be prepared; the day may come when the patient will need to be moved to an extended care facility as his/her needs become overwhelming to be handled at home.
- Join a support group or attend an educational program.

Normal Neuron

Neurofilament

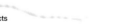

Vacuole

Dendrites

Nucleus

Cell body

Axon

Messages

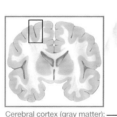

Messages

Synapse

Axon

Neurotransmitters

Neurotransmitters: The Messengers

AD also destroys the way some neurons "talk" to each other. Normally, a neuron receives messages from other neurons at its dendrites. The information passes to the cell body and down its axon as an electrical impulse. This electrical impulse triggers chemicals called neurotransmitters to empty into the small gap (synapse), and the messages continue. AD attacks the neurotransmitter acetylcholine (located at the nucleus basalis of Meynert) and causes a profound effect on memory loss.

Affected Areas of the Brain

Alzheimer's affects the cerebral cortex of the temporal, parietal, and frontal lobes of the brain, gradually impairing their normal functions. The critical structures deep inside the brain that process and relay information to the cerebral cortex and other areas are also affected; these structures include the hippocampus, the amygdala, and the nucleus basalis of Meynert.

Amyloid Plaques (also called senile plaques)
are clumps of beta-amyloid protein that are surrounded by abnormal nerve endings called neurites. These plaques are found between the neurons in the cerebral cortex of the brain. Recent research indicates that random amyloid plaques are seen in normal elderly as well as those with early AD. However, when these plaques occur in clusters, they create a harmful effect and contribute to the development of AD. Researchers are developing medications that would stop or reverse the development of beta-amyloid protein.

Beta amyloid protein core

Neurites

Cerebral cortex (gray matter): thinking

Physical Changes in the Cerebral Cortex

The brain is formed of two tissue types known as the gray and white matter. The gray matter in the cerebral cortex is the outer brain tissue that contains neuron cell bodies. The part of neurons called axons extend deep into the inner tissue, or white matter, to form pathways connecting the different functional areas of the brain. When large numbers of neurons are damaged, gaps occur in communication severely limiting one's ability to think and remember. In AD, the greatest loss of neurons occurs in the cortex of the temporal and parietal lobes, causing the gray matter of that area to shrink or atrophy.

White matter

Neuron cell body

Axon

Alzheimer's

Normal

Abnormal Cellular Structures Involved in Alzheimer's Disease

How and why neurons die in AD is largely unknown. However, several characteristic abnormal cellular structures in the neurons and brain, which scientists believe cause cell malfunction or cell death, are found in the brains of many AD patients. These structures include excessive granulovacuoles, neurofibrillary tangles, and amyloid plaques.

Granulovacuolar Degeneration
is found inside the neurons of the hippocampus. An abnormally high number of fluid-filled spaces, called vacuoles, enlarge the cell's body possibly causing the cell to malfunction or die.

Vacuoles

Neurofibrillary Tangles
are bundles of filaments inside the neurons that abnormally twist around one another. Many neurofibrillary tangles are found in areas of the brain associated with memory and learning (hippocampus), fear and aggression (amygdala), and thinking (cerebral cortex). Scientists believe the neurofibrillary tangles play a role in the memory loss and personality changes seen in AD.

Tangles

 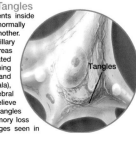 Wolters Kluwer Published by Anatomical Chart Company, Skokie, IL. Developed in consultation with John P. Kachoris, MD.

Understanding Major Depressive Disorder

How Does Depression Affect the Brain?

Depression makes some areas of the brain become less active, while others become more active than normal. Most of these changes take place in an area of the brain called the limbic system. The limbic system is associated with motivation, emotion, learning, sexual arousal, and memory as well as the body's response to stress.

Changes in Parts of the Limbic System Can Affect Mood and Behavior

- The **amygdala** becomes active when we remember especially vivid or disturbing memories. The amygdala of someone who is sad or depressed is very active, and this high level of activity continues even after recovery from depression.
- The **thalamus** relays information from our senses (eyes, ears, nose, and skin) to other parts of the brain that direct behavior and thinking. The thalamus links sensory input to pleasant and unpleasant feelings.
- The **hypothalamus** sends a "fight-or-flight" command to our brain. It does this by releasing and controlling levels of stress hormones, such as adrenaline and cortisol.

Signs of major depressive disorder warrant evaluation and treatment by a health care provider.

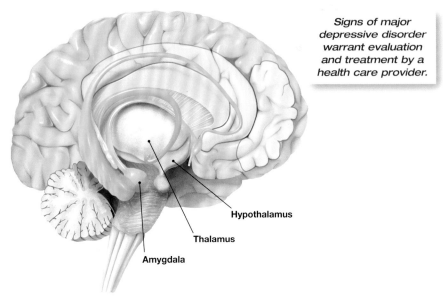

Hypothalamus

Thalamus

Amygdala

What Is Depression?

Feeling depressed can be a normal reaction to loss or to a stressful event or series of stressful events. When depressed feelings are marked by helplessness, hopelessness, and worthlessness, lasting days and affecting daily life and functioning, it can be a treatable medical condition known as major depressive disorder.

Several Factors Can Contribute to Depression

- Problems in the way the brain regulates emotions
- Traumatic events
- Pain
- Medical problems
- Certain medicines
- Genetic structure

These causes seem to come together in different ways that trigger depression in some people.

Signs and Symptoms of Major Depressive Disorder

A person may have major depression if five or more of the following symptoms are present for more than 2 weeks:

- Feeling helpless, hopeless, guilty, or worthless most of the day, particularly in the morning
- Day-long fatigue
- Impaired concentration, indecisiveness, memory loss
- Sleep disturbance (too much or too little)
- Significant weight loss or gain
- Constant, decreased interest or pleasure in activities
- Recurring thoughts of death or suicide
- A sense of restlessness

Treatment

Depression can almost always be treated effectively. If depression is diagnosed, treatment may include one or more of the following:

- **Antidepressants**—These medications restore neurotransmitter levels in the brain. They may take time to work as the brain develops new neurons. Your health care provider may try different antidepressants before finding the treatment that works best for you.
- **Counseling (psychotherapy)**—Counseling involves talking with a trained mental health professional. It helps people gain insight into their feelings and learn how to deal with them, change behaviors, and resolve problems.
- **Exercise**—Regular exercise can ease the symptoms of mild depression. Research suggests that physical activity can help to restore neurotransmitter levels and can improve mood and sense of well-being.
- **Alternative therapies,** such as herbal therapy, may have a beneficial effect on mild cases of depression. Always talk to your health care provider before taking an herbal or dietary supplement.

Does a Chemical Imbalance Cause Depression?

These factors relate to the interaction of chemicals in the brain, but hundreds of millions of chemical interactions take place when we see, think, hear, speak, and feel. It is nearly impossible to point to an imbalance of any chemical or chemicals and identify it as the cause of depression. This is also partly why a treatment that works for one person may not work for another, even if their symptoms are similar. We know, however, that increasing levels of certain chemicals called **neurotransmitters,** especially norepinephrine and serotonin, can help to treat depression in many people.

The Role of Neurotransmitters

Neurotransmitters carry signals between nerve cells **(neurons)** in our brain. Neurons send and receive these signals continuously as our brain carries out functions of daily life, including our behavior, mood, and thought.

Neurons send and receive these signals through openings **(channels)** in a film or membrane.

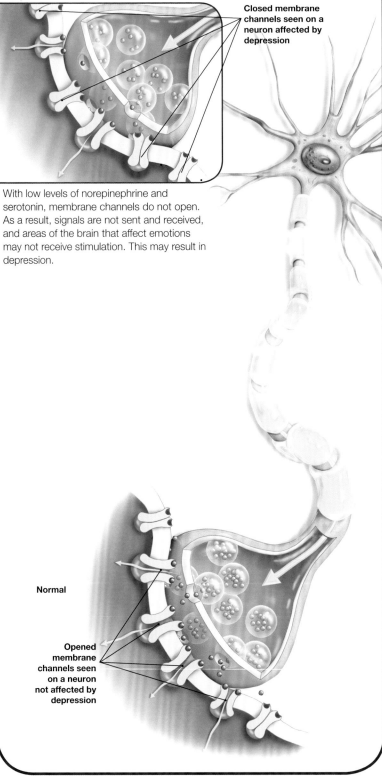

Abnormal

Closed membrane channels seen on a neuron affected by depression

With low levels of norepinephrine and serotonin, membrane channels do not open. As a result, signals are not sent and received, and areas of the brain that affect emotions may not receive stimulation. This may result in depression.

Normal

Opened membrane channels seen on a neuron not affected by depression

UNDERSTANDING EPILEPSY

What Is Epilepsy?
Epilepsy is a common neurological condition that affects millions of people throughout the world. The term "epilepsy" is a general name that refers to many different disorders in which people tend to experience seizures. Other conditions, such as high fever, the use of or withdrawal from drugs or alcohol, or a blow to the head, can cause an isolated seizure. Only those people who have had two or more seizures are diagnosed as having epilepsy.

What Causes Epilepsy?
Many cases of epilepsy are said to be symptomatic. This means they are the result of other conditions such as a birth injury, head injury, stroke, brain tumor, infection, or congenital abnormality. Genetic factors may also play a role in the cause of epilepsy. Some cases of epilepsy, however, remain idiopathic, meaning they develop for reasons that we presently cannot determine.

How the Brain Works
Although it appears to be solid, the brain is made up of billions of cells, including a network of cells called neurons. These neurons branch out, much like branches on a tree. This neural network enables communication within the brain and between the brain and the rest of the body.

Neurons

When a neuron "fires," it sends small electrical impulses along its branches toward surrounding cells. At the end of each branch is a small gap or synapse, which the impulse must overcome in order to continue its journey.

When an impulse reaches the end of a branch, chemicals called neurotransmitters are released to flood the synapse. Some are excitatory, stimulating the neighboring cell to fire. Others are inhibitory, making the next cell less likely to fire.

The brain's ability to turn electrical impulses "on" and "off" allows it to control messages and work effectively. Since normal behavior is the result of many neurons working together, a fine balance of excitatory and inhibitory factors is needed to ensure that the correct neurons fire at the appropriate times. In people with epilepsy, however, this fine balance is upset, making the brain unable to limit the spread of electrical activity. When too many neurons fire at once, an electrical storm is created within the brain.

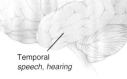

Frontal
motor control, some aspects of personality

Parietal
sensation, some aspects of language

Occipital
— vision

Temporal
speech, hearing

The brain is divided into two hemispheres. The right half controls the left side of the body, and the left half controls the right side of the body. Each hemisphere is divided into four lobes. Within the lobes there are even smaller areas, each associated with specific functions.

Vesicles release neurotransmitters, which flood the synapse.

What Is a Seizure?
A seizure is an excessive discharge of electrical activity within the brain, which leads to a change in movement, sensation, experience, or consciousness. There are many types of seizures. The effects they have on the body vary greatly, depending on where in the brain the seizure starts and where it spreads.

Seizures Can Cause:
- A twitching muscle
- Convulsive movements
- A tingling sensation
- Sweating
- The perception of an unusual smell or taste
- Hallucinations
- Fear or anxiety
- Changes in awareness
- Loss of consciousness
- Other changes

This illustration shows a seizure originating in the left motor strip, affecting movement of the fingers, hand, and arm.

Phases of a Seizure
Aura: an unusual sensation or peculiar feeling often felt prior to a more widespread seizure. Can also be called a simple partial seizure.

Ictus: the whole seizure, including the aura.

Postictus: time after a seizure; may experience muscle weakness or deep sleep.

If Someone Has a Seizure
Although big seizures may be frightening to witness, they are usually not medical emergencies. In most cases the seizure itself is not harmful to the individual who is having it and therefore should be allowed to run its course. An ambulance is usually not necessary unless the seizure lasts longer than 5 minutes, there are multiple, repeated seizures, or the person is injured, diabetic or pregnant. There is nothing family or friends can do to stop a seizure, but certain steps can be taken to prevent further injury.

You Should:
- Stay calm
- Help the person lie down and roll onto one side to prevent choking
- Loosen tight, restrictive clothing and remove eyeglasses
- Protect the person's head with a soft object such as a pillow or jacket
- Gently guide a conscious but confused person away from hazards
- Remain with the person until s/he is awake and alert
- Be comforting and reassuring

You Should Not:
- Put anything into the person's mouth
- Try to restrain the person

Generalized Seizures
These seizures affect both hemispheres of the brain at the same time. Abnormal activity is not focused in one specific area and there generally is no aura at the start.

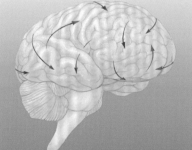

Partial Seizures
These seizures begin in a part of one hemisphere, generally in the temporal or frontal lobe. The two types of partial seizures, called simple and complex, are based on whether a person remains fully conscious during a seizure.

Simple

Complex

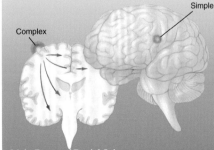

Diagnosing Epilepsy
There is no single test for epilepsy. The doctor will make a diagnosis based on a description of past seizures. Since those who have had a seizure are often unaware of what took place, the doctor may rely on others who witnessed the event. Details about how the patient felt before the attack and how it took place are very useful. The doctor will also review the patient's personal and family medical history, and will give a physical exam to check for other conditions that may have caused the attack.

There are tests designed to gather information about a patient's condition. The most commonly used test is an electroencephalogram (EEG). An EEG involves attaching a series of metal discs called electrodes to the patient's head to measure the brain's electrical activity. Most types of seizures are detectable with the EEG, but some abnormal activity may affect too small an area on the brain's surface or be located too deep to be detected. Other tests such as computed tomography (CT), positron emission tomography (PET), and magnetic resonance imaging (MRI) can provide additional information about the brain. A doctor may order these tests to look for causes of the attack, such as a tumor, congenital malformation, or other changes in the brain.

Main Forms of Generalized Seizures
Absence seizures:
- **Typical** absence seizures (formerly called "petit mal")—result in brief episodes of impaired awareness. There also may be small motor movements, changes in muscle tone, or automatic behaviors.
- **Atonic** seizures—also called drop seizures; associated with a sudden loss of muscle tone in a limb or throughout the entire body. The person having the seizure will often drop things or fall to the ground.
- **Myoclonic** seizures—sudden shocklike jolt to one or more muscles that increases muscle tone and causes movement. These sudden jerks are like those that occur in healthy people as they fall asleep.
- **Tonic-clonic** seizures (formerly called "grand mal")—begin with simultaneous loss of consciousness and the tonic phase (stiffening of the body). The person falls to the ground and often emits a loud cry as the chest muscles stiffen. Next comes the clonic phase, during which the muscles rhythmically jerk.

Main Forms of Partial Seizures
Simple partial seizures (sometimes called "auras"):
Seizure activity is focused in a specific area of the brain. A person remains alert and afterward is able to remember what happened. An aura or simple partial seizure may constitute the entire seizure or may precede a complex partial or generalized seizure. Symptoms vary depending on the area of the brain involved.

- Motor seizures cause a change in muscle activity and may involve jerking or stiffening of a part of the body.
- Sensory seizures may cause abnormal function in any of the five senses.
- Autonomic seizures affect involuntary functions and may cause a rapid heartbeat or breathing rate, sweating, or an unpleasant sensation in the abdomen, chest, throat, or head.
- Psychic seizures may affect perception and memory or stimulate emotions such as fear.

Complex partial seizures:
Seizure is accompanied by impaired consciousness and recall. It may also involve staring, automatic behaviors such as lip smacking, chewing, fumbling, picking, walking, grunting, repetition of words or phrases, or other symptoms and signs.

 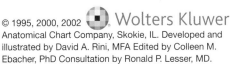

Migraines and Headaches

Primary Headaches are not due to an organic underlying condition but are biological disorders. There are three main types of primary headaches: migraine, cluster, and tension-type.

Migraine Headache

Although individuals experience migraine differently, this type of headache is characterized by throbbing pain, usually on one side of the head. Sufferers may also experience nausea or vomiting and sensitivity to light and sound, all of which may cause inability to perform daily activities. Less than one-third of migraineurs suffer from an "aura," which are visual disturbances such as light flashes, blind spots, or zigzag lines.

Migraine attacks vary from person to person, lasting anywhere from 4 to 72 hours. They usually occur in three phases: 1) preheadache, 2) headache, and 3) postheadache. Pre- and postheadache phases can last from hours to days, and sufferers may experience muscle tenderness, fatigue, and mood changes. Migraines are often hereditary and are more common in women.

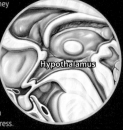

Hypothalamus

Cluster Headache

Cluster headache is named for the grouping of attacks. These relatively short (30-120 minutes) attacks start suddenly with severe pain on one side of the head or neck. Headache periods can last several weeks or months and then disappear for months or even years. Primarily affecting men, cluster headaches generally occur in spring and autumn and are often erroneously associated with seasonal allergies or stress.

Like migraines, the pain of cluster headaches is related to an inflammatory process that develops from the interaction of the trigeminal nerve and blood vessels in the covering of the brain. It is believed that the deep area of the brain, called the hypothalamus, is responsible for the pattern of cluster headaches.

Tension-type Headache

Tension-type headache is the most common form of headache. Sufferers can experience "hat band" or generalized pain over the entire head. It is believed that the underlying cause of tension-type headache is due to chemical and neuronal imbalances in the brain or due to muscle tightening in the head or back of the neck.

There are three categories of tension-type headache based on how frequently they occur.
1. Episodic tension-type headaches occurs less than once per month and is usually triggered by temporary stress, anxiety, fatigue, or anger.
2. Frequent tension-type headaches occurs 1-15 days per month and can occur with a migraine headache.
3. Chronic tension-type headache, also called chronic daily headache, occurs 15 or more days per month; this type is associated with depression, anxiety, and other emotional problems of unknown origin.

Areas Involved in Tension-type Headaches
Temple: Temporalis muscle
Back of the neck: Trapezius muscle / Levator scapulae muscle

Secondary Headaches, also called "organic headaches," may be due to recent head injury or another disorder.

Secondary (Organic) Headache

A secondary headache, also called organic, is not a disease by itself; it is a symptom of another disease or disorder. Sufferers of secondary headache can experience loss of ability to focus, confusion, loss of consciousness, and pain that becomes progressively worse or becomes the worst headache ever experienced.

Some of the underlying diseases/disorders of organic headache can include tumors, high blood pressure, infections, and other head diseases and disorders. Because the underlying cause of secondary headache can be life-threatening, it is important to see your health care provider right away.

Healthy Lifestyle Strategies to Avoid Headaches
- Avoid headache triggers whenever possible.
- Pay close attention to your diet.
- Get adequate and regular sleep.
- Practice relaxation techniques.
- Exercise regularly.

It is very important to follow your health care provider's instructions and to take any medications as prescribed.

The Pathways of a Migraine Attack
1. The migraine starts deep within the brain.
2. Electrical impulses spread to other regions of the brain.
3. Changes in the nerve cell activity and blood flow may result in symptoms such as visual disturbances, numbness or tingling, and dizziness.
4. Chemicals in the brain, such as serotonin, cause blood vessel dilation and inflammation of surrounding tissue.
5. The inflammation irritates the trigeminal nerve, resulting in severe or throbbing pain. These kinds of pain are symptoms of peripheral sensitization.
6. Pain processing centers can become overloaded by the pain signals, causing them to simultaneously fire. This can cause skin sensitivity in the head/scalp, a condition called cutaneous allodynia. This kind of pain is a symptom of central sensitization and may prolong symptoms of migraine, emphasizing the need for early abortive treatment. Note: some people do not develop central sensitization or cutaneous allodynia.

Headache Diagnostic Guide

	Frequency	Duration	Onset	Pain area	Pain characteristic	Associated symptoms	Triggers	Gender
MIGRAINE	2-8 times per month	4-72 h	Gradual	One or both sides of head	Throbbing, pulsating; moderate to severe	Nausea, sensitivity to light and sound	Diet, activity, environment, emotions, medications, hormones	75% female
CLUSTER	1-4 times per day	Pain is felt for 30-120 min	Sudden	Usually one-sided and in the eye region	Mild burning sensation	Tearing of eye on same side as "runny nose"	Alcohol	90% male
TENSION-TYPE	Episodic: 1 per month Frequent: 1-15 days per month Chronic: More than 15 days per month			Both sides of head	Bandlike sensation around neck and/or head; mild to moderate	None	Stress, anxiety, fatigue, anger	Slightly more females are affected
SECONDARY (ORGANIC)	Varied	Usually progressive	Varied	Varied	Varied	Varied	Organic disease/disorder or head injury	Equal distribution

Headache Treatments Guide

	MEDICATION:			NON-DRUG TREATMENT:		
	Abortive medications	Preventative medications	OTC medications	Biofeedback	Oxygen therapy	Alternative therapies
MIGRAINE	X	X	X	X		X
CLUSTER			X		X	
TENSION-TYPE			X	X		

Note: Secondary (Organic) headache treatment is determined by the underlying condition causing the headache. It is important to consult your health care provider to determine the best course of treatment for you.

Abortive medications, also called acute medications, treat the symptoms of the migraine after the attack begins. Many medications of this type must be taken as soon as the attack occurs; otherwise they are not as effective. Examples include triptans and serotonin antagonists.

Preventive medications, also known as prophylactic treatments, are used to reduce the number, severity, and length of attacks. Examples include antiepileptic, antiseizure, and anticonvulsant medications, beta-blockers, calcium channel blockers, antidepressants, and nonsteroidal anti-inflammatory drugs (NSAIDs).

Other pain medications such as over-the-counter or "OTC" medications can help relieve pain and some symptoms associated with headaches. OTC medications include NSAIDs such as aspirin, acetaminophen, ibuprofen, or naproxen sodium; these are sometimes combined with caffeine to enhance effectiveness.

Biofeedback treatment uses a special equipment to monitor the body's responses to pain, thus helping the headache sufferer to refine relaxation techniques. This helps the patient gain more control over the physiological responses to pain.

Oxygen therapy involves inhaling oxygen through a facial mask at the first signs of an attack; this can help stop an acute cluster headache.

Alternative therapies to treat migraines and other headaches include acupuncture, acupressure, yoga practice, massage, and herbal therapies. It is very important to talk to your health care provider before proceeding with any alternative therapies.

Keep a headache diary to uncover any triggers and provide information to your health care provider so that the best course of treatment can be planned. The diary should track the date, time, intensity (on a scale from 1 to 10), symptoms before the headache, triggers, any medication/therapy taken, and a rating of relief (complete, moderate, or none).

© 2007 **Wolters Kluwer** Anatomical Chart Company, Skokie, IL | Medical Illustrations by Lik Kwong, MFA and Dawn Scheuerman, MAMS in consultation with Dr. Seymour Diamond, MD, Director and Founder, Diamond Inpatient Headache Unit, Saint Joseph Hospital, Chicago, IL

UNDERSTANDING MULTIPLE SCLEROSIS

Body of nerve cell

Axon

Normal myelin sheath around axon

Normal Nerve Cell

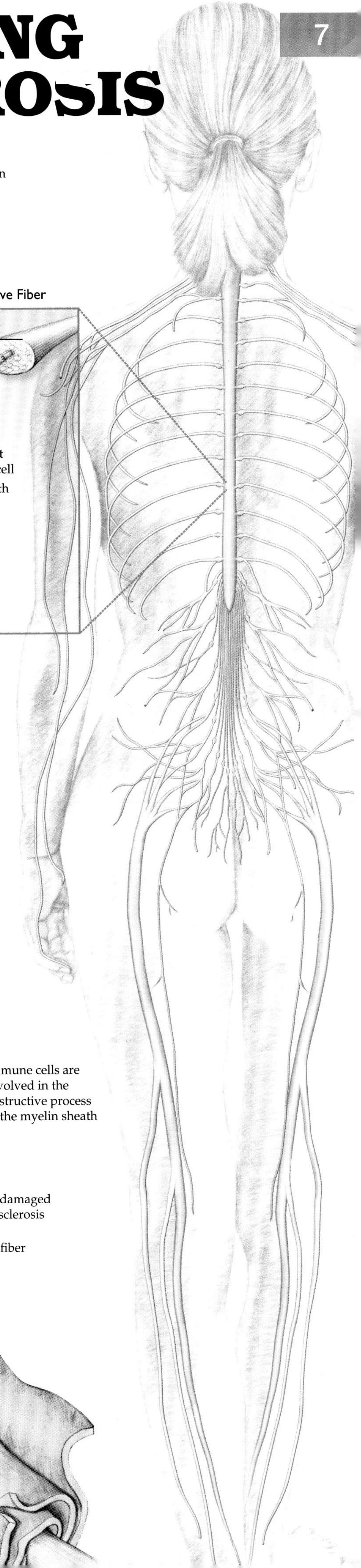

Enlarged View of Nerve Fiber

Nerve fiber from within Central Nervous System

Axon part of nerve cell

Myelin sheath of nerve cell

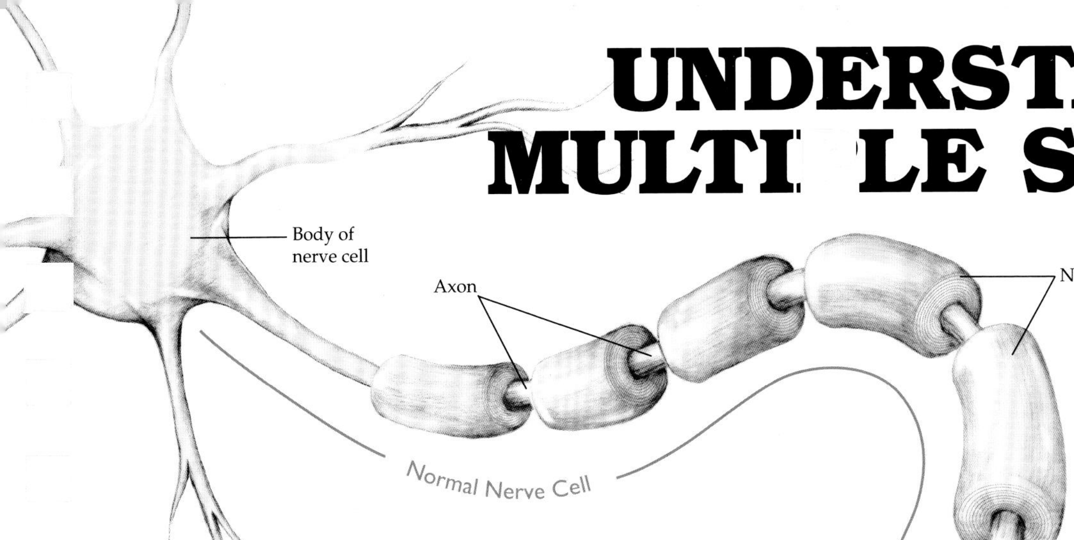

What Is Multiple Sclerosis?

Multiple sclerosis (MS) is an autoimmune disease, which means that the body's immune system attacks its own tissues. In MS, the immune system attacks the protective insulating layer known as the myelin sheath that surrounds the extensions of nerve cells in the brain and spinal cord. Myelin acts like an insulation on a wire. It allows the body to transmit "electrical signals" rapidly from one nerve cell to another and over a long distance. Over time, as myelin is replaced with scar tissue (sclerosis), the brain's ability to transmit signals to the rest of the body is disrupted. The result may be a decrease or a complete loss of control of many neurological functions.

Symptoms and Signs

People with MS experience attacks of symptoms that can last from a few days to several months. These attacks are followed by periods of remission, or symptom-free phases. Early symptoms of MS may include the following:
• Feelings of tingling, burning, numbness, or pain
• Double vision, blurry vision, or blindness
• Weakness, dizziness, and fatigue
During remission the patient may feel better, but there may be lingering stiffness, weakness, numbness, and vision problems. However, the disabilities (symptoms) may be more severe during relapse and include the following:
• Muscle spasms
• Changes in bladder and bowel control
• Slurred speech
• Blindness
• Sexual dysfunction
• Paralysis
• Confusion and forgetfulness
Most people with MS do not develop the most severe symptoms, and regain enough function to continue to lead a normal life.

Prevention and Management

Currently there is no cure or prevention for MS. However, several drugs exist that can help manage symptoms and reduce the frequency of attacks. Additional therapies for managing symptoms include the following:
• Avoidance of heat—some sufferers may experience temporary worsening of symptoms with heat.
• Practice of healthy lifestyle to cope with fatigue and potential stress:
  • Getting enough rest
  • Exercising regularly
  • Eating a healthy, well-balanced diet with plenty of fiber
  • Practicing relaxation techniques

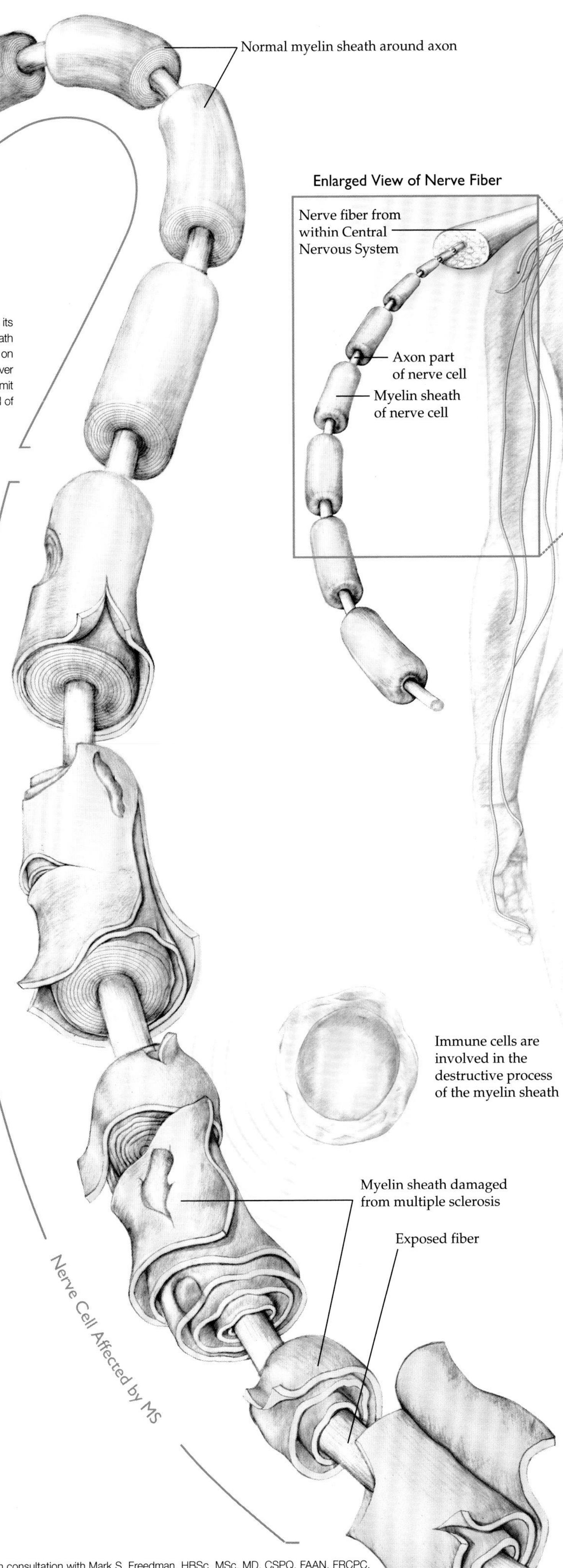

Types of Multiple Sclerosis

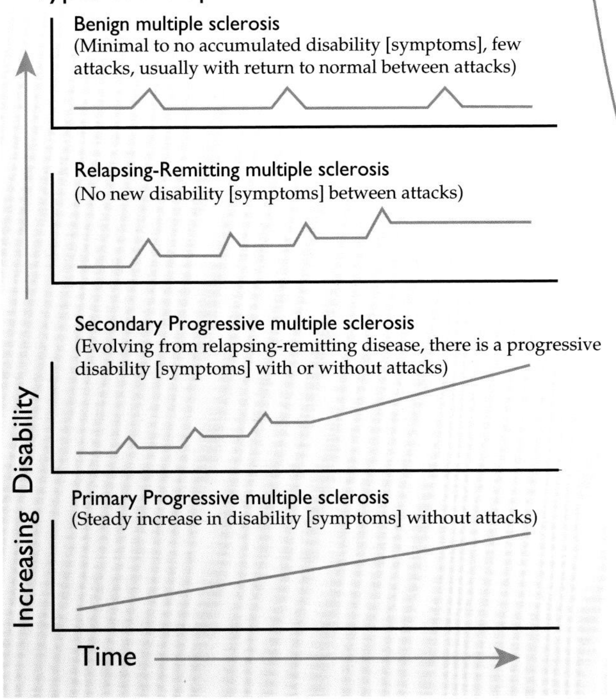

Benign multiple sclerosis
(Minimal to no accumulated disability [symptoms], few attacks, usually with return to normal between attacks)

Relapsing-Remitting multiple sclerosis
(No new disability [symptoms] between attacks)

Secondary Progressive multiple sclerosis
(Evolving from relapsing-remitting disease, there is a progressive disability [symptoms] with or without attacks)

Primary Progressive multiple sclerosis
(Steady increase in disability [symptoms] without attacks)

Increasing Disability

Time

Nerve Cell Affected by MS

Immune cells are involved in the destructive process of the myelin sheath

Myelin sheath damaged from multiple sclerosis

Exposed fiber

Wolters Kluwer · © 2006 Anatomical Chart Company, Skokie, IL. Medical illustrations by Dawn Scheuerman, MAMS, in consultation with Mark S. Freedman, HBSc, MSc, MD, CSPQ, FAAN, FRCPC.

How Pain Works

3 Brain processes the message and alerts the body of pain.

Brain

Spinal cord

Nerves

2 Nerves pick up the injury and send the message to the brain.

- *Red dashed line shows message flow from pain site to brain.*
- *Blue dotted line shows message going from brain to pain site.*

1 Injury occurs in the body.

Understanding Pain

What Is Pain?

It is an unpleasant sensation occurring in varying degrees of severity associated with injury, disease, or emotional disorder.

2 Types of Pain

1. ACUTE PAIN

occurs as a result of injury to the body and generally disappears when the physical injury heals. Acute pain is linked to tissue injury. Anxiety is common with acute pain.

Examples include the following:
- Surgical pain
- Muscle strains
- Orthopedic-type injuries
- Labor and delivery

Symptoms: Patient is able to point to site of pain.
- Sharp
- Burning
- Cramping
- Aching
- Pressure

2. CHRONIC (PERSISTENT) PAIN

lasts beyond the normal healing period—usually at least 3 months. The pain may be multifocal and vague. There may be no signs on x-rays or scans to indicate the source of the pain since some pain may be generated by tissue injury. Depression is common with chronic pain.

Neuropathic chronic pain is a type of pain that is caused by injury to a nerve. Patients describe the pain as having tingling, numbness, or burning sensation. Neuropathic pain is difficult to treat.

Common types of neuropathic chronic pain include the following:
- Diabetic neuropathy—nerve damage as a result of high blood sugar.
- Postherpetic neuralgia—pain from shingles after the blisters have healed.
- HIV/AIDS—pain from the viral illness or the drugs used to treat the disease.
- Peripheral vascular disease—pain in legs, usually during activity, from lack of blood supply to the extremities. The legs may be discolored and/or cold, and the skin may be shiny.

Symptoms:
- Painful itching
- Strange sensations
- Extreme sensitivity to normal touch and temperature
- Burning
- Electriclike sensation
- Painful numbness
- Pins and needles

Nonneuropathic chronic pain is pain that is not caused by injury to a nerve.

The most common types include the following:
- Low back pain—pain in the lower back from muscles, ligaments, tendons, arthritis, or damaged discs
- Osteoarthritis—arthritis resulting from wear and tear of the joints and with normal aging
- Rheumatoid arthritis—an autoimmune disorder resulting in pain, stiffness, and inflammation of the joints

Symptoms: Poorly localized pain (patient may not be able to point to site of pain).
- Gnawing
- Pounding
- Deep aching

Unknown: There are many common chronic pain syndromes that are neither known to be chronic nonneuropathic nor neuropathic.

These include the following:
- Fibromyalgia syndrome—diffuse body pain with tenderness in the muscles
- Tension headache—pressure-type headache lasting days to weeks and often not severe
- Migraine headache—episodic headache that persists for hours to days with nausea and is often severe
- Irritable bowel syndrome (IBS)—abdominal pain with cramping, bloating, and constipation often alternating with diarrhea
- Some low back pain—back pain that is not muscular, not related to disc injury, and without a known cause

Symptoms: May be a combination of chronic non-neuropathic and neuropathic symptoms.

Treatment

Specific treatment options need to be tailored to the individual patient. Be sure to consult with your health care professional to determine the right treatment for you.

Prevention techniques:
- Regular exercise
- Healthy body weight
- Safe techniques when lifting heavy objects

Right   Left

Where Do You Feel Pain?

Left   Right

Pain Scale

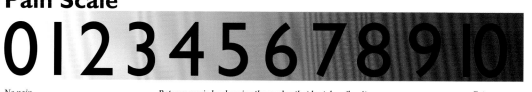

0 1 2 3 4 5 6 7 8 9 10

No pain

Rate your pain by choosing the number that best describes it.

Extreme pain

Wolters Kluwer   Anatomical Chart Company, Skokie, IL. Consultation with Bill McCarberg, MD and Yvonne D'Arcy, MS CRNP, CNS.

Understanding Parkinson's Disease

Parkinson's disease (PD) is a slowly progressive, degenerative disease of the brain. It affects nerve cells in the areas of the brain called the basal ganglia, which are important in determining how your body moves.

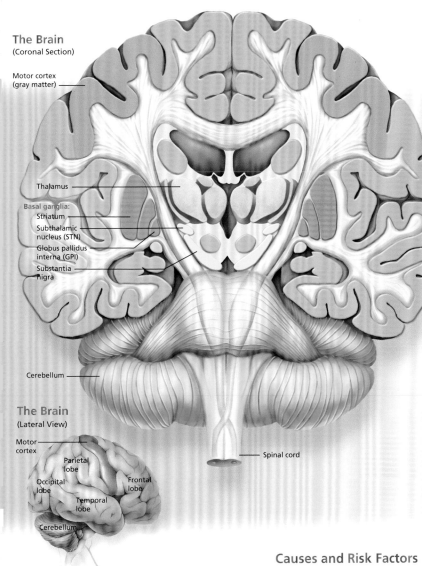

The Brain
(Coronal Section)

- Motor cortex (gray matter)
- Thalamus
- Basal ganglia:
  - Striatum
  - Subthalamic nucleus (STN)
  - Globus pallidus interna (GPI)
  - Substantia nigra
- Cerebellum
- Spinal cord

The Brain
(Lateral View)

- Motor cortex
- Parietal lobe
- Occipital lobe
- Frontal lobe
- Temporal lobe
- Cerebellum

The Role of Neurotransmitters

1. A neuron receives the message from other neurons at its dendrites.
2. The information is passed down its axon as an electrical impulse.
3. In the axon, sacs containing dopamine are stimulated to release into the synapse.
4. Dopamine crosses the synapse to bind to dopamine receptors on the receiving cell.
5. Dopamine stimulates the receptors to open, transmitting the message to the next nerve cell.
6. After the message is sent, the receptors release the dopamine back into the synapse where it is either reabsorbed into the axon or broken down by a chemical called MAO-B.

The Brain and Body Movement

- The impulse for movement is generated in the motor cortex of the brain.
- The cluster of nerve cells called the basal ganglia and the cerebellum ensure that movement is carried out in a smooth coordinated manner.
- These clusters of nerves are interconnected to each other in complex feedback loops. They are also interconnected with the motor cortex and another structure close to the basal ganglia called the thalamus, which acts as a relay center for sensory information and movement.
- The basal ganglia are found on both sides of the brain and are responsible for activating and inhibiting specific motor circuits. The basal ganglia are made up of smaller components called the striatum, globus pallidus, subthalamic nucleus (STN), and substantia nigra.
- Nerve cells in the substantia nigra produce dopamine, a neurotransmitter that acts as a chemical messenger in brain circuits important for planning and controlling body movement.
- The action of dopamine is balanced with another neurotransmitter called acetylcholine; both neurotransmitters ensure smooth, coordinated movement.

Signs and Symptoms

PD does not affect everyone the same way and progresses at different rates. However, most cases begin on only one side of the body and may worsen and spread to the other side as the disease progresses. The main signs and symptoms include the following:

- Tremors: involuntary shaking (predominately of the hands) is usually the first symptom. The jaw or lips are also commonly involved; less often involved are the arms, legs, tongue, and face. In most cases, tremors will occur at rest and may not interfere with daily activities or become bothersome to the patient.
- Bradykinesia: slowness of movement, which is the major cause of disability in PD and tends to be interpreted by patients as "weakness." It can eventually lead to difficulty with walking manifested by a stooped posture, inability to initiate gait, and short shuffling steps. PD patients may also lack facial expression and blink less often.
- Rigidity: stiffness in the limbs and trunk of the body caused by increase in muscle tone; this is seen in about 90% of the patients.
- Postural instability: impairment of the reflexes controlling the posture, leading to a sense of imbalance with an increased tendency to fall; this symptom usually does not occur until late in the disease process.

Related Symptoms Include

- Masklike expression
- Stooped posture
- Rigidity
- Tremors
- Short shuffling steps

- Decreased or lost sense of smell (may precede all other symptoms)
- Increased risk of dementia with age, onset, and severity of PD
- Depression
- Sleep problems
- Trouble chewing, swallowing, or speaking
- Difficulty writing legibly (very small compact handwriting)
- Hallucinations (side effect of medications)
- Urinary and constipation problems

Tremor impulse

Causes and Risk Factors

- For reasons not yet understood, the nerve cells in the substantia nigra that produce dopamine are dying. When 60%-80% of dopamine is lost, symptoms such as tremor, slowness of movement, stiffness, and balance problems occur.
- Gender. Parkinson's occurs only slightly more commonly in men than women.
- Age. The disease usually begins between the ages of 50 and 60 years, but can occur earlier.
- Scientists are still studying the genetic and environmental factors that may lead to PD.

Management and Treatments

Currently there is no cure for PD, but many people with Parkinson's enjoy an active lifestyle and a normal life expectancy. The main categories of management of PD include medication and surgery. Certain lifestyle changes may also help make living with PD easier.

Medications

Medication is the first line of defense for PD patients. There are many options that may be used alone or in combination to control symptoms.

- Levodopa/Carbidopa is a combination drug that once ingested, passes into the brain and is converted to dopamine. It is recognized as the most effective treatment for motor symptoms of the disease. Over time, however, this treatment can have a "wearing-on/wearing-off" effect or patients may notice dyskinesias, which are involuntary jerking or swaying movements of the body that typically occur at peak doses of the drug.
- Dopamine agonists are medications that mimic the effect of dopamine on the brain.
- MAO-B (Monoamine oxidase B) inhibitors help prevent the breakdown of the body's natural and levodopa dopamine level.
- COMT (Catechol-*O*-methyltransferase) inhibitors optimize the delivery of levodopa by blocking COMT, an enzyme that breaks down dopamine in the digestive tract.
- Antidepressants and/or antianxiety medications may be prescribed as needed.

Therapy

Although specific exercise cannot stop the progression of PD, improving muscle strength can help patients feel more confident and capable.

- Physical therapy may be advised to help improve mobility, gait and balance, range of motion, and muscle tone.
- Speech therapy or a speech pathologist may improve problems with speaking and swallowing.

Surgery

When management with medications fails due to fluctuations in the response, lack of effectiveness, or development of side effects such as dyskinesias, surgical options may be considered.

Deep-Brain Stimulation (DBS) is the most common surgical procedure to treat PD and is most often used for those who have advanced PD. It involves implanting an electrode in the desired area of the brain (globus pallidus, thalamus, or subthalamus). The electrode is connected to a pacemaker implanted under the skin below the collarbone, where it sends electrical signals to regulate movement activity. Unfortunately, deep-brain stimulation is not beneficial for patients who do not respond to levodopa/carbidopa treatment.

Pallidotomy—The internal part of the globus pallidus interna (GPI) is destroyed by passing high-frequency energy current through it. This procedure is useful in controlling dyskinesias.

Thalamotomy—The same high-frequency energy current is used to destroy a small area in the thalamus. This procedure is useful in controlling tremors.

- Electrode brain implant
- Generator

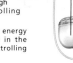

UNDERSTANDING SLEEP DISORDERS

What Is Sleep?

Sleep is a natural, reversible state of decreased responsiveness to the environment. During sleep, usually the eyes are closed and the body is relaxed and almost motionless. We think of sleep in contrast to wakefulness, when the body and mind are active. Although sleep provides important rest and restoration for the brain and body, the brain is very active during the portions of sleep when we are dreaming.

Why Does the Body Need Sleep?

Sleep is important for survival and appears to have specific functions for the endocrine, immune, cardiovascular, and nervous systems. It also has been suggested that sleep is important for bodily restoration, energy conservation, and memory consolidation. Not having an appropriate amount of normal, restful sleep may seriously affect daily functioning.

What Does the Suprachiasmatic Nucleus Do?

The suprachiasmatic nucleus (SCN) is an area of the hypothalamus that initiates signals to other parts of the brain that control hormones, body temperature, and other functions that play a role in making you feel sleepy or wide awake. The SCN works like a biological clock that sets off a regulated pattern of activities that affect the whole body. The SCN controls the production of melatonin in the pineal gland. During the day the melatonin level is very low, but it increases in the evening and is elevated throughout the night, when you normally sleep. The functioning of the SCN normally helps you sleep for about 8 hours at night and remain awake for about 16 hours in the daytime and evening.

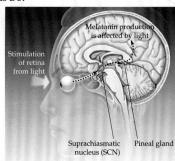

Melatonin production is affected by light

Stimulation of retina from light

Suprachiasmatic nucleus (SCN)   Pineal gland

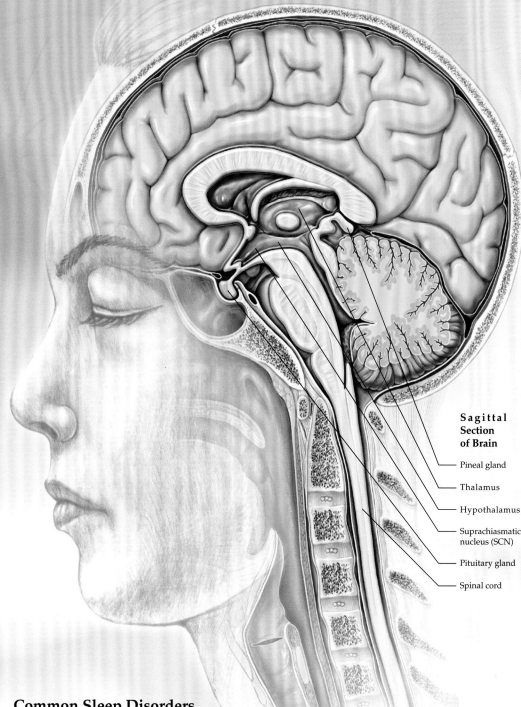

Sagittal Section of Brain

- Pineal gland
- Thalamus
- Hypothalamus
- Suprachiasmatic nucleus (SCN)
- Pituitary gland
- Spinal cord

Stages of Sleep

People usually cycle through different stages of sleep. Time spent in these stages may vary with age.

Non-REM 75%-80% of sleep	As you fall asleep, you enter non-REM sleep, which comprises of Stages 1-4*
Stage 1*	Drowsiness and light sleep.
Stage 2*	This stage takes up a majority of a night's total sleep. It is defined by unique EEG characteristics.
Stages 3 & 4*	Deepest and most restorative sleep: Blood pressure drops, breathing slows down, and hormones are released for growth and development in youths.
REM (Rapid Eye Movement) 20%-25% of sleep	Occurs in episodes beginning about 90 minutes after onset of sleep and recurring with lengthening episodes about every 90 minutes. Most REM sleep is during the latter half of the night. The brain is active, and dreams occur as the eyes dart back and forth. The body becomes relaxed and immobile. Breathing and heart rate may become irregular.

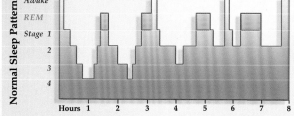

Normal Sleep Pattern — Awake, REM, Stage 1, 2, 3, 4 — Hours 1 2 3 4 5 6 7 8

Tips for a Good Night's Sleep

- Try to keep a regular bedtime and wakeup time.
- Avoid napping if you can't sleep well at night.
- Don't lie in bed awake if you can't sleep.
- Try to relax before going to bed.
- Exercise regularly, but not close to bedtime.
- Avoid caffeine, nicotine, and alcohol before bed.
- Maintain a comfortable room temperature.
- See a doctor if sleep problems continue.
- Limit screen time throughout the day and avoid at least 1 hour prior to bedtime.

Common Sleep Disorders

Sleep disorders can interfere with the ability to sleep or remain awake at the appropriate times. Some sleep disorders involve behaviors or experiences that occur in association with sleep. Some of the most common sleep disorders are shown below.

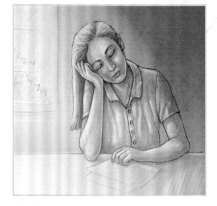

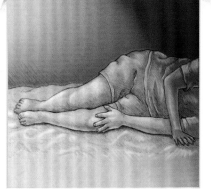

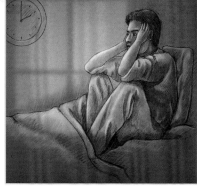

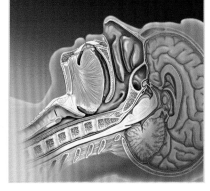

Narcolepsy

People with narcolepsy feel sleepy throughout their waking time, in spite of having sufficient opportunity for sleep at nighttime. They may nap several times a day but feel refreshed only for short periods. At times, sleep seems irresistible. They often have problems concentrating. Inattention and sleepiness can interfere with normal daily functioning. People with narcolepsy may experience cataplexy (sudden muscle weakness during emotional situations) and, when falling asleep, a brief sense of muscle paralysis or dreamlike hallucinations.

Restless Legs Syndrome

Restless legs syndrome (RLS) is a disorder that causes a very unpleasant crawling sensation, mostly in the legs. The natural response is an urge to move them for relief. It usually is worse in the evening and when someone is at rest. It often interferes with the ability to sleep and may cause involuntary kicking during sleep. Someone with severe RLS may feel very uncomfortable sitting for a prolonged period of time in a theater or riding long distances in a car. RLS symptoms can begin at any age.

Insomnia

Insomnia is the most common sleep problem. It may include difficulty falling asleep and staying asleep, as well as a sense of light or unrefreshing sleep. Most commonly it is due to stress, but it also may result from psychiatric (mental), medical, and other sleep disorders. Poor sleep habits can contribute to insomnia. For most people, insomnia lasts just a few days or weeks, but for others it may be a chronic condition lasting years. The daytime consequences are fatigue, lack of energy, difficulty concentrating, and irritability.

Obstructive Sleep Apnea

Obstructive sleep apnea is a recurrent interruption in breathing during sleep. It results from sleep-related muscle relaxation in the upper airway, which leads to a decrease or complete blockage of airflow for brief periods. The blood oxygen level may fall, causing arousals or awakenings that can disturb sleep. People with severe sleep apnea may be dangerously sleepy during the daytime. Those who are obese or snore loudly are at the greatest risk for sleep apnea, but others may have sleep apnea due to large tonsils or other features of their airway anatomy.

© 2005 Wolters Kluwer Anatomical Chart Company, Skokie, IL. Medical illustrations by Lik Kwong, MFA, in consultation with David N. Neubauer, MD.

Understanding Stroke

What Is Stroke?

Stroke refers to the sudden death of brain tissue caused by a lack of oxygen resulting from an interrupted blood supply. An **infarct** is the area of the brain that has "died" because of this lack of oxygen. There are two ways that brain tissue death can occur. **Ischemic stroke** is a blockage or reduction of blood flow in an artery that feeds that area of the brain. It is the most common cause of an infarct. **Hemorrhagic stroke** results from bleeding within and around the brain causing compression and tissue injury.

Ischemic Stroke

This type of stroke results from a blockage or reduction of blood flow to an area of the brain. This blockage may result from atherosclerosis and blood clot formation.

Atherosclerosis is the deposit of cholesterol and plaque within the walls of arteries. These deposits may become large enough to narrow the lumen and reduce the flow of blood while also causing the artery to lose its ability to stretch.

A **thrombus**, or blood clot, forms on the roughened surface of atherosclerotic plaques that develop in the wall of the artery. The thrombus can enlarge and eventually block the lumen of the artery.

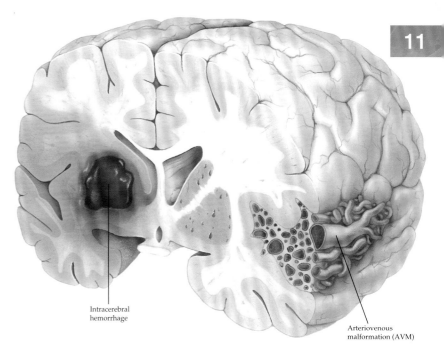

Intracerebral hemorrhage

Arteriovenous malformation (AVM)

Lumen

Plaque

Thrombus

Common Sites of Plaque Formation
(indicated by yellow circles)

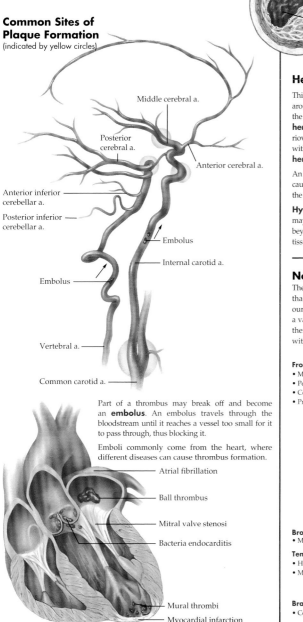

Middle cerebral a.

Posterior cerebral a.

Anterior cerebral a.

Anterior inferior cerebellar a.

Posterior inferior cerebellar a.

Embolus

Internal carotid a.

Embolus

Vertebral a.

Common carotid a.

Part of a thrombus may break off and become an **embolus**. An embolus travels through the bloodstream until it reaches a vessel too small for it to pass through, thus blocking it.

Emboli commonly come from the heart, where different diseases can cause thrombus formation.

Atrial fibrillation

Ball thrombus

Mitral valve stenosi

Bacteria endocarditis

Mural thrombi

Myocardial infarction

Hemorrhagic Stroke

This type of stroke is caused by bleeding within and around the brain. Bleeding that fills the spaces between the brain and the skull is called a **subarachnoid hemorrhage**. It is caused by ruptured aneurysms, arteriovenous malformations, and head trauma. Bleeding within the brain tissue itself is known as **intracerebral hemorrhage** and is primarily caused by hypertension.

An **aneurysm** is a weakening of the arterial wall that causes it to stretch and balloon. It usually occurs where the artery branches.

Hypertension is an elevation of blood pressure that may cause tiny arterioles to burst causing the tissue beyond the rupture to die. Blood vessels in the dead tissue then leak causing more bleeding.

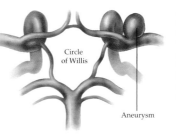

Circle of Willis

Aneurysm

An **arteriovenous malformation** (AVM) is an abnormality of the brain's blood vessels in which arteries lead directly into veins without first going through a capillary bed. The pressure of the blood coming through the arteries is too high for the veins, causing them to dilate in order to transport the higher volume of blood. AVMs may burst and also cause symptoms by putting pressure on sensitive areas causing seizures, or pain.

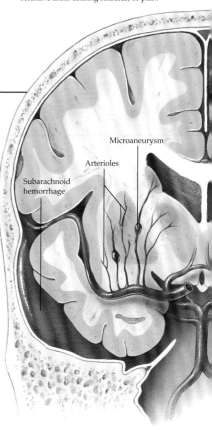

Microaneurysm

Arterioles

Subarachnoid hemorrhage

Normal Functional Areas of Brain

The brain has two sides: a right hemisphere that controls the left side of the body and a left hemisphere that controls the right side of the body. Each hemisphere has four lobes and a cerebellum that control our daily functions. Depending on what part of the brain has been affected, stroke victims experience a variety of neurological deficits. Rehabilitation is crucial to the stroke patient's recovery. Physical therapists and speech therapists help patients "relearn" their lost functions and devise ways to cope with the loss of those they cannot regain.

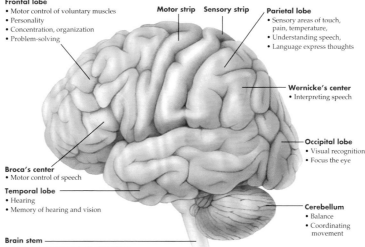

Frontal lobe
• Motor control of voluntary muscles
• Personality
• Concentration, organization
• Problem-solving

Motor strip   **Sensory strip**

Parietal lobe
• Sensory areas of touch, pain, temperature,
• Understanding speech,
• Language express thoughts

Wernicke's center
• Interpreting speech

Broca's center
• Motor control of speech

Temporal lobe
• Hearing
• Memory of hearing and vision

Occipital lobe
• Visual recognition
• Focus the eye

Cerebellum
• Balance
• Coordinating movement

Brain stem
• Controls heart rate and rate of breathing

Events Leading to Stroke

Stroke victims often have small strokes or "warning signs," before a large permanent attack.

Transient Ischemic Attacks (TIAs) are brief attacks that last anywhere from a few minutes to 24 hours. The symptoms resolve completely, and the person returns to normal. It is possible to have several TIAs before a large attack.

Complete Infarction (CI) is an attack that leaves permanent tissue death and results in serious neurological deficits. Recovery is usually not total and takes longer than 3 weeks.

Common Neurological Deficits After Stroke

Left-sided stroke
• Right-sided paralysis
• Speech/language deficits
• Slow, cautious behavior
• Hemianopsia of right visual field
• Memory loss in language
• Right-sided dysarthria
• Aphasia
• Apraxia

Right-sided stroke
• Left-sided paralysis
• Spatial/perceptual deficits
• Quick, impulsive behavior
• Hemianopsia of left visual field
• Memory loss in performance
• Left-sided dysarthria

Related Terms

Paralysis—Loss of muscle function and sensation

Hemiparesis—Weakness of muscles on one side of body

Hemianopsia—Loss of sight in half of visual field

Aphasia—Difficulty with oral communication; reduced ability to read or write

Apraxia—Inability to control muscles; movement is uncoordinated and jerky

Dysarthria—Slurring of speech and "mouth droop" on one side of face due to muscle weakness

Risks for Stroke

Hypertension
Heart disease
Atherosclerosis
Previous TIAs
High cholesterol
High alcohol consumption
Obesity
Diabetes
Bruit noise in carotid artery
Cigarette smoking
Oral contraceptive use
Family history of stroke

Understanding
Schizophrenia

Schizophrenia is a psychiatric illness that often begins when a person is in his or her late teens, 20s, or 30s. As with any illness, the symptoms can differ from person to person and can change over time. When the disease is active, most patients experience the hallmark symptoms of psychosis in the form of delusions and hallucinations. When the disease is inactive, many patients still experience trouble with concentration and motivation.

What Causes Schizophrenia?

Genes and Environment—While schizophrenia is found in only 1% of the population, 10% of those who have the disease also have a first-degree relative (parent, brother, or sister) or second-degree relative (aunt, uncle, grandparent, cousin) with the disorder, which leads researchers to believe that genetics play some part in the illness. While genes are clearly involved, no single gene can cause schizophrenia. It is very likely that genes interacting with the environment (such as exposure to viruses or malnutrition before birth, problems during birth, subsequent drug use, or head injury) cause schizophrenia.

Different Brain Chemistry and Structure—Scientists believe there is an imbalance in the delicate chemical reactions of the brain, specifically with the neurotransmitters dopamine and glutamate. Neurotransmitters are substances that allow brain cells to communicate with each other.

Causes of Psychosis Other Than Schizophrenia—Schizophrenia is only one cause of psychosis. Therefore, schizophrenia is only diagnosed if other causes of psychosis have been excluded:

- **Medical Illnesses**—(eg, Brain infections, like syphilis or AIDS)
- **Intoxications**—(eg, Illicit drugs, toxins, and medications)
- **Other Psychiatric Illnesses**—(eg, Bipolar disorder, delusional disorder, personality disorders)

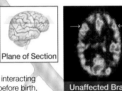
Plane of Section

Unaffected Brain

Affected Brain

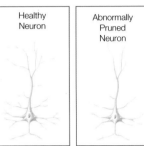
Gray Matter Deficit in Schizophrenia

Average Deficit
0%
-10%
-20%

Onset of Illness

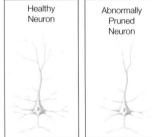
Illness After 5 Years

Healthy Neuron

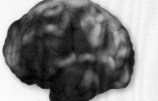
Abnormally Pruned Neuron

Stages of Illness

Premorbid Phase—This phase is associated with a cognitive decline that precedes the onset of the illness by several years occurring during pre-post natal, childhood, and puberty.

Prodromal Phase—A prodrome refers to the early symptoms and signs of an illness that precede the fully developed illness. For schizophrenia, this is the period from the first change in a person until the development of the first psychotic symptoms.

Acute Psychotic Episode—Patient shows symptoms of psychotic episodes, and these may be present for up to 2 years before treatment. Symptoms include the following:
- Positive symptoms (hallucinations, delusions, etc.)
- Negative systems (emotional and behavioral changes)
- Depression and suicidality

Post-psychotic Phase (Unspecific Symptoms)—Once treatment (medication and psychotherapy) begins, it can take up to three months to see whether the treatment is effective. When treatment is effective, positive symptoms remit and the levels of depression are low or may disappear. For other patients, symptoms may persist or emerge and they may need to try other medications or treatment interventions.

Depressive symptoms are particularly important in the postpsychotic period, as they have been associated with an increased risk of suicide. They can also be warning signs of a relapse.

Maintenance Phase—The prognosis of schizophrenia varies from complete recovery (after a period of acute illness) to severe, ongoing symptoms that require institutionalization. Even when the symptoms are successfully treated, function often remains impaired. For most patients, having schizophrenia means living in the community with varying degrees of symptoms and varying needs for support.

Some people may have a relapse—their symptoms come back or get worse. Usually, relapses happen when people stop taking their medication, or when they only take it sometimes. Some people stop taking their medication because they feel better or they may feel they do not need it anymore. But no one should stop taking an antipsychotic medication without talking to his or her doctor first.

Symptoms of Schizophrenia Fall Into Four Broad Categories

Positive Symptoms are often the most obvious signs of the illness.

- **Hallucinations** are unusual perceptions of things that are not there; such as seeing things, hearing voices, smelling odors, and feeling sensations on the skin. People with schizophrenia may hear voices for a long time before family and friends notice the problem. The voices may talk to the person about his or her behavior, order the person to do things, or warn the person of danger.
- **Delusions** are false beliefs that are persistent and that do not go away after receiving logical or accurate information. People with schizophrenia may believe that neighbors can control their behavior or that radio stations are broadcasting their thoughts. Or, they may believe that others are trying to harm them by cheating, poisoning, or spying on them.
- **Disorganized speech** is speech that is unclear or confused. People have difficulties expressing themselves.

Negative Symptoms are harder to recognize as part of the disorder and can be mistaken for depression or lack of motivation.

- "Flat affect" (a person's face does not move or he or she talks in a dull, monotonous voice)
- Lack of pleasure in everyday life (anhedonia)
- Lack of interest in beginning planned activities (avolition)
- Speaking little, even when encouraged to elaborate (alogia)

Mood Symptoms are important since they reduce the quality of life and may increase a patient's risk of suicide. Some mood symptoms include the following:
- Depression
- Demoralization (hopelessness, loss of meaning in life, feeling incompetent)
- Dysphoria (a state of being ill at ease)
- Irritability
- Euphoria or mania (frantic, hyperactivity or overexcited thoughts and speech)

Cognitive Symptoms are subtle, and like negative symptoms, they can be difficult to recognize. Because cognition includes "executive functioning" such as goal setting and figuring out steps to flexibly achieve those goals, cognitive symptoms often make it hard to be independent and earn a living.
- Inability to understand information and use it to make decisions or solve problems
- Trouble focusing and paying attention
- Poor verbal learning (difficulties learning new material in a class or from a book)
- Problems with "working memory" (the ability to hold information "on-line" briefly, like dialing a phone number)

Medial View of Brain

Limbic Cortex

Medial Prefrontal Cortex (mPFC)

Dopamine System Pathways

Brain Stem

Spinal Cord

Cerebellum

Lateral View of Brain

Dorsolateral Prefrontal Cortex (dlPFC)

Ventrolateral Prefrontal Cortex (vlPFC)

Anterior Prefrontal Cortex (aPFC)

Superior Temporal Gyrus (STG)

Wernicke's Area

Cerebellum

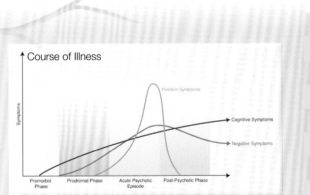
Course of Illness

Symptoms

Positive Symptoms
Cognitive Symptoms
Negative Symptoms

Premorbid Phase | Prodromal Phase | Acute Psychotic Episode | Post-Psychotic Phase

Treatment and Management

Antipsychotic Medications are the mainstay of treatment for schizophrenia; they are most effective in the treatment of acute psychosis and the prevention of relapse. Antipsychotics do not work well for negative symptoms and cognitive problems.

While all antipsychotics (except clozapine) have similar efficacy with regards to treating psychosis, people respond in different ways to antipsychotic medications and no one can tell beforehand how a person will respond. Sometimes a person needs to try several medications before finding the right one. Medications can greatly differ with regards to side effects. Concerning side effects include persistent abnormal movements (called tardive dyskinesia), which are more likely with the older drugs. Weight gain and diabetes are also concerns with most antipsychotics.

Psychosocial Treatments are as important as medications. Patients who receive regular psychosocial treatment also are more likely to keep taking their medication, and they are less likely to have relapses or be hospitalized.

- **Cognitive Behavioral Therapy (CBT)** is a type of psychotherapy that focuses on thinking and behavior. CBT helps patients with symptoms that do not go away even when they take medication. The therapist teaches people with schizophrenia how to test the reality of their thoughts and perceptions, how to "not listen" to their voices, and how to manage their overall symptoms.

- **Integrated Treatment for Substance Abuse**—Substance abuse is the most common co-occurring disorder in people with schizophrenia. When schizophrenia treatment programs and drug treatment programs are used together, patients get better results.

- **Rehabilitation Programs** can include job counseling and training, money management counseling, help in learning to use public transportation, and opportunities to practice communication skills. Programs like these help patients hold jobs, remember important details, and improve their functioning.

- **Family Education**—People with schizophrenia are often discharged from the hospital into the care of their families, so it is important that family members know as much as possible about the disease.

© 2010 Wolters Kluwer

Published by Anatomical Chart Company, Skokie, IL. Developed in consultation with Oliver Freudenreich, MD.

CANCER (ONCOLOGY)

- Understanding Breast Cancer
- Understanding Cervical Cancer
- Understanding Ovarian Cancer
- Understanding Colorectal Cancer
- Understanding Leukemia
- Understanding Lung Cancer
- Non–Small Cell Lung Cancer
- Multiple Myeloma
- Understanding Liver Cancer
- Understanding Kidney Cancer
- Understanding Pancreatic Cancer
- Understanding Prostate Cancer
- Understanding Skin Cancer

Understanding Breast Cancer

What Is Breast Cancer?

Breast cancer is the most common form of cancer in women and is the number 2 killer (after lung cancer) of women aged 35-54. It can also occur in men, though incidence is rare. The survival rate has improved because of earlier diagnosis and the variety of treatments now available. The most common location for breast cancer is the upper outer quadrant (the upper part of the breast closest to the arm), although it may occur in any part of the breast. The size at which a cancer can be felt varies based on its location in the breast and the characteristics of both the cancer and the normal breast tissue. Breast cancer may spread by way of the lymphatic system to the underarm lymph nodes or by the bloodstream to the lungs, liver, bones, and other organs, or directly to the skin or surrounding tissues.

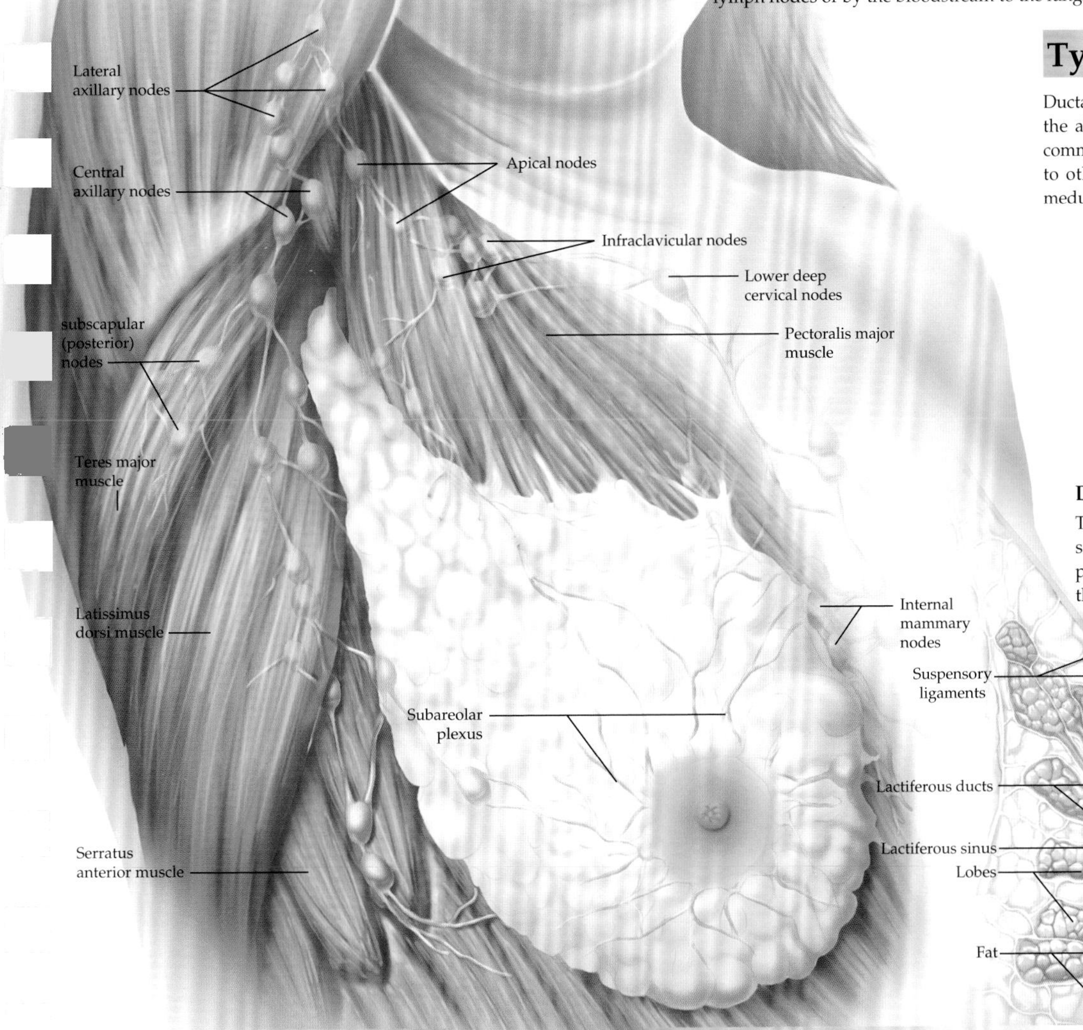

Types of Breast Cancer

Ductal carcinoma in situ (DCIS) is the most common type of in situ cancer. In situ cancers lack the ability to spread outside of the breast. Infiltrating ductal carcinoma (IDC) is the most common type of invasive breast cancer. Invasive or infiltrating cancers have the ability to spread to other parts of the body. Others invasive cancers include infiltrating lobular carcinoma, medullary carcinoma, tubular cancer, and mucinous cancer.

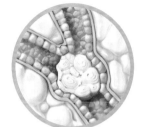

Ductal Carcinoma In Situ
This is breast cancer at its earliest stage. It is confined to the ducts (milk passage). Nearly 100% of women at this cancer stage can be cured.

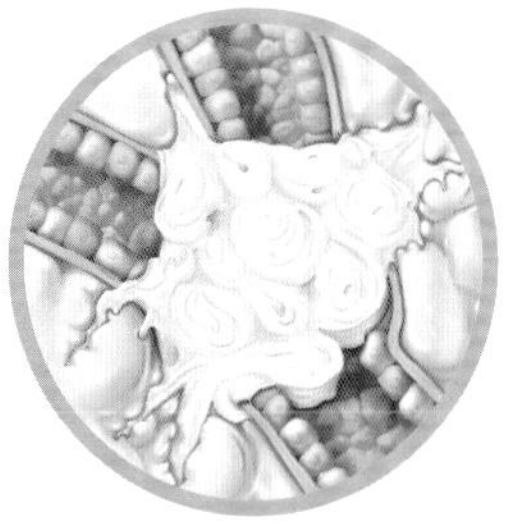

Infiltrating (Invasive) Ductal Carcinoma
This cancer starts in a duct, then breaks through the duct wall, and invades the fatty tissue of the breast. IDC is the most common type of breast cancer, accounting for nearly 80% of cases.

Breast Self-Examination (BSE)

The best time to perform a self-examination is about 1 week after your period ends. If you do not have regular periods, perform a self-examination on the same day every month.

- Stand before a mirror. Compare both breasts, noticing the shape and size. It is not unusual for one breast to be larger than the other. Check for unusual signs such as puckering, dimpling, scaling of skin, or change in size or shape. Look at the same things with your arms in different positions.
- Raise your left arm. Using the pads of three fingers of your right hand, feel your left breast firmly, carefully and slowly. Begin at the outer edge, pressing in small circles moving slowly around the breast. Be sure to cover the entire breast. Also be sure to examine from your armpit to the collar bone, as well as below your breast.
- Repeat the steps above on your right breast.
- While lying down, repeat the steps above on both breasts. Lie flat on your back, with your arm over your head. Place a pillow or folded towel under the shoulder of the breast that you are going to examine. This position flattens the breast and makes it easier to check.

BSE Patterns

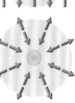

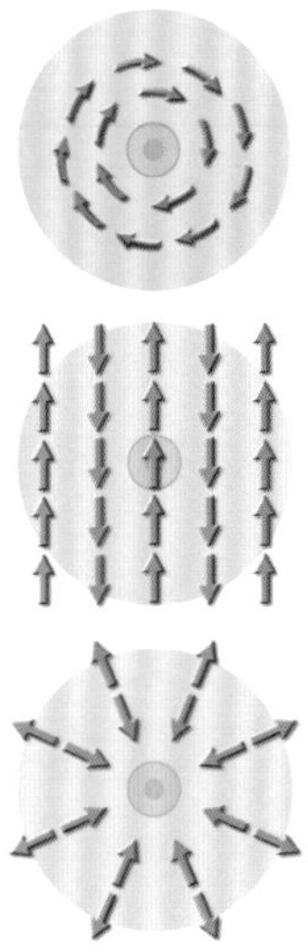

Lymph node / anatomy labels (left illustration)

- Lateral axillary nodes
- Central axillary nodes
- Apical nodes
- Infraclavicular nodes
- Lower deep cervical nodes
- Pectoralis major muscle
- subscapular (posterior) nodes
- Teres major muscle
- Latissimus dorsi muscle
- Internal mammary nodes
- Suspensory ligaments
- Subareolar plexus
- Serratus anterior muscle
- Lactiferous ducts
- Lactiferous sinus
- Lobes
- Fat

Signs and Symptoms

- A lump or mass in the breast
- Change in shape or size of the breast
- Change in the skin, such as thickening or dimpling, scaly skin around the nipple, an orange-peel-like appearance, or ulcers
- Discharge from the nipple that occurs without squeezing the nipple
- Change in the nipple, such as itching, burning, erosion, or retraction
- Swelling of the arm
- Pain (with an advanced tumor)
- Change in skin temperature or color (a warm, hot, or pink area)

Risk Factors for Breast Cancer

The cause of breast cancer isn't known, but its higher incidence in women suggests that estrogen is a cause or contributing factor. Women who are at increased risk include those who

- have a family history of breast cancer in close relatives (mother, sister, daughter)
- have a long menstrual history (began menstruating at an early age or experienced menopause late)
- have had cancer in one breast
- have had breast biopsy showing atypical hyperplasia (increased cell production)
- were first pregnant after age 31
- have never been pregnant
- were exposed to low-level ionizing radiation

Staging

Clinical staging is a part of the pretreatment evaluation and is performed based on physical examination and x-ray studies. The final (pathologic) stage is determined by microscopic examination of the biopsied tissue and axillary specimen to assess the size of the cancer and the presence of lymph node involvement, and the possibility of systemic metastasis (spread of cancer outside of the breast and lymph nodes). The most commonly used system is the **Tumor-Nodes-Metastasis system (TNM)**. **T** represents the tumor, **N** the lymph node involvement, and **M** the metastasis if any.

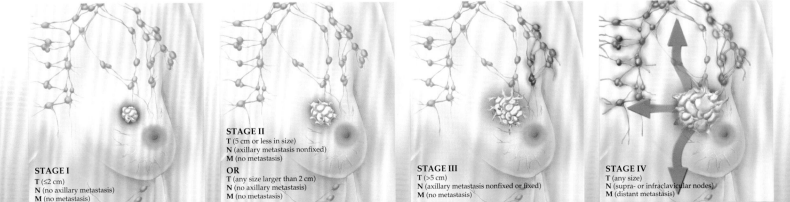

STAGE I
T (≤2 cm)
N (no axillary metastasis)
M (no metastasis)

STAGE II
T (5 cm or less in size)
N (axillary metastasis nonfixed)
M (no metastasis)
OR
T (any size larger than 2 cm)
N (no axillary metastasis)
M (no metastasis)

STAGE III
T (>5 cm)
N (axillary metastasis nonfixed or fixed)
M (no metastasis)

STAGE IV
T (any size)
N (supra- or infraclavicular nodes)
M (distant metastasis)

Published by Anatomical Chart Company, Skokie, IL | Medical illustrations by Liana Bauman, MAMS, in consultation with Ruth O'Regan, MD, William E. Burkel, PhD, University of Michigan Medical School and Monica Morrow, MD, FACS.

Fallopian Tube

Uterus

Fallopian Tube

Ovary

Ovary

Body of Uterus

Understanding
CERVICAL CANCER

The cervix is the lower, narrow end of the uterus. Cervical cancer is a disease in which cancer cells form in the tissues of the cervix. The most common types of cervical cancers are squamous cell cancer, adenosquamous cancer, and adenocarcinoma.

THE CERVIX AS VIEWED THROUGH A SPECULUM ON A PELVIC EXAM

Cervix

Ectocervical lesion

Vaginal wall

RISK FACTORS

Persistent human papillomavirus (HPV) infection, a sexually transmitted disease, is the major risk factor for developing cervical cancer. Other risk factors include the following:

- Smoking cigarettes
- History of sexually transmitted disease
- Many sexual partners
- First sexual intercourse at a young age
- Multiple children (Multiparous)
- Long-term use of oral contraceptives
- Weakened immune system

SIGNS AND SYMPTOMS

There are usually no signs or symptoms early in the disease, although cervical cancer can be detected with yearly checkups.
Some possible signs, which may appear as the disease progresses, include the following:

- **Abnormal vaginal bleeding**
  (bleeding between periods, after intercourse, or after menopause)
- **Unusual vaginal discharge**
  (may be pale, watery, red, or foul-smelling)
- **Pelvic pain at rest or during intercourse**

Note: Many other conditions may cause these same symptoms.

DIAGNOSIS/SCREENING

Tests that are used to detect and diagnose cervical cancer include the following:

- **Pelvic examination:** The doctor uses a speculum to visually examine the cervix and one or two fingers to feel for abnormalities.
- **Pap smear:** Cells from the cervix and vagina are collected and examined under a microscope to identify any abnormalities.
- **Colposcopy:** A colposcope, an instrument with a magnifying lens, is used to examine the vagina and cervix more closely.
- **Biopsy:** If abnormalities are found on colposcopy, a sample of tissue from the cervix is taken to view under a microscope.
- **Endocervical curettage:** Cells from the cervical canal are collected using a spoon-shaped instrument called a curette.
- **Cone biopsy (conization):** A cautery loop or a scalpel is used to remove the outer part of the cervix; this may also cure very early stage cervical cancer.

TREATMENT

Treatment options depend on the following:

- Stage of the cancer
- Size of the tumor
- Patient's desire to have children
- Patient's age and other medical problems

Treatment options include the following:

- **Surgery:** an operation to remove cancer; may include radical hysterectomy or more limited procedures to preserve fertility in very early stage cancer
- **Radiation therapy:** use of high-energy x-rays or other types of radiation to kill cancer cells
- **Chemotherapy:** use of drugs to stop the growth of cancer cells, either by killing the cells or by stopping the cells from dividing

Two or more methods may be used to treat cervical cancer in the same patient.

DETECTED EARLY, CERVICAL CANCER HAS A BETTER CHANCE TO BE CURED.

PREVENTION

- Having yearly checkups, including Pap smear examination.
  - HPV testing may be helpful for some Pap smear abnormalities and in women over age 30.
  - For patients who have had cervical cancer in the past, your doctor may recommend more frequent testing for the first few years after treatment.
- Talking to your doctor about a HPV vaccination. To be most effective, vaccination should occur before becoming sexually active.
- The risks of developing cervical cancer can be reduced by the following:
  - Regular pelvic and Pap smear examinations
  - Limiting the number of sexual partners
  - Avoiding sex with people who have had multiple sexual partners
  - Delaying the date of first sexual intercourse
  - Not smoking
  - HPV vaccination in appropriate patients

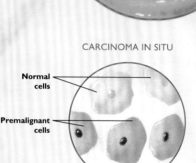

CARCINOMA IN SITU

Normal cells

Premalignant cells

SQUAMOUS CELL CARCINOMA

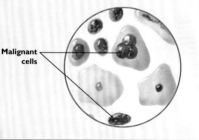

Malignant cells

STAGING

After the cervical cancer is diagnosed, the stage of the cancer (how far the cancer has spread) is determined. The following stages are used for cervical cancer:

STAGE 0: (Carcinoma in Situ): Cancer is found only in the outer layer of cells lining the cervix.
STAGE I: Cancer has invaded past the surface layer but is found only in the cervix.
STAGE II: Cancer has spread beyond the cervix but not to the pelvic wall nor to the lower third of the vagina.
STAGE III: Cancer has extended to the lower third of the vagina; it may have spread to the pelvic wall and/or blocked kidney functions.
STAGE IV: Cancer has spread to the bladder, rectum, or other parts of the body.

Common tests used to determine the stage of the cancer include the following:
- Pelvic examination
- Imaging tests:
  - X-rays of the chest and urinary system
  - Barium enema to assess the rectum
Additional tests used to determine treatment options include the following:
- CT scan (CAT scan)—Computerized tomography or computerized axial tomography
- MRI—Magnetic resonance imaging
- PET scan—Positron emission tomography

STAGE 0-1

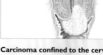

Carcinoma confined to the cervix.

Carcinoma confined to the cervix, "cauliflower" lesion.

Bulky endocervical barrel-shaped lesion.

STAGE 2

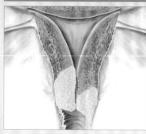

Carcinoma extends into the upper vagina.

Carcinoma extends into the parametrium (fibrous tissue that separates the cervix from the bladder) but does not extend to the pelvic sidewall.

STAGE 3

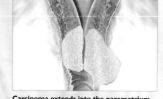

Carcinoma involves the anterior (front) vaginal wall, extending to the lower third of the vagina.

The parametrium is completely invaded and the carcinoma extends to the pelvic sidewall.

STAGE 4

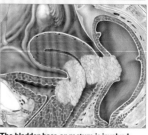

The bladder base or rectum is involved; distant metastasis may also be present.

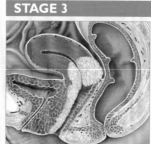

© 2007 Wolters Kluwer Published by Anatomical Chart Company, Skokie, IL. In consultation with Eric L. Eisenhauer, MD.

Understanding Ovarian Cancer

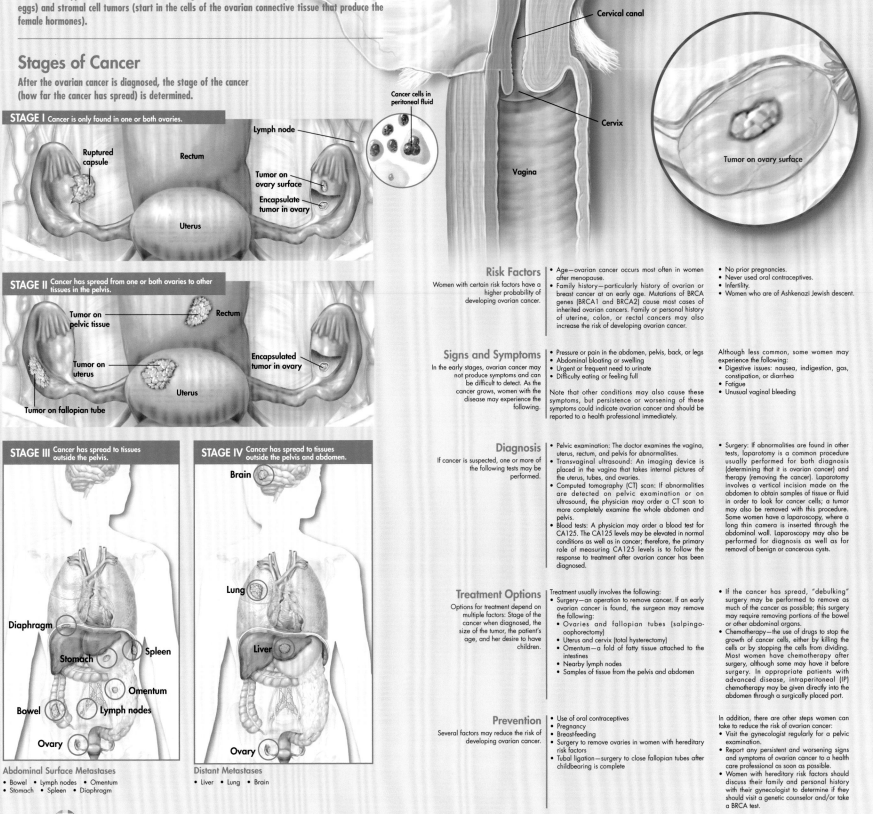

Round ligament

Uterine (Fallopian) tube

Broad ligament

Fundus of uterus

Ovarian ligament

Ovary

Ovarian artery and vein

Body of uterus

Cervical canal

Cervix

Cancer cells in peritoneal fluid

Vagina

Tumor on ovary surface

What Is Ovarian Cancer?

Ovaries are almond-sized reproductive organs that release eggs and make hormones. The most common form of ovarian cancer starts on the surface of the ovary and is called epithelial ovarian cancer. Rare types of ovarian cancers include germ cell tumors (develop in the cells that produce eggs) and stromal cell tumors (start in the cells of the ovarian connective tissue that produce the female hormones).

Stages of Cancer

After the ovarian cancer is diagnosed, the stage of the cancer (how far the cancer has spread) is determined.

STAGE I Cancer is only found in one or both ovaries.

Ruptured capsule

Rectum

Lymph node

Tumor on ovary surface

Encapsulate tumor in ovary

Uterus

STAGE II Cancer has spread from one or both ovaries to other tissues in the pelvis.

Tumor on pelvic tissue

Rectum

Tumor on uterus

Encapsulated tumor in ovary

Uterus

Tumor on fallopian tube

STAGE III Cancer has spread to tissues outside the pelvis.

Diaphragm

Stomach

Spleen

Bowel

Omentum

Lymph nodes

Ovary

Abdominal Surface Metastases
- Bowel • Lymph nodes • Omentum
- Stomach • Spleen • Diaphragm

STAGE IV Cancer has spread to tissues outside the pelvis and abdomen.

Brain

Lung

Liver

Ovary

Distant Metastases
- Liver • Lung • Brain

Risk Factors

Women with certain risk factors have a higher probability of developing ovarian cancer.

- Age—ovarian cancer occurs most often in women after menopause.
- Family history—particularly history of ovarian or breast cancer at an early age. Mutations of BRCA genes (BRCA1 and BRCA2) cause most cases of inherited ovarian cancers. Family or personal history of uterine, colon, or rectal cancers may also increase the risk of developing ovarian cancer.
- No prior pregnancies.
- Never used oral contraceptives.
- Infertility.
- Women who are of Ashkenazi Jewish descent.

Signs and Symptoms

In the early stages, ovarian cancer may not produce symptoms and can be difficult to detect. As the cancer grows, women with the disease may experience the following.

- Pressure or pain in the abdomen, pelvis, back, or legs
- Abdominal bloating or swelling
- Urgent or frequent need to urinate
- Difficulty eating or feeling full

Note that other conditions may also cause these symptoms, but persistence or worsening of these symptoms could indicate ovarian cancer and should be reported to a health professional immediately.

Although less common, some women may experience the following:
- Digestive issues: nausea, indigestion, gas, constipation, or diarrhea
- Fatigue
- Unusual vaginal bleeding

Diagnosis

If cancer is suspected, one or more of the following tests may be performed.

- Pelvic examination: The doctor examines the vagina, uterus, rectum, and pelvis for abnormalities.
- Transvaginal ultrasound: An imaging device is placed in the vagina that takes internal pictures of the uterus, tubes, and ovaries.
- Computed tomography (CT) scan: If abnormalities are detected on pelvic examination or on ultrasound, the physician may order a CT scan to more completely examine the whole abdomen and pelvis.
- Blood tests: A physician may order a blood test for CA125. The CA125 levels may be elevated in normal conditions as well as in cancer; therefore, the primary role of measuring CA125 levels is to follow the response to treatment after ovarian cancer has been diagnosed.

- Surgery: If abnormalities are found in other tests, laparotomy is a common procedure usually performed for both diagnosis (determining that it is ovarian cancer) and therapy (removing the cancer). Laparotomy involves a vertical incision made on the abdomen to obtain samples of tissue or fluid in order to look for cancer cells; a tumor may also be removed with this procedure. Some women have a laparoscopy, where a long thin camera is inserted through the abdominal wall. Laparoscopy may also be performed for diagnosis as well as for removal of benign or cancerous cysts.

Treatment Options

Options for treatment depend on multiple factors: Stage of the cancer when diagnosed, the size of the tumor, the patient's age, and her desire to have children.

Treatment usually involves the following:
- Surgery—an operation to remove cancer. If an early ovarian cancer is found, the surgeon may remove the following:
  - Ovaries and fallopian tubes (salpingo-oophorectomy)
  - Uterus and cervix (total hysterectomy)
  - Omentum—a fold of fatty tissue attached to the intestines
  - Nearby lymph nodes
  - Samples of tissue from the pelvis and abdomen

- If the cancer has spread, "debulking" surgery may be performed to remove as much of the cancer as possible; this surgery may require removing portions of the bowel or other abdominal organs.
- Chemotherapy—the use of drugs to stop the growth of cancer cells, either by killing the cells or by stopping the cells from dividing. Most women have chemotherapy after surgery, although some may have it before surgery. In appropriate patients with advanced disease, intraperitoneal (IP) chemotherapy may be given directly into the abdomen through a surgically placed port.

Prevention

Several factors may reduce the risk of developing ovarian cancer.

- Use of oral contraceptives
- Pregnancy
- Breast-feeding
- Surgery to remove ovaries in women with hereditary risk factors
- Tubal ligation—surgery to close fallopian tubes after childbearing is complete

In addition, there are other steps women can take to reduce the risk of ovarian cancer:
- Visit the gynecologist regularly for a pelvic examination.
- Report any persistent and worsening signs and symptoms of ovarian cancer to a health care professional as soon as possible.
- Women with hereditary risk factors should discuss their family and personal history with their gynecologist to determine if they should visit a genetic counselor and/or take a BRCA test.

© 2008 Wolters Kluwer Published by Anatomical Chart Company, Skokie, IL. In consultation with Eric Eisenhauer, MD.

UNDERSTANDING · colorectal cancer

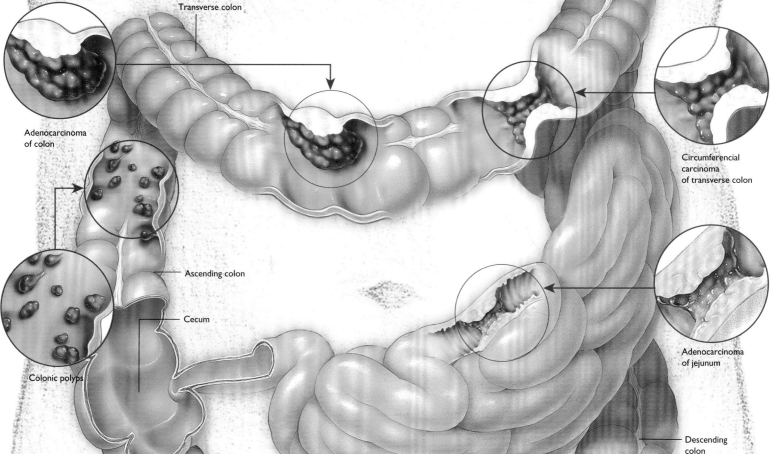

Transverse colon

Adenocarcinoma
of colon

Ascending colon

Cecum

Colonic polyps

Vermiform appendix

Circumferencial
carcinoma
of transverse colon

Adenocarcinoma
of jejunum

Descending
colon

Adenocarcinoma of
rectosigmoid region

Rectum

Anus

Sigmoid
colon

What Is Colorectal Cancer? Cancer that begins in the colon is called colon cancer, and cancer that begins in the rectum is called rectal cancer. Cancers affecting either of these organs is also called colorectal cancer.

Colorectal cancer occurs when some of the cells that line the colon or the rectum become abnormal and grow out of control. The abnormal-growing cells create a tumor, which is the cancer.

Who Is at Risk for Colorectal Cancer? Everybody is at risk for colorectal cancer. Colorectal cancer is the 3rd leading type of cancer causing deaths in the United States. The majority of people who develop colorectal cancer have no known risk factors.

The exact cause of colorectal cancer is not yet known. Below are some factors that could increase a person's risk of developing this disease.

• **Age**—The disease is more common in people over 50. The chance of getting colorectal cancer increases with each decade of life. However, it has also been detected in younger people.
• **Gender**—Overall the risks are equal, but women have a higher risk for colon cancer and men are more likely to develop rectal cancer.
• **Polyps**—Beginning as noncancerous growths on the inner wall of the colon or rectum, these are fairly common in people over 50 years of age. Adenomas are one type of noncancerous polyps that can mutate and are the potential precursors of colon and rectal cancer.
• **Personal history**—Research shows that women who have a history of ovarian or uterine cancer have a slight increased risk of developing colorectal cancer. In addition, people who have ulcerative colitis or Crohn's disease also are at higher risk.
• **Family history**—Parents, siblings, and children of a person who has had colorectal cancer are more likely to develop the disease themselves. A family history of familial polyposis, adenomatous polyps, or hereditary polyp syndrome also increases the risk.
• **Diet**—A diet high in fat and calories and low in fiber may be linked to a greater risk.
• **Lifestyle factors**—Alcohol, smoking, lack of exercise, and overweight status are additional risk factors.
• **Diabetes**—Diabetics have a 30%-40% increased risk.

Signs and Symptoms

Colorectal cancer may not cause any symptoms in early stages. However the following signs should raise suspicion:

• Change in bowel habits: Diarrhea or constipation or a change in the consistency of stool
• Narrow, pencil-thin stools
• Rectal bleed or blood in stool
• Persistent abdominal discomfort such as gas, pain, or cramps
• Feeling bowel does not empty completely
• Unexplained weight loss
• Constant fatigue

Screening tests

• **Fecal Occult Blood Test (FOBT)**—Checks for hidden blood in the stool.
• **Sigmoidoscopy**—Sigmoidoscope is a long, flexible tube with a tiny video camera at the tip that is inserted into the rectum to allow the doctor to view the lower part of the colon—the rectum, the descending colon, and the sigmoid colon.
• **Colonoscopy**—Colonoscope is a long, flexible tube with a tiny video camera at the tip that is inserted into the rectum to allow the doctor to view the inside of the entire colon. The doctor may also biopsy the tissue and remove polyps during a colonoscopy.
• **Barium enema**—Chalky white liquid called barium is released into the colon (through the rectum) and then an x-ray is performed.
• **Digital rectal examination.**

Diagnostic tests

If the screening tests or symptoms indicate the possibility of colorectal cancer, patients will undergo a diagnostic workup. These will help determine if colorectal cancer is present and the stage of the disease. Tests may include the following:

• **Medical history.**
• **Physical examination.**
• **Blood tests.**
• **Biopsy**—abnormal tissue is removed and examined during a screening test to check for cancer cells.
• **Imaging tests.**
• **Ultrasound.**
• **Computed tomography (CT).**
• **Magnetic resonance imaging (MRI).**
• **Chest x-ray** (to see if the cancer has spread to the lungs).

Treatments

Choice of treatment(s) depends on the location of the tumor (colon or rectum) and the stage of the disease. Common types of treatments include the following:

• **Surgery**—This is the most common treatment. It is used for removal of polyps and tumors and to check for the spread of the disease. Common types include laparoscopy and open surgery. After removal of part of the colon or rectum, the healthy parts are usually reconnected. When reconnection is not possible, a colostomy may be performed.
• **Chemotherapy**—Drug therapy that prevents the spread of cancer cells.
• **Radiation therapy**—Also known as radiotherapy; uses high energy-rays to kill cancer cells.
• **Biological therapy**—Patients receive a monoclonal antibody through a vein that binds to colorectal cancer cells, interfering with their cell growth and spread in the body.

The Stages of Cancer

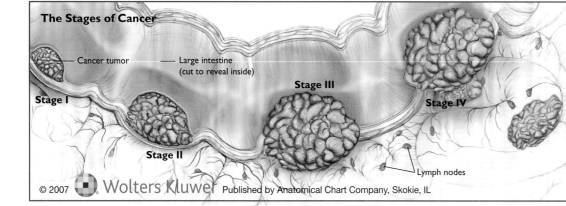

Cancer tumor

Large intestine
(cut to reveal inside)

Stage I

Stage II

Stage III

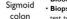

Stage IV

Lymph nodes

The earlier cancer is found and treated, the better the chances of getting well. The diagnosis of cancer is made by a microscopic test (biopsy) of a piece of tissue. Medical imaging techniques are used to measure how much the cancer has spread (grown)—this is known as staging.
The doctors often decide on the treatment based on the stage of cancer.

Doctors identify the stages of cancer as follows:
Stage I: The cancer has grown into the inner wall of the colon or rectum. The tumor has not yet reached the outer wall of the colon or extended outside the colon. Dukes' A is another name for Stage I colorectal cancer.

Stage II: The tumor extends more deeply into or through the wall of the colon or rectum. It may have invaded nearby tissue, but cancer cells have not yet spread to the lymph nodes. Dukes' B is another name for Stage II colorectal cancer.

Stage III: The cancer has spread to nearby lymph nodes, but not to other parts of the body. Dukes' C is another name for Stage III colorectal cancer.

Stage IV: The cancer has spread to other parts of the body, such as the liver or lungs. Dukes' D is another name for Stage IV colorectal cancer.

What Is Leukemia?

Leukemia is a cancer of the blood or bone marrow characterized by an abnormal production of white blood cells in the body. The leukemic cells generally look different from normal blood cells, and they do not function properly. Over time, leukemic cells may crowd out other types of blood cells, thereby affecting the production of normal red and white blood cells, and platelets.

Blood Cell Development

Blood cells are produced inside the bone in a spongy space called the bone marrow. The process of blood cell formation is called hematopoiesis. All blood cells have a common origin called a stem cell. Stem cells develop into specific mature blood cells by a process called differentiation. Early immature cells are called blasts, which grow into mature blood cells. Once the cells are matured, they are released into the blood where they circulate throughout the body and perform their respective functions.

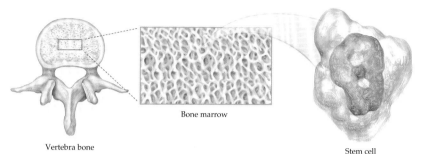

Vertebra bone

Bone marrow

Stem cell

What Is the Function of Blood?

Blood is continuously circulating through the blood vessels carrying vital elements to every part of the body. The blood plays an important role in transporting nutrients from the digestive tract to the body tissues. Oxygen is transported from the lungs to other cells of the body. Waste from cells is carried to the respiratory and excretory organs through the blood. Hormones are transported from the endocrine glands to target tissues via blood. White blood cells participate in the body's immune system to help fight infections and diseases.

What Are the Causes and the Risk Factors?

The exact cause of leukemia is still unknown, but it is influenced by both genetic and environmental factors such as:

- Genetic predisposition
- Environmental exposure to chemicals and/or radiation
- Immunologic factors
- Myelodysplastic syndrome (disease of the blood)

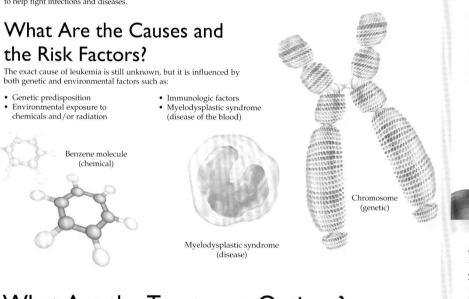

Benzene molecule (chemical)

Myelodysplastic syndrome (disease)

Chromosome (genetic)

What Are the Treatment Options?

A person with **acute lymphoblastic leukemia** or **acute myeloid leukemia** needs to be treated right away with chemotherapy (drugs that destroy cancer cells).

Acute lymphoblastic leukemia (ALL)—chemotherapy involves multiple phases, which can vary according to protocols.
- Induction phase—large doses of anticancer drugs are used (4-5 drugs given over 1 month).
- Consolidation phase—new combinations of drugs are used to destroy any leukemia cells that are still "hiding" within the body.
- Delayed intensification phase—the goal is to give intense chemotherapy when the amount of leukemia cells is low.
- Maintenance phase—used to keep the leukemia in remission (can last 18 months to 2.5 years).
- CNS prophylactic (preventive) therapy—since ALL may spread to the coverings of the brain and spinal cord, medication is given directly into the spinal fluid using a lumbar puncture (spinal tap).

Chronic lymphocytic leukemia (CLL)—therapy options include the following:
- Observation or "watchful waiting" for a patient who has no symptoms, large lymph nodes, and normal red cell and platelet counts.
- Chemotherapy—single or combination of drugs are used.
- Monoclonal antibodies—created in the lab to specifically react with certain types of cancer cells. This can help the patient's immune system to respond and destroy these cancer cells.

Acute myeloid leukemia (AML)—chemotherapy involves the following:
- Induction phase—usually 2 chemotherapy drugs are used and sometimes a third drug is added.
- Consolidation phase—usually involves 2-4 cycles of additional chemotherapy.
- Maintenance phase—not used in AML, except in a variant known as acute promyelocytic leukemia.

Chronic myeloid leukemia (CML)—initial therapy involves the following:
- Imatinib—an oral drug specifically designed to target and interfere with the growth of a protein made by CML cells.

Allogeneic stem cell transplantation (SCT)—is a procedure where healthy bone marrow (stem cells) from a donor are transplanted into a leukemia patient. This treatment may be used for all types of leukemia, but it is done only after chemotherapy has been initiated.
Stem Cell Transplant...
- Is seldom used in pediatric ALL, but it is used in adult ALL
- Is rarely used in CLL patients, since this type of leukemia usually occurs in older patients and the course is often prolonged with multiple therapeutic options
- Is considered at early stages of AML
- May still be considered for young CML patients with a matched sibling or for patients who are not responding well to imatinib

Bone marrow biopsy (SCT procedure)

Types of Leukemia

Leukemias are grouped by how quickly the disease develops and progresses:
- **Acute leukemia**—gets worse quickly as the production of abnormal cells increases rapidly
- **Chronic leukemia**—gets worse slowly and symptoms may not appear for a long time

Leukemias are also grouped by the type of white blood cells that are affected.
- When leukemia affects lymphoid cells, it is called **lymphocytic leukemia**.
- When myeloid cells are affected, the disease is called **myeloid** or **myelogenous leukemia**.

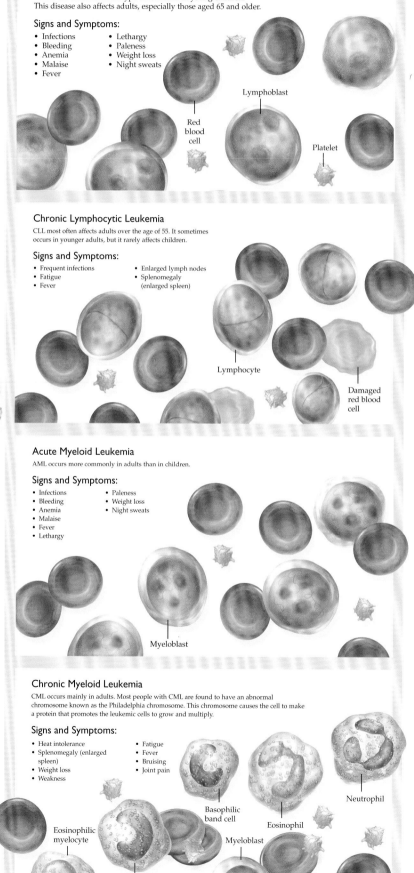

Acute Lymphoblastic Leukemia

ALL is the most common type of leukemia in young children. This disease also affects adults, especially those aged 65 and older.

Signs and Symptoms:
- Infections
- Bleeding
- Anemia
- Malaise
- Fever
- Lethargy
- Paleness
- Weight loss
- Night sweats

Lymphoblast

Red blood cell

Platelet

Chronic Lymphocytic Leukemia

CLL most often affects adults over the age of 55. It sometimes occurs in younger adults, but it rarely affects children.

Signs and Symptoms:
- Frequent infections
- Fatigue
- Fever
- Enlarged lymph nodes
- Splenomegaly (enlarged spleen)

Lymphocyte

Damaged red blood cell

Acute Myeloid Leukemia

AML occurs more commonly in adults than in children.

Signs and Symptoms:
- Infections
- Bleeding
- Anemia
- Malaise
- Fever
- Lethargy
- Paleness
- Weight loss
- Night sweats

Myeloblast

Chronic Myeloid Leukemia

CML occurs mainly in adults. Most people with CML are found to have an abnormal chromosome known as the Philadelphia chromosome. This chromosome causes the cell to make a protein that promotes the leukemic cells to grow and multiply.

Signs and Symptoms:
- Heat intolerance
- Splenomegaly (enlarged spleen)
- Weight loss
- Weakness
- Fatigue
- Fever
- Bruising
- Joint pain

Basophilic band cell

Neutrophil

Eosinophilic myelocyte

Eosinophil

Myeloblast

Basophil

UNDERSTANDING Lung Cancer

Lung cancer is the rapid growth of abnormal (malignant) cells in one or both of the lungs. It can invade nearby tissues and may spread (metastasize) to other areas of the body.

Trachea

Lymph nodes

Metastasis to paratracheal lymph nodes

Bronchus

Tumor projecting into bronchi

Metastasis to carinal lymph nodes

LEFT UPPER LOBE

Tumor projecting into bronchi

LEFT LOWER LOBE

APPROXIMATELY 90% OF LUNG CANCER DEATHS ARE RELATED TO SMOKING

There are 2 major types of lung cancer:
Non–small cell lung cancer and small cell lung cancer

Non–small cell lung cancer (NSCLC) is more common than small cell lung cancer, accounting for about 85% of all lung cancers; it generally grows and spreads more slowly. The three most common type of non–small cell lung cancer are as follows:
1. **Adenocarcinoma** is the most common subtype of NSCLC. It is usually found in the outer part of the lung.
2. **Squamous cell carcinoma** is a tumor found near a bronchus.
3. **Large cell carcinoma** is a fast-growing form that can develop in any part of the lung.

NSCLC is staged according to the size of the tumor, the level of lymph node involvement, and the extent to which the cancer has spread. Stages include the following:

Stage 0	Cancer is limited to the lining of the air passages and has not yet invaded the lung tissue.
Stage I	Cancer has invaded the underlying lung tissue, but has not yet spread to the lymph nodes.
Stage II	Cancer has spread to the neighboring lymph nodes or has spread to the chest wall, or the diaphragm, or the pleura between the lungs, or membranes surrounding the heart.
Stage III	Cancer has spread from the lung to either the lymph nodes in the center of the chest or the collarbone area. The cancer may have spread locally to areas such as the heart, blood, vessels, trachea, and esophagus.
Stage IV	Cancer has spread to other parts of the body, such as the liver, bones, or brain.

Small cell lung cancer (SCLC), also known as oat cell cancer, is the less common form of lung cancer. It is a fast-growing cancer that forms in the tissues of the lungs and spreads to other parts of the body.

SCLC is staged differently from non–small cell types. Rather than using numbers, it is classified as either limited or extensive.

Limited	Cancer is confined to one lung and to its neighboring lymph nodes.
Extensive	Cancer has spread beyond one lung and nearby lymph nodes; it may have invaded both lungs, more remote lymph nodes, or other organs.

How Is Lung Cancer Diagnosed?
The tests used to diagnose whether a patient has lung cancer varies depending on the patient's symptoms.
Chest x-ray—Most patients undergo this test to see if there are any abnormalities.
Chest CT scan—If an abnormality is discovered in the chest x-ray, a computerized tomography (CT) scan is performed to provide a series of detailed pictures of parts inside the body, taken from different angles.
Biopsy—There are several different types of biopsy procedures. The choice of procedure, which may involve surgery, will depend on what is discovered via the chest x-ray and/or chest CT scan.
Sputum cytology—A sample of phlegm is examined under a microscope.

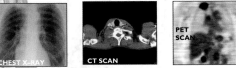

CHEST X-RAY   CT SCAN   PET SCAN   MRI

How Is Lung Cancer Staged?
If cancer is diagnosed, more tests are done so the doctor can plan a treatment.
These tests help discover the stage (extent) of the cancer. Common tests include the following:
Positron emission tomography (PET) scan—After a small amount of radioactive glucose (sugar) is injected into a vein of a patient, a special camera makes computerized pictures highlighting potential cancer cells.
PET/CT scan—PET scan information is combined with the anatomical information from a CT scan to reliably determine whether an abnormal growth is cancerous or benign (noncancerous).
Magnetic resonance imaging (MRI) of the head—A powerful magnet linked to a computer produces detailed images of the areas inside the head.
Mediastinoscopy/Mediastinotomy—A lighted instrument (scope) is inserted into the body to examine the chest and nearby lymph nodes.

Risk Factors
- **Smoking cigarettes, cigars, and pipes.**
- **Exposure to:**
  Secondhand smoke.
  Radon—Radioactive gas that occurs naturally in soil and rocks. Mine workers may be exposed to radon. Radon may also be found in homes and buildings.
  Asbestos—Group of naturally occurring fibrous minerals that are used in certain industries.
  Pollution.
- **Having previous lung diseases, such at tuberculosis (TB) and emphysema.**
- **Personal history**—A person with a history of lung cancer is more likely to develop it again than someone who has never had the disease.
- **Heredity**—Genetics seem to play a role in who develops lung cancer.

Signs and Symptoms
- **Cough that does not go away**
- **Constant chest pain**
- **Coughing up blood**
- **Shortness of breath, wheezing, or hoarseness**
- **Problems with pneumonia or bronchitis**
- **Swelling of the neck and face**
- **Loss of appetite and/or weight**
- **Fatigue**

If lung cancer has spread to other organs (metastasized), signs may include headaches, visual changes, strokelike symptoms (if cancer has spread to the brain), and bone pain (if the cancer has spread to the bones).

Treatment Options
Treatment depends on a number of factors including the type of lung cancer, the size/location/stage of the tumor, and the general health and pulmonary function of the patient. Many different types of treatments or combination of treatments may be used, such as the following:
Surgical Resection—A portion of the lung containing the tumor is removed. Depending on the case, the surgeon may remove only a small portion, the entire lobe (lobectomy), or the entire lung (pneumonectomy). Lymph nodes are also sampled at the time of surgery. Lobectomy is the most widely used surgical procedure for lung cancer.
Chemotherapy—The use of anticancer drugs that kill cancer cells throughout the body.
Radiation Therapy—The use of high-energy rays to kill cancer cells. This therapy is directed to a limited area and affects the cancer cells only in that area.
Endobronchial Therapy—A group of therapies used to treat lesions that are accessible in the lung airways. They are primarily used for palliative therapy (to relieve symptoms, not to cure the disease) but may also be used for early stages of the disease.

How Can Lung Cancer Be Prevented?
- **Don't smoke**—If you do smoke, quit. If you stop smoking, the risk of lung cancer decreases each year as normal cells replace abnormal cells. After 10 years, the risk drops to a level that is one-third to one-half of the risk of people who continue to smoke.
- **Avoid secondhand smoke.**
- **Test your home for radon.**
- **Avoid carcinogens**—People who are exposed to large amounts of asbestos should use protective equipment.

 Wolters Kluwer   Published by Anatomical Chart Company, Skokie, IL.

Non–Small Cell Lung Cancer

Non–small cell lung cancer (NSCLC) includes
- Adenocarcinoma (most common)
- Squamous cell carcinoma
- Large cell neuroendocrine lung cancer
- Carcinoids
- Sarcomatoid carcinomas

Signs and Symptoms
- Chest discomfort or pain
- Trouble breathing
- Wheezing
- Swelling in the face and/or veins in the neck
- Cough—A cough that doesn't go away or gets worse over time
- Coughing up blood
- Hoarseness
- Dyspnea

Early-stage lung cancers may be asymptomatic and detected by x-rays done for other reasons.

Diagnosis/Screening
- Lung cancer screening using a low-dose CT scan is recommended in patients aged 55-74 years with a >30-pack/year smoking history who are actively smoking or who quit <15 years ago
- Annual screening for 3 years in this patient population decreased lung cancer mortality by 20%.

NSCLC screening tests include the following:
- Chest x-ray
- CT scan
- Sputum cytology
- Bronchoscopy
- Thoracoscopy
- Thoracentesis
- Light and electron microscopy
- Immunohistochemistry
- Fine-needle aspiration biopsy of the lung

Staging
Non-small cell lung cancer is staged based on the size of the primary tumor and where it has spread (lymph nodes, distant organs).

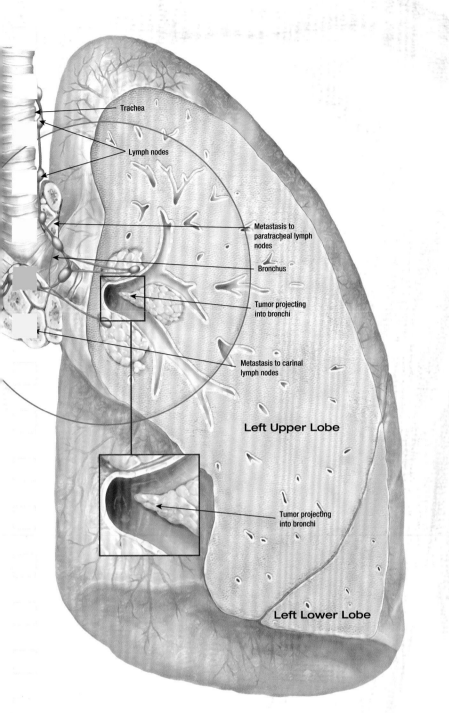

Trachea

Lymph nodes

Metastasis to paratracheal lymph nodes

Bronchus

Tumor projecting into bronchi

Metastasis to carinal lymph nodes

Left Upper Lobe

Tumor projecting into bronchi

Left Lower Lobe

Stages of Non–Small Cell Lung Cancer

Occult (Hidden)	• Cannot be detected by normal imaging, but is found in mucus coughed up from the lungs or cells taken from the airways leading to the lungs
Stage 0	• Abnormal cells found in airways leading to the lungs
Stage IA	• Tumor size is ≤3 cm in diameter and only found in the lung
Stage IB	• Has not spread to lymph nodes • Is <5 cm • Has spread to main bronchus below trachea • Has spread to membrane that covers the lung • Causes partial collapse of lung or pneumonitis develops
Stage II	• Any size tumor that invades the chest wall, diaphragm, lining of the lungs/heart, or main bronchus. • This includes separate tumors in the same lobe, and a tumor that has spread to local lymph nodes. • Divided into IIA and IIB depending on size and location of tumor.
Stage III	• Tumor that has spread to more distant lymph nodes in the chest. Any size tumor that invades the center of the chest, heart, great vessels, windpipe, esophagus, or spine. • This includes separate tumors in different lung lobes on the same side of the chest. • Divided into IIIA and further into sections 1, 2, and 3, and IIIB and further into sections 1 and 2 depending on size, location, and lymph nodes affected.
Stage IV	• Spreads to distant organ (adrenal gland, bone, brain, liver, opposite lung) or tumor cells are found in fluid around the lung or heart

Treatment Options

Chemotherapy	• Used to kill tumor cells that have spread throughout the body • Toxic to normal cells so patients may experience hair loss, numbness of the hands/feet, and/or nausea/diarrhea
Immunotherapy	• Harnesses the ability of the immune system to kill tumor cells throughout the body. • Side effects are principally inflammatory and include diarrhea, pneumonia, and thyroid problems. • Medications are given by intravenous infusion every 2-3 weeks to stimulate the immune system to kill tumor cells throughout the body more effectively.
Targeted Therapy	• Uses drugs that specifically block tumor proteins that cause cancer in specific populations, avoiding many of the side effects of chemotherapy, which targets normal and cancerous cells nonspecifically

Surgery	• Surgical options include
	  ◆ Resection
	  ◆ Endoscopy
	  ◆ Lobectomy
	• Combinations of surgery and the above therapies

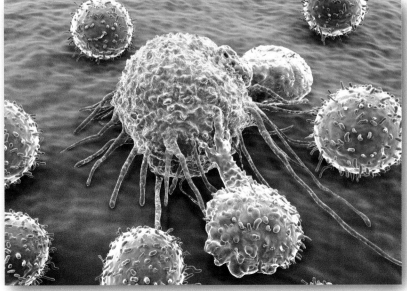

Immunotherapy unleashes the body's natural ability to attack and kill tumor cells

 Wolters Kluwer Medical illustrations by Dawn Gorski, MAMS, in consultation with Curtis R. Chong, MD, PhD, M.Phil, FACP, Massachusetts General Hospital, Boston, MA.

Multiple Myeloma

- Multiple myeloma is a cancer of the white blood cells (B cells) that produce antibodies.
- Cancerous B cells are trapped in an immature state and divide rapidly.
- Multiple myeloma is distinguished from smoldering or asymptomatic myeloma by the presence of damage to organs (ie, elevated blood calcium levels, renal failure, anemia, and bony lesions).
- There are approximately 30,000 new cases of myeloma in the US each year.
- The median age of diagnosis is 66 years.
- African Americans are twice as likely to have this disease.
- The most common symptom of multiple myeloma is bone pain, weakness, and/or fracture.

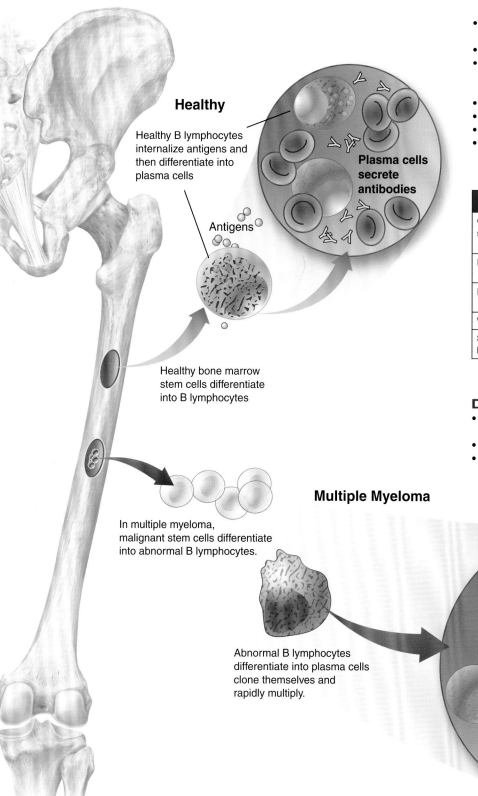

Healthy

Healthy B lymphocytes internalize antigens and then differentiate into plasma cells

Plasma cells secrete antibodies

Antigens

Healthy bone marrow stem cells differentiate into B lymphocytes

In multiple myeloma, malignant stem cells differentiate into abnormal B lymphocytes.

Multiple Myeloma

Abnormal B lymphocytes differentiate into plasma cells clone themselves and rapidly multiply.

Damaged plasma cells do not fight infection

Signs and Symptoms

Common symptoms	Symptoms due to high blood calcium levels caused by degrading bones	Less common symptoms
Bone pain	Loss of appetite	Swelling of lymph nodes, liver, or spleen
Fatigue	Nausea	Increased infections such as pneumonia or urinary tract
Weight loss	Confusion	Back pain
Shortness of breath		

Diagnosis/Screening

- Blood and urine tests to look for evidence of increased antibodies and damage to bone or kidneys
- Bone marrow biopsy
- X-rays of the spine and long bones

Treatment

- Patients with myeloma who are healthy enough may undergo a bone marrow transplant.

Drug Treatments

Most patients with signs or symptoms of multiple myeloma are treated with regimens that involve drug combinations that may include one of the following.

Drug class	What they treat
Proteasome inhibitor	Inhibit the ability of cancer cells to degrade proteins
Angiogenesis inhibitor	Causes degradation of proteins necessary for survival of multiple myeloma cells
Glucocorticoid	Steroid that works on the immune system to minimize inflammation and swelling
Monoclonal antibody (mAb)	Antibodies that bind to the surface of the myeloma cells
Alkylating agent	Conventional chemotherapy agents used to kill rapidly dividing myeloma cells
Bisphosphonates	Strengthen bones and prevent fractures

Staging

Stage I Least aggressive	Stage II	Stage III Aggressive
Small number of myeloma cells are found	Moderate number of myeloma cells are present	Large number of myeloma cells
Hemoglobin slightly below normal		Low hemoglobin levels
Calcium levels normal		High blood calcium
Small amount of monoclonal immunoglobulin in blood or urine		Large amount of monoclonal immunoglobulin in blood or urine
Normal bone structure		Areas of bone are destroyed —more than three lesions

© 2017 Wolters Kluwer Medical illustrations by Jennifer Smith, in consultation with Curtis Chong, MD, PhD, M.Phil, FACP, Massachusetts General Hospital, Boston, MA.

Understanding
Liver Cancer

Liver cancer is a cancer that starts in the liver, the largest organ found in your body. The liver removes toxic waste from the body, produces enzymes and bile to help food digestion, and converts food into substances your cells use to live and grow.

Signs and Symptoms

Liver cancer does not usually cause any symptoms in its early stages. When the cancer grows larger, it can cause some of the following symptoms:
• Weight loss
• Loss of appetite and feeling of fullness
• Nausea and vomiting
• Fever
• Pain in the upper abdomen on the right side
• Swollen abdomen (bloating)
• Weakness and lack of energy
• Yellow skin and eyes, pale stools, and dark urine (jaundice)

How Is Liver Cancer Diagnosed?

If symptoms suggest liver cancer, the following tests may be done to come to a diagnosis:
• Physical examination: The organs in the abdomen, including the liver and spleen, will be carefully felt through the skin to check for lumps or abnormal areas.
• Blood tests: The blood is tested for high levels of a protein called alpha-fetoprotein (AFP), which can be a sign of liver cancer. Other tests can show whether the liver is functioning properly.
• Ultrasound: Sound waves are used to make an image of the liver.
• CT scan: A series of x-rays are taken of the liver and other organs in the abdomen. Patients may receive an injection of contrast material so that the liver shows up more clearly in the images.
• MRI: Radio waves and strong magnets are used to take a series of images of the liver and other organs in the abdomen.
• Biopsy: In some cases, a doctor may remove a sample of liver tissue and look at it under a microscope. Biopsies can be done through the skin with a needle, or during laparoscopic or open surgery.

Stages of Cancer

In order to plan treatment, the physician must understand the extent (stage) of the disease. The stage is based on the size and spread of the tumor; the higher the stage, the more advanced the cancer. To determine if the cancer has spread, imaging tests such as a bone scan, CT scan, or MRI may be performed. Recurrent cancer is cancer that has come back after a period of being undetectable following treatment. The most commonly used staging system is the Tumor-Nodes-Metastasis system (TNM). T represents the primary tumor, N describes lymph node involvement, and M describes metastasis (spread away from the primary site of the tumor), if any.
• Stage I (T1, N0, M0): A single tumor that has not grown into any blood vessels and has not spread to nearby lymph nodes or other parts of the body.
• Stage II (T2, N0, M0): One or more tumors, none larger than 5 cm, may have grown into small blood vessels but have not spread to lymph nodes or other parts of the body.
• Stage IIIA-B (T3 or T4, N0 or N1, M0): One or several tumors have grown into a major liver blood vessel, are growing into a nearby organ, or are growing into the outer covering of the liver. The cancer has not spread to lymph nodes or distant parts of the body. Some patients with stage III liver cancer have tumors that are larger than 5 cm.
• Stage IIIC (Any T, N1, M0): Tumors have spread to nearby lymph nodes.
• Stage IV (Any T, Any N, M1): Tumors have spread to distant parts of the body.

In addition, several other staging systems have been developed that define the extent of liver cancer and liver function. At this time there is no single staging system used by all doctors. Other systems include the following:
• Barcelona-Clinic Liver Cancer (BCLC) system
• Cancer of the Liver Italian Program (CLIP) system
• Okuda system

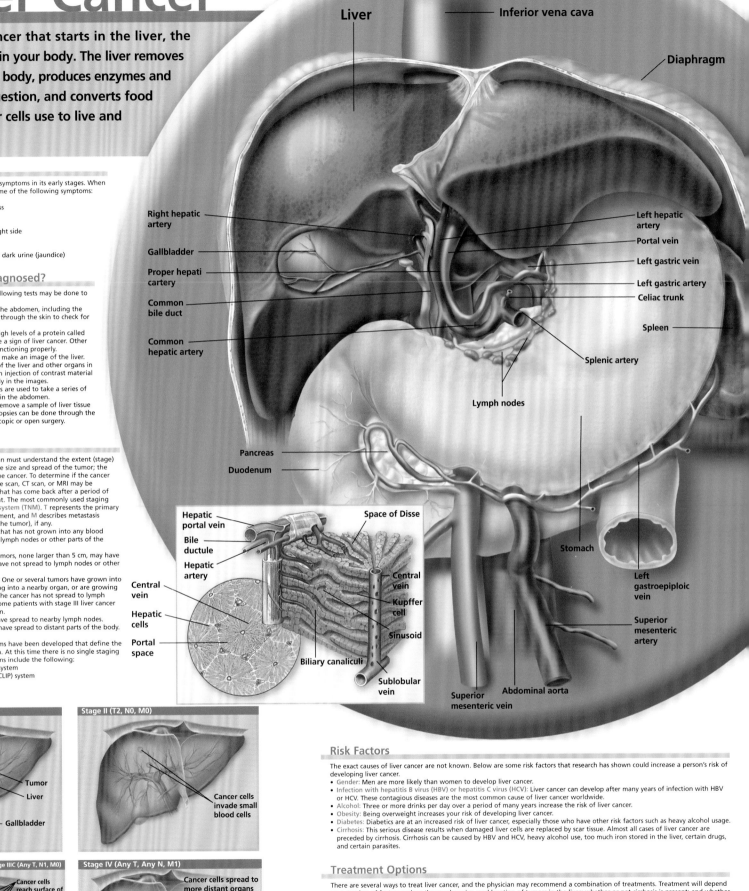

Liver — Inferior vena cava — Diaphragm
Right hepatic artery — Left hepatic artery — Portal vein
Gallblader — Left gastric vein
Proper hepatic cartery — Left gastric artery — Celiac trunk
Common bile duct — Spleen
Common hepatic artery — Splenic artery
Lymph nodes
Pancreas
Duodenum — Stomach — Left gastroepiploic vein
Superior mesenteric artery
Abdominal aorta
Superior mesenteric vein

Hepatic portal vein — Space of Disse
Bile ductule
Hepatic artery — Central vein
Central vein — Kupffer cell
Hepatic cells — Sinusoid
Portal space — Biliary canaliculi
Sublobular vein

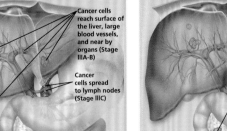

Stage I (T1, N0, M0)
Tumor
Liver
Gallbladder

Stage II (T2, N0, M0)
Cancer cells invade small blood cells

Stage IIIA-B (T3 or T4, N0 or N1, M0), Stage IIIC (Any T, N1, M0)
Cancer cells reach surface of the liver, large blood vessels, and near by organs (Stage IIIA-B)
Cancer cells spread to lymph nodes (Stage IIIC)

Stage IV (Any T, Any N, M1)
Cancer cells spread to more distant organs

Risk Factors

The exact causes of liver cancer are not known. Below are some risk factors that research has shown could increase a person's risk of developing liver cancer.
• Gender: Men are more likely than women to develop liver cancer.
• Infection with hepatitis B virus (HBV) or hepatitis C virus (HCV): Liver cancer can develop after many years of infection with HBV or HCV. These contagious diseases are the most common cause of liver cancer worldwide.
• Alcohol: Three or more drinks per day over a period of many years increase the risk of liver cancer.
• Obesity: Being overweight increases your risk of developing liver cancer.
• Diabetes: Diabetics are at an increased risk of liver cancer, especially those who have other risk factors such as heavy alcohol usage.
• Cirrhosis: This serious disease results when damaged liver cells are replaced by scar tissue. Almost all cases of liver cancer are preceded by cirrhosis. Cirrhosis can be caused by HBV and HCV, heavy alcohol use, too much iron stored in the liver, certain drugs, and certain parasites.

Treatment Options

There are several ways to treat liver cancer, and the physician may recommend a combination of treatments. Treatment will depend on a number of factors such as the number, size, and location of tumors in the liver; whether or not cirrhosis is present; and whether or not the cancer has spread. The physician will first determine whether your cancer can be completely removed through a surgical procedure. If your cancer cannot be removed through surgery, then he or she will recommend treatments to shrink your cancer for as long as possible.

Resectable—
For early-stage patients, a surgery can be performed to remove all of the visible sites of cancer. These surgeries include the following:
• Partial resection: This procedure involves removal of the part or parts of the liver that contain cancer.
• Liver transplant: If your cancer is present only in the liver but cannot be removed by a partial resection, the physician may recommend removal of the entire liver and replacement with healthy liver tissue through a liver transplant.

Unresectable—
For advanced-stage patients or patients who cannot undergo a partial resection or liver transplant for health reasons, a number of local and systemic treatments can be given to control the growth of the cancer. These include the following:
• Ablation: Heat (radiofrequency ablation) or alcohol (percutaneous ethanol injection) is used to kill cancer cells.
• Embolization: In this procedure, blood vessels to the tumor are blocked causing the tumor to die.
• Radiation therapy: Radiation uses high-energy rays to kill cancer cells.
• Chemotherapy: Drugs are given by mouth or IV (intravenously) and spread throughout the body to kill cancer cells.
• Targeted therapy: Newer drugs can focus on killing only cells within liver cancer tumors, while sparing the healthy cells of the body.

Stages of Kidney Cancer

To plan the best treatment, your doctor needs to know the stage (extent) of the disease. Staging may involve additional tests.

Stage I An early stage of kidney cancer where the tumor measures up to 7 cm. The cancer is confined to the kidney only.

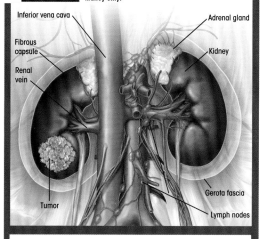

Inferior vena cava
Fibrous capsule
Renal vein
Adrenal gland
Kidney
Gerota fascia
Tumor
Lymph nodes

Stage II The tumor measures more than 7 cm but is still confined to the kidney.

Tumor

Stage III Characterized by any of the following:
- The tumor has not spread beyond Gerota fascia and may have involvement of the adrenal gland.
- Renal vein or vena cava involvement.
- The tumor is spreading to one of the nearby lymph nodes.

Tumors

Stage IV Characterized by any of the following:
- The tumor extends beyond Gerota fascia.
- Metastases to more than one lymph node.
- Cancer spreads to other organs.

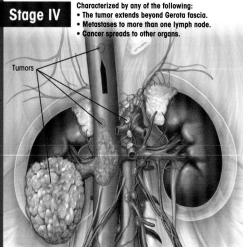

Tumors

UNDERSTANDING
Kidney Cancer

Your kidneys are two bean-shaped organs, each about the size of your fist, that are part of the urinary tract. Their primary function is to remove waste and extra water from the blood as urine. They also help stimulate the production of red blood cells and play a role in blood pressure regulation. Like any other organ in your body, your kidneys can develop a tumor (abnormal growth), which may be benign (noncancerous) or malignant (cancerous). Renal tumors are most commonly seen in adults but can also be found in children. The most common type of kidney cancer in adults is clear renal cell carcinoma (clear RCC).

Adrenal gland
Minor calyx
Kidney
Major calyx
Cortex
Renal column
Medulla (pyramid)
Perirenal fat in renal sinus
Fibrous capsule
Renal pelvis
Ureter

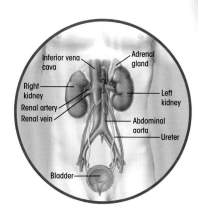

Inferior vena cava
Adrenal gland
Right kidney
Left kidney
Renal artery
Renal vein
Abdominal aorta
Ureter
Bladder

What Are the Risk Factors?

Generally, your risk of renal cell carcinoma increases as you age and occurs most commonly in people over 50. Men are twice as likely to develop renal cell carcinoma, the reasons for which remain unknown. There are several known risk factors for development of renal cell carcinoma such as the following:

Smoking—People who smoke are twice as likely to develop kidney cancer as nonsmokers.
Obesity—People who are obese have an increased risk of kidney cancer.
Long-term dialysis—Dialysis is a treatment for those whose kidneys do not work well.

Chemicals in the workplace—Such as asbestos, cadmium, or those found in the iron/steel industry.
Certain hereditary (genetic) disorders—May predispose patients to form renal tumors.

Signs and Symptoms

Kidney cancer rarely causes symptoms in its early stages, and most are diagnosed incidentally (during studies for unrelated complaints or findings). However, the following signs or symptoms may alert the clinician to search for kidney cancer:

- Blood in the urine (making the urine slightly rusty to deep red)
- A lump or mass in the side of the abdomen
- Back or side pain that does not go away
- Weight loss

- Anemia (too few red blood cells)
- Intermittent fever or sweats
- Fatigue

How Is Kidney Cancer Diagnosed?

Unfortunately, there are no blood or urine tests that directly detect the presence of kidney tumors, and oftentimes early stages of kidney tumors do not produce symptoms. However, your physician may recommend some of the following tests:

- **Urinalysis**—A test to check for presence of blood in the urine.
- **Blood tests**—To check for anemia (too few red blood cells).
- **Magnetic resonance imaging (MRI) or computed tomography (CT)**—To generate cross-sectional pictures of your body.
- **Ultrasound**—May help to differentiate solid masses (more likely to be cancerous) from cystic masses (fluid filled and less likely to be cancerous) in the kidneys.

- **Intravenous pyelogram (IVP)**—Dye is injected into a blood vessel, and x-rays are taken of the kidneys as the dye circulates through them. IVP used to be the most common imaging technique before the era of MRI or CT.
- **Biopsy**—In some cases, your doctor may recommend a kidney biopsy to obtain a tissue sample.

Treatments

The best treatment approach will depend on various factors including your general health, the kind of kidney cancer you have, whether the cancer has spread, and your own preferences for treatment.

Surgery—Tumor removal is the standard mode of treatment; it is done through a procedure that removes the entire affected kidney (nephrectomy) or removes only the part that contains the tumor (partial nephrectomy). Most patients can live a normal life with a single, adequately functioning kidney. Even in cases when the remaining kidney is functioning suboptimally, the patient may still be able to live a normal life.
Tumor ablation—Destroys the tumor without surgically removing it; this can be done through cryotherapy (freezing), interstitial radiofrequency ablation—also known as RFA or RITA (heating tumors with radio waves), laser coagulation (electromagnetic

energy), and microwave thermotherapy (controlled heat). The risk of tumor recurrence is somewhat higher with these approaches and is generally reserved for older or frail patients.
Observation—Means there is no intervention other than periodic surveillance with imaging. In selected patients, when the renal tumors are small or patients are older with multiple comorbidities, observation may be a reasonable option.
Embolization—Blocks the blood flow to an actively bleeding tumor (forcing the tumor to die) and may be considered in patients who cannot tolerate surgery.

Prevention
- Quit smoking.
- Maintain a healthy diet by eating more fruits and vegetables.
- Exercise. Aim for 30 minutes on most days.

- Control high blood pressure through exercise, diet, weight loss, and medication (if prescribed).
- Reduce or avoid exposure to toxins by wearing a mask and heavy gloves.

Understanding
Pancreatic Cancer

The pancreas is an important part of your digestive system. It produces digestive juices to help your body digest food, and it releases hormones, including insulin, to help your body process sugar. Pancreatic cancer occurs when cells in the pancreas develop genetic mutations. These mutations cause the cells to grow uncontrollably and continue living after normal cells would die. These accumulating cells can form a tumor. The majority of pancreatic cancers are adenocarcinomas, found in the cells that line the pancreas ducts where digestive juices are produced.

Signs and Symptoms

Pancreatic cancer is sometimes called a **"silent disease"** because early pancreatic cancer often does not cause symptoms. But, as the cancer grows, symptoms may include the following:

- Pain in the upper abdomen or upper back
- Yellowing of the skin and the white of the eyes (jaundice)
- Weakness
- Loss of appetite and weight loss
- Nausea and vomiting
- Depressed mood

Risk Factors

- **Smoking.**
- **Age**—Pancreatic cancer occurs most often in adults age 55 and over.
- **Race**—African Americans have the highest pancreatic cancer rate.
- **Gender**—More men than women are diagnosed with pancreatic cancer.
- **Chronic Pancreatitis**—Inflammation of the pancreas.
- **Family History**—Pancreatic cancer is more common in families with a history of pancreatic cancer or pancreatitis.
- **Environmental Factors**—Exposure to asbestos, pesticides, dyes, chemicals.
- **Pancreatic Cysts**—Intraductal papillary mucinous neoplasm (IPMN), a type of pancreatic cyst, is thought to be a common precursor to pancreatic cancer.

Diagnosis

- **CT Scan**—(computerized tomography) uses x-ray images to help your doctor visualize your internal organs.
- **ERCP**—(endoscopic retrograde cholangiopancreatography). This procedure uses a dye to highlight the bile ducts in your pancreas. A flexible tube (endoscope) is gently passed down your throat, through your stomach, and into the upper part of the small intestine. A dye is then injected into the ducts through a small hollow tube (catheter) that is passed through the endoscope. X-rays are then taken of the ducts.
- **Biopsy**—A small sample of tissue is obtained for examination under a microscope.
- **Laparoscopy**—determines the extent or the stage of the cancer, once cancer is confirmed. The surgeon passes a laparoscope through an incision in your abdomen. The camera on the end of the scope transmits video to a screen in the operating room. This allows your doctor to look for signs cancer has spread within your abdomen.

Stages of Cancer

Resectable (Stage I and II)—This means the cancer can likely be removed with surgery.

Locally Advanced (Stage III)—These cancers may not be able to be removed with surgery because they have spread into major blood vessels or nearby organs.

Metastatic (Stage IV)—These cancers spread to distant parts of the body such as the liver, abdominal cavity, or lungs.

Managing Cancer, Managing Life

- Learn all you can about pancreatic cancer.
- Explore your options for pain management: medications, heat/cold, acupuncture, massage, meditation.
- Maintain proper nutrition to promote strength and healing.
- Consider dietary (caloric and enzyme) supplements.
- Drink plenty of fluids.
- Build a strong support system.

Tumor on Tail of Pancreas

Common Hepatic Artery
Aorta
Pancreas
Bile Duct
Celiac Trunk
Hepatic Portal Vein
Splenic Artery
Tail
Body
Head
Spleen
Inferior Mesenteric Vein
Small Intestine
Superior Mesenteric Vein and Artery

Tumor on Head of Pancreas

Location of Pancreas and Surrounding Organs

Lung
Liver
Stomach (cut)
Spleen
Gallbladder
Large Intestines (cut)
Small Intestines (cut)
Pancreas

Treatment Options

Treatment for pancreatic cancer depends on the stage and location of the cancer as well as the patient's age, overall health, and personal preferences. The first goal of pancreatic cancer treatment is to eliminate the cancer. When surgery is not an option, the focus may be on preventing the pancreatic cancer from growing or causing more harm.

Local Therapy—Treatment that affects cells in the tumor and the area close to it.

- Surgery—Your physician will discuss the type of surgical procedure required based on where the tumor is located. The most common surgery is the Whipple procedure, which removes the head of the pancreas, the bile duct and gallbladder, and parts of the stomach and the small intestine. Sometimes a distal pancreatectomy can be used, which removes half the pancreas as well as the spleen.
- Radiation Therapy—Radiation therapy uses high-energy beams to destroy cancer cells. It is often combined with chemotherapy to treat patients after surgery to prevent the recurrence of pancreatic cancer. It also can be used to treat some patients whose cancer is too advanced to be removed surgically.
- Endoscopic Stent Placement—A stent is a device inserted into an organ to treat an obstruction caused by a cancerous tumor. It is open at both ends so that food, liquid, or body liquids can pass through. Stents are commonly used to treat symptomatic jaundice caused by obstruction of the bile duct, and can be used when the cancer blocks the passage of food out of the stomach.

Systemic Therapy—Treatment using medications that travel through the bloodstream, reaching and affecting cells all over the body.

- Chemotherapy—Chemotherapies are drugs that help to kill cancer cells, and may be used to reduce the rate of tumor growth, relieve symptoms, and extend survival. They also are sometimes used after surgery or in combination with radiation therapy in an effort to slow tumor growth or prevent the recurrence of pancreatic cancer.
- Targeted Therapy—Refers to a medication or drug that is designed to target a specific pathway in the growth and development of a tumor.
- Supportive Therapy—These are medications that treat symptoms caused by the cancer, such as pain, nausea, weight loss, and depression. Controlling cancer-related symptoms is an important way to maintain your strength in order to receive anticancer therapies.

© 2010 **Wolters Kluwer** Published by Anatomical Chart Company, Skokie, IL. Developed in consultation with Dr. Geoffrey R. Oxnard.

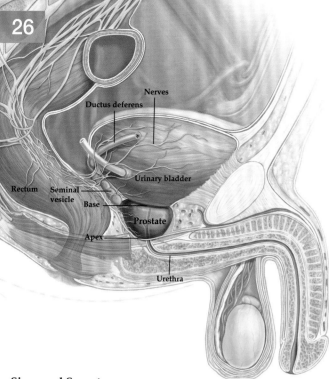

UNDERSTANDING PROSTATE CANCER

What is Prostate Cancer?
Prostate cancer is cancer of the walnut-sized gland of a man's reproductive system that makes part of the seminal fluid, which carries sperm out of the body.

Risk Factors
The causes of prostate cancer are not known. Below are some factors, which research has shown could increase a man's risk of developing prostate cancer.
Age—The primary risk of prostate cancer increases with age.
Family history—The risk of prostate cancer increases if a close male family member (father or brother) has had the disease.
Race or ethnicity—African American men are more likely to develop prostate cancer.
Geographic location—There is a higher incidence of prostate cancer in men residing in North America, Northwest Europe, and Australia, in part due to prescreening. There is a lower incidence in men residing in Asia and in some developing countries.
Diet—A diet high in fat and red meat may increase a man's risk of developing prostate cancer. Although the data are limited, eating cruciferous vegetables (such as broccoli), tomatoes, and soybeans may decrease the risk of this disease.

Staging and Gleason Score
To plan treatment, the physician must understand the extent (stage) and how fast the cancer will grow and spread (which is best determined by the Gleason score).

Gleason Score—The system of grading the aggressiveness of the cancer is the Gleason Pathologic Scoring System, which scores or grades the cancer from 1 to 5. To get a Gleason score, the two most common areas of cancer are scored individually and added together for a Gleason score between 2 and 10. A lower score indicates a less aggressive cancer, and a higher score indicates a more aggressive cancer.

Gleason Pathologic Scoring System
How your cells look under a microscope determines the Gleason score. Based on appearance, the pathologist can identify which cells are normal, which are cancer cells, and how aggressive those cells are.

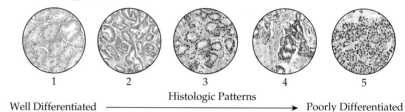

1   2   3   4   5

Histologic Patterns

Well Differentiated ⟶ Poorly Differentiated

Staging—The cancer stage is based on the size and spread of the tumor; the higher the stage, the more advanced the cancer. The most commonly used system is the Tumor-Nodes-Metastasis system (TNM).
T = the size and location of the primary **Tumor**
N = the number of lymph **Nodes** to which the cancer has spread
M = the spread away from the primary site of the tumor to other parts of the body is **Metastasis**

Signs and Symptoms
Many men with prostate cancer do not experience any symptoms when they are diagnosed. While the symptoms listed below may be due to prostate cancer, they can also be associated with other non cancerous conditions.
- Erection difficulties
- Blood in semen
- Pain in lower back, hips, upper thighs
- Urinary problems, which can include the following:
  - Difficulties starting or stopping the flow of urine
  - Urine flow that starts and stops
  - Needing to urinate often, especially at night
  - Weak urine flow
  - Pain or burning sensation during urination
  - Blood in the urine

Screening and Diagnosis
Screening can help find and treat cancer early. Men may want to see their doctor to discuss prostate cancer screening if they are over the age of 50, have any of the risk factors, or are experiencing any of the symptoms. Some common screening tests include the following:

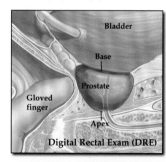

Digital Rectal Exam (DRE)

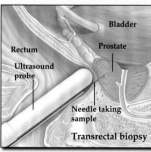

Transrectal biopsy

Blood test for prostate-specific antigen (PSA)—PSA is a substance produced by the prostate that helps keep semen liquid. A blood test is performed to test the level of PSA. Although high levels of PSA could indicate cancer, other causes could include inflammation of the prostate or benign prostatic hyperplasia (BPH).

Digital rectal examination (DRE)—Most tumors arise in the area of the prostate (peripheral zone), which can be detected by the DRE.

Depending on the results of the screening test(s), the physician will perform additional diagnostic tests, which may include the following:

Transrectal ultrasound—A probe inserted into a man's rectum can better determine the exact size and location of the abnormal areas.

Transrectal biopsy—By inserting a needle through the rectum into the prostate, tissue is removed to look for cancer cells.

Endorectal MRI—A probe inserted into a man's rectum can obtain sharp images of the prostate and identify suspicious areas.

Other imaging tests such as a bone scan, CT scan, or MRI may be performed to determine if the cancer has spread to other parts of the body.

Treatments
There are several ways to treat prostate cancer and a combination of treatments may be recommended by the physician. Treatment will depend on a number of factors such as the PSA level, the Gleason score (indicates how aggressive the cancer is), spread (stage) of the cancer, as well as the age, symptoms, and health of the patient.

Common treatment options include the following:

Surgery—The procedure can include removal of all or part of the prostate gland.

Radiation therapy—Radiation treatment can be external, which uses a high-powered x-ray machine outside the body to kill cancer cells. Radiation can also be internal, by implanting small radioactive "seeds" inside the prostate tissue.

Hormone therapy—Medication is used to stop or block the production of male sex hormones that stimulate the growth of cancer cells.

Active surveillance or "watchful waiting" (because prostate cancer can be very slow growing)— If the risks or possible side effects of the treatment options above outweigh the benefits, the physician may recommend close monitoring of the cancer to determine growth rate. If disease characteristics get worse or symptoms occur, then the above treatment options may be considered.

Prognostic Factors
Like other forms of cancer, the prognosis for prostate cancer stage depends on how far the cancer has spread at the time it's diagnosed. Gleason score, PSA, stage, and volume of disease (determined by biopsy information) are the main factors that affect the outcome. Talk to your cancer specialist if you are trying to find out about your prognosis.

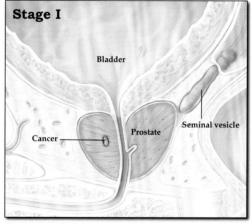

Stage I
The cancer is not found during a digital rectal examination (T1), but found when doing a biopsy for increased PSA or surgery for another reason. It is located only in the prostate.
T1, N0, M0, PSA <10, Gleason ≤6

Stage II
The tumor is not felt on the digital rectal examination (T1) but the PSA or Gleason score is higher than stage 1, or the tumor can be felt but is confined to the gland.
Stage IIA : T1, N0, M0, PSA 10-20, Gleason 6
OR   T1, N0, M0, PSA <20, Gleason 7
OR   T2a-b (tumor felt on one side only) N0, M0, PSA <20, Gleason ≤7
Stage IIB : T1-2, N0, M0, PSA ≤20 and/or Gleason ≤8
OR   T2c (tumor felt on both sides) N0, M0

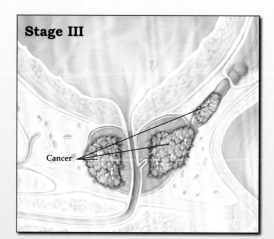

Stage III
The cancer has spread outside the prostate, perhaps to the seminal vesicles, but not to the lymph nodes
T3, N0, M0, any PSA, any Gleason

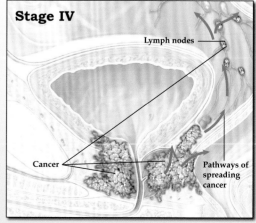

Stage IV
The cancer may have spread to nearby muscles, organs, lymph nodes, or other parts of the body.
T4, N1, M1, any PSA, any Gleason

 Wolters Kluwer   Published by Anatomical Chart Company | In consultation with James L. Gulley, MD, PhD, FACP.

Understanding Skin Cancer

Skin cancer is the uncontrolled growth of abnormal skin cells. There are different types of skin cancer. Basal cell carcinoma is the most common, followed by squamous cell carcinoma. Melanoma is less common, but more dangerous. Currently there are between 2 and 3 million nonmelanoma skin cancers and 132,000 melanoma skin cancers that occur globally each year.

Risk Factors:
- Fair skin
- Increasing age
- Numerous and/or atypical moles
- Precancerous skin lesions
- A history of excessive sun exposure and/or sunburns
- A family or personal history of skin cancer
- Use of tanning devices
- Sunny or high-altitude climates
- A weakened immune system
- Prior exposure to certain toxins or x-ray treatment

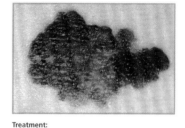

Epidermis
Dermis
Subcutaneous layer
Rete ridges
Rete pegs
Hair follicle
Sebaceous gland
Arrector pili muscle
Eccrine sweat gland
Sensory nerve
Artery
Vein
Reticular layer
Papillary layer
Subcutaneous fat
Vater-Pacini corpuscle

Precancerous Growths

Actinic keratoses (AKs) or solar keratoses are the most common sun-related **precancerous skin growths** noted in fair-skinned individuals. They are benign (nonmalignant). If left untreated, AKs have the potential to develop into squamous cell carcinoma, a type of skin cancer.

- AKs appear as crusty, "dry" scaly bumps that are rough textured and sandpaperlike to the touch.
- They can be skin colored, reddish, or yellowish; they may also be tan or dark brown in color (pigmented AKs).
- AKs can gradually enlarge, thicken, and become more elevated and form "cutaneous horns."
- They appear mainly on the face, especially on the nose, ears, temples, forehead, neck, and sometimes on or around the lips. They also commonly arise on the top of the forearms and hands and on the scalps of bald men.

Treatments include the following:
- Cryosurgery: freezing with liquid nitrogen that is applied to individual AKs.
- Biopsy, followed by electrodesiccation (electrocautery) or electrodesiccation alone
- Topical chemotherapy with a prescription cream or lotion
- Laser surgery, photodynamic therapy, or chemical peeling

Actinic keratoses

Atypical Moles

Atypical nevus, also called **dysplastic nevus, atypical mole, or Clark nevus,** is a **benign skin growth.** While it can sometimes look like a melanoma, it's not a melanoma or a skin cancer. Such atypical nevi are often inherited.

- They are usually larger than a common mole.
- They often have an irregular coloration (tan, brown, black, pink, or red), but the center may be raised giving it a "sunny side egg" appearance.

Sometimes atypical nevi are considered to be precursors or predictors of malignant melanoma, especially when found on individuals who have:
- A first-degree relative (parent, sibling, or child) or second-degree relative (grandparent, grandchild, aunt, uncle) with malignant melanoma
- A large number of moles (nevi), often more than 50, some of which are atypical nevi

Treatments include the following:
- Shave excision: A small blade cuts around and beneath the mole. This technique is often used for smaller moles and doesn't require sutures.
- Excisional surgery: The mole and a surrounding margin of normal healthy skin are cut out with a scalpel or a sharp punch device. Sutures are used to close the skin.

Atypical nevus (plural: nevi)

Types of Skin Cancer (Nonmelanoma)

Basal cell carcinoma (BCC) is the most **common type of skin cancer.** It's often easily treated and cured in most cases. Although BCC qualifies as a cancer, its harmful effects, if recognized and treated early, are usually minor.

- Frequently found on the head and neck; also on the trunk and lower limbs.
- Resembles a shiny pimple or sore that does not heal.
- It's usually a dome-shaped bump with a pearly appearance.
- It may have a small scab on its surface or simply look like a flat red patch.
- BCCs are slow growing and very rarely metastasize (spread); however, if they are ignored, they can extend below the skin and cause considerable damage to nerves, cartilage, and bone.
- Diagnosis is generally made by a skin biopsy.

Treatments include the following:
- Electrodessication and curettage (ED and C): The surface of the skin cancer is removed with a scraping instrument (curette) and then the base of the tumor is seared with an electric needle.
- Surgical excision: In this procedure, which is used for both new and recurring tumors, the cancerous tissue and a surrounding margin of healthy skin is cut out.
- Cryosurgery: Freezing with liquid nitrogen.
- Mohs micrographic surgery: During this procedure, an experienced Mohs surgeon removes the tumor layer by layer, examining each layer under the microscope until no abnormal cells remain.
- Radiation therapy.
- Topical chemotherapy with creams or ointments.
- Laser surgery.

Basal cell carcinoma (BCC)

Squamous cell carcinoma (SCC) is the second most common type of skin cancer. In most cases, it arises in an AK. If not treated, this cancer can metastasize (spread). As with BCCs, SCCs are highly curable with both surgical and nonsurgical therapy, especially if treated early.

- They begin as a firm, red nodule or a scaly, crusted flat lesion.
- SCCs can appear as a nonhealing sore, bump, or ulcer.
- As with AKs, SCCs are found mainly on sun-exposed areas of the face especially on the nose, ears, temples, forehead, neck, and sometimes on or around the lips. They also commonly arise on the top of the forearms and hands and on the scalps of bald men.
- They are more common in men, particularly those who work in outdoor occupations.

Other predisposing factors include the following:
- Radiation exposure.
- Immunosuppression by medications, organ transplantation, or disease such as HIV/AIDS.
- Larger and deeply penetrating SCCs and those found next to or on mucous membranes (eg, on lips), are considered more dangerous and must be treated more thoroughly.
- Diagnosis is generally made by shave or excisional biopsy.

Treatments include the following:
Most SCCs can be completely removed with relatively minor surgery. Depending on the size, location, and aggressiveness of the tumor, treatment may include one or more of the following:

- Electrodesiccation and curettage (ED and C): The surface of the skin cancer is removed with a scraping instrument (curette), and then the base of the tumor is seared with an electric needle.
- Surgical excision.
- Cryosurgery: Freezing with liquid nitrogen.
- Mohs micrographic surgery.
- Radiation therapy: This may be an option for treating large cancers on the eyelids, lips and ears—areas that are difficult to treat surgically—or for tumors too deep to cut out.
- Topical chemotherapy with creams or ointments.
- Laser therapy.

Squamous cell carcinoma (SCC)

Malignant Melanoma

Malignant melanoma (MM) is the **most serious type of all skin cancers.** It can arise on normal skin or from an existing mole. **If not treated promptly,** it **can metastasize (spread)** downward into other areas of the skin, lymph nodes, or internal organs.

Melanocytes are found throughout the lower part of the epidermis. They make melanin, the pigment that gives skin its natural color. When skin is exposed to the sun, melanocytes make more pigment, causing the skin to tan, or darken. MM is a disease in which malignant (cancer) cells form from these melanocytes.

Malignant melanoma may have some or all of the following **"ABCDE"** features:

A—Asymmetry One half is unlike the other half.
B—Border that is irregular or notched like a jigsaw puzzle piece.
C—Color that is varied (brown, black, pink, blue-gray, white, or mixtures of these colors).
D—Diameter that is >6 mm (diameter of a pencil eraser), but can be smaller.
E—Evolving, or change in a preexisting mole. Any change—in size, color, elevation, or any new symptoms such as itching, bleeding, or crusting; particularly, a mole that looks different from the rest.

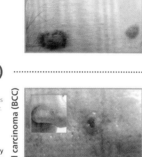

Treatment:
- Surgical excision is the treatment of choice, and follow-up should be performed by a dermatologist or surgeon who has experience in dealing with MMs.

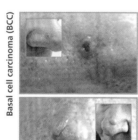

Asymmetry | Border | Color | Diameter | Evolving

Skin Cancer Prevention

- Avoid sun exposure during the hours between 10 AM and 4 PM, when the sun is strongest.
- Wear protective headgear such as a hat with a wide brim or a baseball cap.
- Wear special clothing made of tightly woven or knitted fabrics that allow less sunlight to pass through.
- Choose a broad-spectrum sunscreen that blocks both ultraviolet B (UVB, the burning rays) and ultraviolet A (UVA, the more penetrating rays that promote wrinkling and aging).
- Apply sunscreen even on cloudy, hazy days. Ultraviolet (UV) rays can still bounce off sand, water, and snow.
- Avoid tanning beds.
- Wear UV-blocking sunglasses.
- All first-degree relatives of individuals who have a MM or multiple atypical nevi should undergo a dermatologic examination; also, the need to protect children (beginning at an early age) from excessive sun exposure should be emphasized.
- Anyone who has had a history of melanoma needs lifelong skin surveillance.

Self-Examination

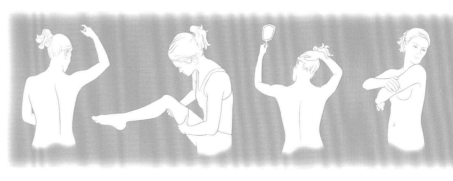

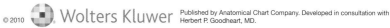 Wolters Kluwer — Published by Anatomical Chart Company. Developed in consultation with Herbert P. Goodheart, MD.

© 2010

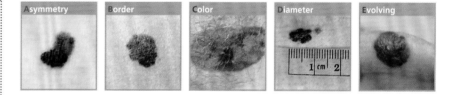

CARDIOVASCULAR AND VENOUS DISEASES & DISORDERS

- Cardiovascular Disease
- Understanding High Cholesterol
- Deep Vein Thrombosis
- Heart Disease
- Understanding Hypertension
- Understanding High Blood Pressure
- Heart Failure
- Peripheral Artery Disease
- Understanding Valve Stenosis

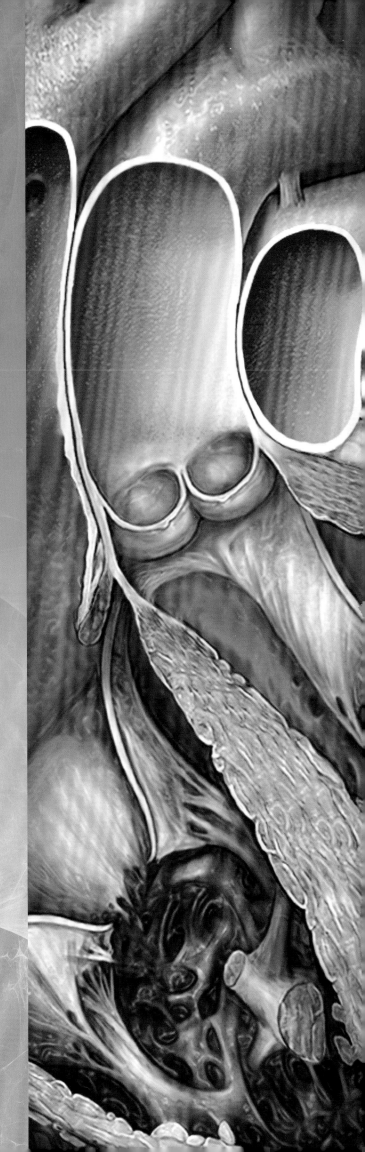

Cardiovascular Disease

Posterior View

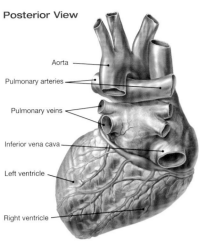

- Aorta
- Pulmonary arteries
- Pulmonary veins
- Inferior vena cava
- Left ventricle
- Right ventricle

Anterior View

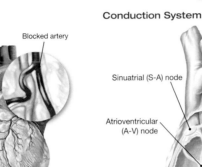

- Superior vena cava
- Aorta
- Right atrium
- Pulmonary trunk
- Left auricle
- Right ventricle
- Left ventricle
- Inferior vena cava

Coronary Arteries

(Anterior View)
Coronary arteries supply blood to heart tissue. They originate from the aorta.

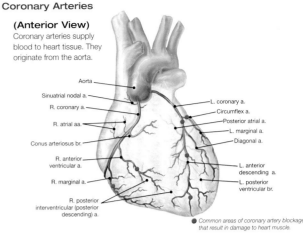

- Aorta
- Sinuatrial nodal a.
- R. coronary a.
- R. atrial aa.
- Conus arteriosus br.
- R. anterior ventricular a.
- R. marginal a.
- R. posterior interventricular (posterior descending) a.
- L. coronary a.
- Circumflex a.
- Posterior atrial a.
- L. marginal a.
- Diagonal a.
- L. anterior descending a.
- L. posterior ventricular br.

● *Common areas of coronary artery blockage that result in damage to heart muscle.*

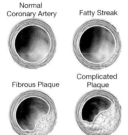

- Normal Coronary Artery
- Fatty Streak
- Fibrous Plaque
- Complicated Plaque

Coronary Artery Disease

- The arteries can accumulate fatty deposits called **plaques**, most commonly in people who smoke cigarettes or who have high levels of "bad" cholesterol, high blood pressure, diabetes, and/or a family history of coronary disease.
- This buildup, leads to hardening of the arteries, called **atherosclerosis**, which causes the vessels to narrow or become obstructed.
- Coronary artery disease results as atherosclerotic plaque develops in the coronary arteries and obstructs blood flow to the heart. This results in diminished supply of oxygen to the heart muscle.

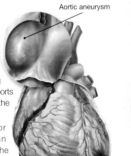

Blocked artery

Angina

- The coronary arteries supplying the heart can become narrowed over time, due to atherosclerotic plaque.
- The narrowed blood vessels limit the amount of blood flow to the heart.
- When the oxygen needs of the heart muscle exceed the supply through the narrowed or obstructed arteries (such as during physical exertion), pain or discomfort in the chest, called **angina**, results.

Conduction System

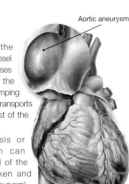

- Sinuatrial (S-A) node
- Atrioventricular (A-V) node
- Atrioventricular bundle (Bundle of His)
- Right bundle branch
- Left bundle branch
- Purkinje fibers

Electrocardiogram (ECG)

Repeating electrical impulses travel through the heart, controlling the rhythmic contraction of the heart muscle. The normal impulse is displayed and is composed of three distinct waves: P, QRS, and T.

The Cardiac Cycle

① Atrial Systole
The atria contract, emptying blood into the ventricles.

② Ventricular Systole
Shortly after atrial systole, the ventricles contract, ejecting blood from the heart to the lungs and the rest of the body.

③ Diastole
Atria and ventricles dilate, and blood refills each chamber.

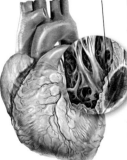

Infarction

Myocardial Infarction (Heart Attack)

- Myocardial infarction is a life-threatening type of acute coronary emergency that can complicate the course of patients with coronary artery disease at any time.
- It occurs most commonly when atherosclerotic plaque within a coronary artery becomes disturbed, causing a blood clot to form at that site, further reducing blood flow and oxygen supply to the heart muscle.
- As a result, part of the heart muscle is either damaged (infarction) or ceases to function and becomes scar tissue. The damaged part of the heart loses its ability to contract and pump blood.

Aortic Aneurysm

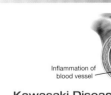

Aortic aneurysm

- The aorta is the largest blood vessel in the body. It arises from the top of the heart's main pumping chamber and transports blood to the rest of the body.
- Atherosclerosis or degeneration can cause the wall of the aorta to weaken and balloon out (aneurysm).
- The aortic aneurysm may suddenly rupture or tear, often leading to death.

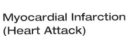

Blood clot

Cerebrovascular Accident (Stroke)

- A **cerebrovascular accident (CVA)**, also known as a stroke, is a sudden impairment of cerebral circulation in one or more blood vessels.
- In one form of stroke, a blood clot forms, or clotlike material travels from a different point in the circulation, and blocks an artery feeding the brain.
- This interrupts or diminishes oxygen supply often causing the brain tissues to become damaged, either temporarily or permanently.

Left Ventricular Hypertrophy

Thickened heart muscle

- Left ventricular hypertrophy (LVH) is an abnormal thickening of the walls of the main pumping chamber of the heart.
- It can develop as a result of long-standing high blood pressure, from cardiac valve abnormalities, and also from certain genetic conditions.
- LVH causes increased stiffness of the heart muscle that can lead to symptoms of heart failure, including shortness of breath and swollen legs.

Heart Failure

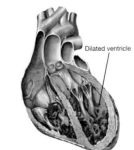

Dilated ventricle

- Heart failure is a common debilitating condition.
- In some cases the main heart pumping chamber enlarges and contracts poorly as shown here; in other cases the heart muscle becomes abnormally thick or stiffened.
- Symptoms of heart failure result from reduced blood output from the heart, and/or backup of fluid into the lungs and other body organs and tissues, with fatigue, weakness, shortness of breath, and often swelling (edema) of the legs.

Kawasaki Disease

Inflammation of blood vessel

- Also known as **mucocutaneous lymph node syndrome**, Kawasaki disease is a multi-organ illness affecting children.
- It generally starts with high fever, followed by the development of redness and swelling of the hands, feet, eyes, lips, and tongue; swollen lymph glands; and sores in the mouth.
- Acute complications involving the heart include inflammation of the heart muscle and accumulation of fluid around the heart.
- Fatal heart attacks may occur due to inflammation of the blood vessels (coronary arteries) of the heart, causing blood clots to form and obstruct the arteries.
- Chronic complications include aneurysms of the coronary arteries that can rupture in adulthood.

© 2017 Wolters Kluwer   Anatomical Chart Company, Philadelphia, PA. Medical illustrations by Lik Kwong, MFA, in consultation with Leonard S. Lilly, MD, Harvard Medical School, Brigham and Women's Hospital, Boston, MA.

Understanding High Cholesterol

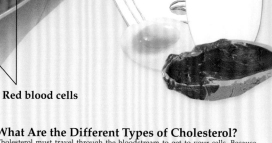

Phospholipid (other fats)

LIPOPROTEIN

Protein

Cholesterol

What Is High Cholesterol?

Cholesterol is a waxy, fatlike substance found in all of your body's cells. Cholesterol comes from two sources, your body and your food. Cholesterol is made in the liver and other cells and is also found in food from animals, like dairy products, eggs, and meat. You can end up with high cholesterol because of the foods you eat and the rate at which your body breaks down cholesterol. Your body needs a certain amount of cholesterol to build and maintain cells, but too much or too little cholesterol can create a major health risk. Extra cholesterol can build up on your artery walls, and over time, cholesterol deposits, called plaque, may narrow your arteries causing less blood flow or form a clot, putting you at risk for heart disease, heart attack, and stroke.

What Causes High Cholesterol?

- **Eating an unhealthy diet**
  – with too much saturated fat, trans fat, and cholesterol. Saturated fat and cholesterol are in foods that come from animals, such as meats, whole milk, egg yolks, butter, and cheese. Trans fat is found in fried foods and packaged foods, such as cookies, crackers, and chips.
- **Excess body weight.**
- **Lack of physical activity**
- **Age**
  – men over age 45 and women over 55 are at higher risk.
- **Gender**
  – men are more prone to high cholesterol than women—until women reach 50-55 when naturally occurring cholesterol levels in women increase.
- **Family history**
  – some people have a genetic predisposition to high cholesterol. Genes passed down from both sides of your families may cause your body to make too much or too little cholesterol.
- **Some diseases**
  – diabetes, thyroid disease, metabolic disease, and others.
- **Cigarette smoking.**
- **Certain medicines**
  – thiazide diuretics, beta-blockers, retinoids, estrogen, and corticosteroids.

CHOLESTEROL MADE BY YOUR BODY (LIVER)

CHOLESTEROL FROM FOOD YOU EAT

Prevention and Management

- **Get regular cholesterol screenings:**
  The first step in preventing high cholesterol and ultimately, heart disease, heart attack, or stroke is to get a simple blood test to check your cholesterol levels. Healthy adults should have this test done every 5 years. If you are at increased risk for heart disease or if you are a man over 45 or a woman over 55, your doctor might have you tested more often.
- **Adopt a healthier lifestyle including the following:**
  – Do regular aerobic exercise.
  – Don't smoke.
  – Maintain a healthy weight.
  – Eat a nutritious diet low in saturated fat and cholesterol.
- **Lower LDL levels**
  Clinical trials have demonstrated that lowering LDL cholesterol has many benefits and saves lives.
- **Take cholesterol medications, if prescribed by a health practitioner**
  Even after adopting a healthier lifestyle, your cholesterol level may not reach target and a medication may be required.

Cholesterol transport in the blood

Red blood cells

Risks of High Cholesterol

Cholesterol plays a big part in the development of atherosclerosis. Atherosclerosis is the buildup of fatty deposits, including cholesterol, on the inner lining of arteries. This buildup (called plaque) may narrow the arteries causing a decrease in blood flow, or a blood clot may develop that can clog or block the artery. As a result of this, cholesterol may increase the risk of heart disease, stroke, and other vascular diseases.

HDL

HDL   HDL

LDL

LDL

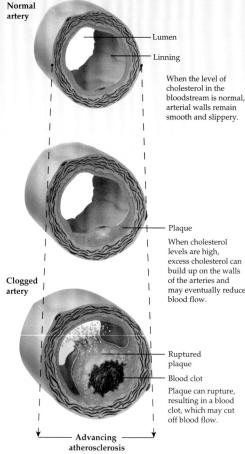

Normal artery

Lumen

Linning

When the level of cholesterol in the bloodstream is normal, arterial walls remain smooth and slippery.

Plaque

When cholesterol levels are high, excess cholesterol can build up on the walls of the arteries and may eventually reduce blood flow.

Clogged artery

Ruptured plaque

Blood clot

Plaque can rupture, resulting in a blood clot, which may cut off blood flow.

Advancing atherosclerosis

What Are the Different Types of Cholesterol?

Cholesterol must travel through the bloodstream to get to your cells. Because cholesterol is a fat, it separates from blood like oil from water; to keep this from happening, cholesterol attaches to a protein. The combination of cholesterol and other lipids (fats and phospholipids) with protein is called a lipoprotein. Although there is only one type of cholesterol, there are several types of lipoproteins that transport cholesterol. Blood tests for cholesterol generally provide results for the following types of lipoproteins:

Low-density lipoprotein (LDL) BAD CHOLESTEROL

- Called "bad cholesterol" because high levels can lead to heart disease and stroke.
- Transports cholesterol from your liver to the cells that need it.
- Leftover LDLs that are not needed release their cholesterol into the blood.

High-density lipoprotein (HDL) GOOD CHOLESTEROL

- Called "good cholesterol" because high levels reduce the risk for heart disease and stroke.
- Scientists think that HDL helps get rid of bad cholesterol in the blood. HDL picks up extra cholesterol and carries it to the liver, which then flushes it from the body.

Triglycerides

- Are not cholesterol, but are a different type of fat. Excess calories, alcohol, or sugars are converted into triglycerides and stored in fat cells throughout the body.
- High levels can raise the risk for heart disease.
- Are often part of a blood test doctors do to check cholesterol levels.

What Levels of Cholesterol Are Healthy?

Knowing your cholesterol levels is an important part of understanding your own risk for heart disease. To determine how much cholesterol is in your body, your doctor will give you a blood test (also called a lipid profile or panel). Cholesterol levels are measured in milligrams (*mg*) of cholesterol per deciliter (dL) of blood in the United States and some other countries. The general guidelines below will help you understand your cholesterol test results.

TYPE	HEALTHY CHOLESTEROL LEVELS*	UNHEALTHY CHOLESTEROL LEVELS*
TOTAL CHOLESTEROL the level of all of the lipids (fats) in your blood, including LDL and HDL cholesterol	<200 mg/dL Generally, a lower total cholesterol level is better.	200-239 mg/dL—borderline high 240 mg/dL and above—high A person with this level has more than twice the risk of heart disease as someone whose cholesterol is below 200 mg/dL.
LDL ("BAD" CHOLESTEROL)	<70 mg/dL—ideal for people at very high risk of heart disease and stroke <100 mg/dL—Lowest risk of heart attack and stroke	100-129 mg/dL—near or above desirable 130-159 mg/dL—borderline high 160-189 mg/dL—high 190 mg/dL and up—very high The more LDL there is in the blood, the greater the risk of heart disease. LDL cholesterol can build up on the walls of your arteries and over time may lead to heart attack or stroke.
HDL ("GOOD" CHOLESTEROL)	40 mg/dL or higher 60 mg/dL and above is considered protection against heart disease.	<40 mg/dL (for men) <50 mg/dL (for women) Low HDL cholesterol is a major risk factor for heart disease.
TRIGLYCERIDES	<150 mg/dL (150 mg/dL is normal)	150-199 mg/dL—borderline high 200-499 mg/dL—high 500 mg/dL and above—very high *Normal triglyceride levels vary by age and sex. High triglyceride levels in your blood can help clog arteries with plaque (cholesterol and fat buildup) and may raise the risk of heart attack and stroke. Above 600 mg/dL increases the risk for pancreatitis.

These levels should be used as a general guideline. Current recommendations might have changed and should be followed instead of what is stated here. Target levels also differ according to the number of risk factors you have for coronary artery disease. Please see your doctor to find out what your target level should be.

Wolters Kluwer Developed in consultation with Dr. Douglas S. Moodie

Vascular Circulation

The circulation of blood through the blood vessels (*arteries, capillaries, and veins*) of the body is driven by the beating action of the heart. The heart beats at a rate of about 70 beats per minute, forcing blood into the arteries, which in turn transports oxygen and nutrients throughout the body. After exchanging oxygen for carbon dioxide and nutrients for waste products, the blood begins its journey back to the heart through a network of veins. On returning to the heart, the nonoxygenated blood is pumped into the arteries of the lungs (*pulmonary arteries*), where the blood regains oxygen. Then the blood reenters the heart through the pulmonary veins for another cycle. The entire cycle takes about a minute to complete.

Enlarged view of lung

Pulmonary arterial circulation shown in blue (*nonoxygenated blood*)

Pulmonary venous circulation shown in red (*oxygenated blood*)

Embolus

Pulmonary artery

Pulmonary Embolism

A pulmonary embolus is a piece of blood clot (*venous thrombus*) that has broken off and traveled into a pulmonary artery of the lungs. If the embolus is very large, it can block blood flow into the pulmonary arteries. This is called pulmonary embolism. This causes severe breathing difficulties and can even cause death. Smaller pulmonary emboli can cause chest pain or cause no symptoms. With time, the smaller emboli are either dissolved or break up and disappear.

External iliac vein

Femoral vein

Tunica intima

Tunica media

Tunica adventitia

Thrombus (*blood clot*) blocking blood flow through a vein

Cross Section of a Vein

○ The circles show locations in the veins commonly affected by DVT (*applies to both legs*).

↑ The arrows show the direction of the venous blood flow back to the heart and then into the lungs.

Posterior tibial vein

Perineal vein

ⓓ Embolus (*a broken-off piece of thrombus*)

Lung

Pulmonary artery

Heart

Abdominal aorta

Inferior vena cava

Common iliac vein

Common iliac artery

Femoral artery

ⓒ Venous thrombus (*blood clot*)

ⓑ Clumping of:
Fibrin
Platelet
Red blood cell

Direction of blood flow

ⓐ Damage to the inner lining of blood vessel

How Does a Thrombus (*Blood Clot*) Form?

1. Under normal circumstances, blood remains fluid because the lining (*endothelium*) of blood vessels contains substances that prevent it from clotting.

2. Blood clotting is important because it prevents excessive blood loss when a vessel is cut. ⓐ There are substances in the inner layer of a blood vessel that stimulate blood clotting (*coagulation*). ⓑ A clot forms when blood is exposed to these substances.

3. Under certain abnormal circumstances, the blood can clot to produce a thrombus, ⓒ even though the blood vessel is not cut. These abnormal circumstances either cause clotting by releasing chemicals into the blood or cause damage to the inner lining of the vessel, thereby removing the inner protective layer.

4. The chance of clotting is increased if the blood flow is sluggish (*stagnant*). Blood flow can become sluggish because of prolonged bed rest or when there is an inherited defect in the body's ability to counteract a tendency to clot.

5. A venous thrombus is made up of a fibrin mesh with trapped blood cells. The thrombus can block the vein, grow, or be dissolved by the body—or a piece of it can break off. The broken-off piece (*embolus*) can travel to the lungs, where it is called a pulmonary embolus. ⓓ

Layers That Makes Up a Vein

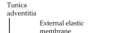

Tunica adventitia

External elastic membrane

Tunica media

Internal elastic membrane

Tunica intima (*endothelium*)

Valve

What Is Deep Vein Thrombosis?

Deep vein thrombosis (DVT), or venous thrombosis, occurs when a blood clot forms in the deep veins of the legs. It usually starts in the calf veins and may extend into the thigh veins. A blood clot is a jellylike mass of congealed blood.

What Causes Deep Vein Thrombosis?

Deep vein thrombosis occurs when blood, which is normally fluid, is stimulated to clot. This happens because the vessel is damaged or substances that trigger blood clotting (*coagulation*) are released into the blood by inflamed or damaged tissues. Blood clotting is encouraged by sluggish blood flow (*venous stasis*).

What Are the Consequences of DVT?

If the blood clot is small, it can be dissolved by the body. On the other hand, it can grow and block the blood flow through the vein. This causes pain and leg swelling. If a piece of the blood clot (*thrombus*) breaks off, it is called an embolus. A pulmonary embolus is a piece of blood clot that has traveled to the lungs.

What Are the Main Risk Factors?

The risk factors for venous thrombosis are:
- Prolonged bed rest and immobility
- Varicose veins
- Major surgery
- Leg trauma
- The hormone estrogen in contraceptive pills or hormone replacement therapy
- Previous venous thrombosis
- Hereditary predisposition because of abnormal anticoagulant proteins
- Cancer (*malignancy*)
- Overweight (*obesity*)

What Are the Symptoms and Complications of DVT and Pulmonary Embolism?

Many venous thrombi cause no symptoms. The common symptoms are the following:
- Pain, tenderness, and/or swelling in the calf or elsewhere in the leg
- Discoloration of the calf
- Symptoms of pulmonary embolism

The symptoms of pulmonary embolism are the following:
- Difficulty breathing
- Sharp chest pain that is aggravated by taking a deep breath
- Blood in sputum
- Rapid heart rate

The complications of DVT are **(1)** chronic pain and swelling of the leg because of scarring of the valves within the vein and blockage of blood flow, and **(2)** pulmonary embolism, which occurs when a blood clot fragment, which has broken off from a venous thrombus, enters and blocks a pulmonary artery. A very large embolus can block blood flow into the pulmonary arteries and cause death. Smaller pulmonary emboli obstruct smaller arteries and can cause damage to the lungs. Many pulmonary emboli do not cause symptoms. With time, most pulmonary emboli are dissolved by the body.

How Are DVT and Pulmonary Embolism Treated?

Treatment of DVT is aimed at relieving symptoms, preventing the blood clot from growing, and preventing pulmonary embolism.

This is achieved by:
- Blood-thinning drugs known as anticoagulants.
- In cases of large pulmonary embolism, clot-dissolving drugs.
- Compression stocking to counteract swelling in the leg, if it is still present after 3 months.
- Surgery can be used to prevent a venous thrombus from traveling to the lungs, but this is rarely necessary.

Anatomical Chart Company, Skokie, IL. Medical illustrations by Lik Kwong, MFA, in consultation with Jack Hirsh, MD, FRCP(C), Hamilton Health Sciences Research, Canada.

Heart Disease

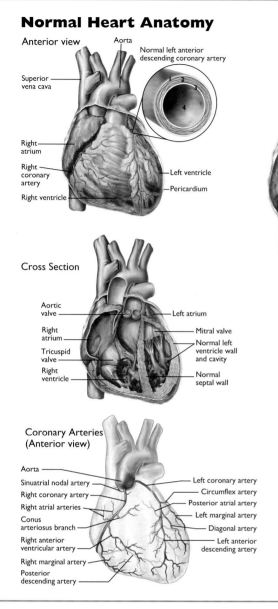

Normal Heart Anatomy

Anterior view

- Aorta
- Normal left anterior descending coronary artery
- Superior vena cava
- Right atrium
- Right coronary artery
- Right ventricle
- Left ventricle
- Pericardium

Cross Section

- Aortic valve
- Right atrium
- Tricuspid valve
- Right ventricle
- Left atrium
- Mitral valve
- Normal left ventricle wall and cavity
- Normal septal wall

Coronary Arteries (Anterior view)

- Aorta
- Sinuatrial nodal artery
- Right coronary artery
- Right atrial arteries
- Conus arteriosus branch
- Right anterior ventricular artery
- Right marginal artery
- Posterior descending artery
- Left coronary artery
- Circumflex artery
- Posterior atrial artery
- Left marginal artery
- Diagonal artery
- Left anterior descending artery

Progression of Heart Disease in Atherosclerosis

Narrow artery leads to—

Ischemia: Lack of blood supply due to narrowing of a coronary artery, resulting in oxygen starvation of heart tissue. This causes symptoms of chest pain and tightness called *angina*.

Narrowed coronary artery

Ischemia may be present without anatomical changes to myocardium

Key to Circular Insets
Coronary Artery

1. Adventitia
2. Media
3. Intima
4. Lumen
5. Advanced plaque
6. Fatty deposits
7. Hemorrhage
8. Thrombus

Blocked artery leads to—

Myocardial Infarction (MI): Heart attack caused by sudden insufficient blood supply commonly due to ruptured plaque and thrombus formation. This occludes the artery lumen, producing an area of necrosis in heart muscle.

Coronary thrombosis

Area of necrosis

Heart Disease in Hypertension

Hypertension is persistent high blood pressure. It can lead to increased incidence and acceleration of atherosclerosis, as well as hypertrophy (thickening) and dilation of the left ventricle.

Hypertrophy of Left Ventricle
(compensated stage)

- Thickened left ventricle wall
- Small left ventricle cavity
- Thickened septal wall

Hypertrophy and Dilation of Left Ventricle
(decompensated stage)

- Enlarged left ventricular cavity and thinned wall

Recovery—
Collateral Blood Supply

Accessory blood supply from adjacent vessels travels to the region affected by the heart attack to provide fresh blood.

Partially occluded coronary artery

Collateral blood supply

Scarred cardiac tissue

Heart Failure

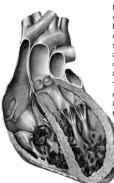

Heart failure is a common debilitating condition defined by the heart's mechanical inability to pump blood effectively. The result is a decrease in blood circulation, which forces blood to back up and oxygen supply to decrease in muscle and lung tissues. Excess accumulation of fluids in tissue throughout the body causes swelling (edema), which impairs the function of affected organs.

The most common type of heart failure is dilated cardiomyopathy, illustrated to the right. The heart muscle is damaged or defective, the walls of the ventricles are typically thinned, and the chambers are dilated.

Common Causes of Heart Failure:
- Heart attacks
- High blood pressure
- Viral infections

Mitral Valve Prolapse
(click-murmur syndrome)

The mitral valve is actually formed by four leaflets (two major and two minor), which lie between the left atrium and left ventricle. Under normal conditions the valve closes when the left ventricle contracts, preventing blood from reentering the atrium. In certain instances, the leaflets bulge (prolapse) into the atrial space, producing a clicking sound. The prolapsed valves may also leak blood back into the atrium, producing a sound called a murmur. Mitral valve prolapse is a benign condition that rarely requires treatment.

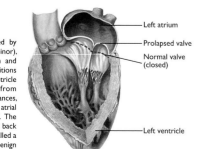

- Left atrium
- Prolapsed valve
- Normal valve (closed)
- Left ventricle

The Aging Heart

The natural progression of aging affects every part of our body including our heart. Just like the changes that happen to the rest of our body, the changes that happen to our heart are an adaption due to our age and lifestyle as we get older. Although these changes can help the older heart work more efficiently, the heart also has its adjustments that can lead to slower resting time, stiffening of the arteries, and thickening of the heart walls.

Cross Section of Aging Aorta

- Media loses elasticity (mural fibrosis)
- Internal elastic membrane is frayed
- Subintima is thickened and fibrous
- Endocardium of left atrium thickened and opaque
- Stenosis of the aortic valve
- Increase in fat deposited within and around the heart
- Development of gray-white areas of fibrosis
- Left ventricle becomes thicker

There is an increase in collagen, elastic tissue, and fat cells in the conduction system with increasing age.

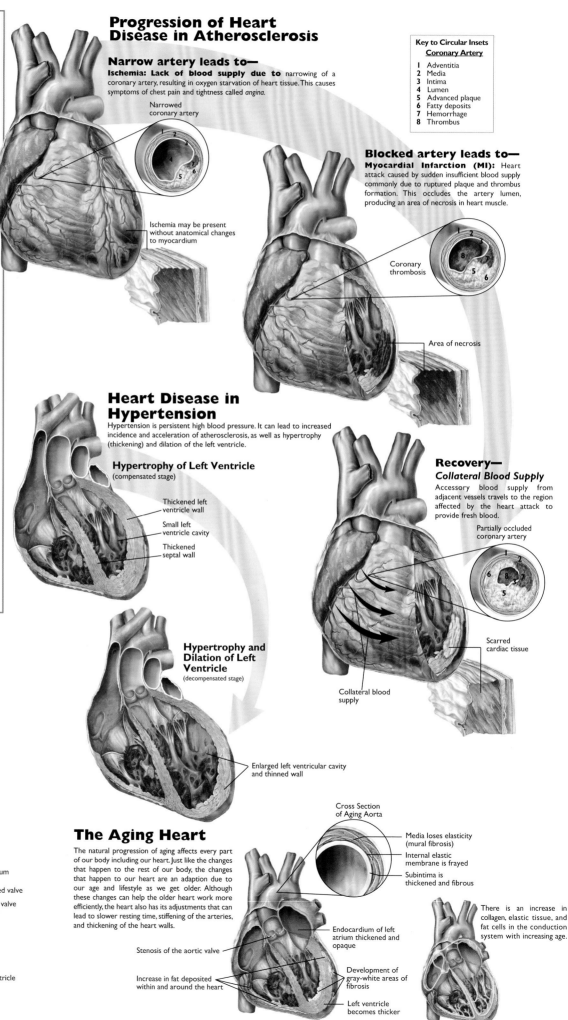

Understanding Hypertension

What Is Hypertension?

- *Hypertension*, or "high blood pressure," is a common, chronic condition that may cause long-term damage to the heart, brain, kidneys, eyes, and blood vessels.
- The entire circulatory system may be affected.
- Multiple blood pressure readings should be taken to establish if hypertension is truly present.

Types of Hypertension

- **White Coat Hypertension**—Elevated blood pressure readings only in a stressful setting, such as a physician's office.
- **Essential Hypertension**—Most common type with no specific cause. It is generally improved by a healthier lifestyle and medication, if needed.
- **Secondary Hypertension**—Result of an underlying disorder or abnormality of the kidney, major arteries, the adrenal gland, or other organs.

Effects in Blood Vessels

Increase in arterial blood pressure can alter and damage the inside artery wall. The wall may become thicker while the space that transports the blood becomes smaller (*vascular hypertrophy*).

Adventitia
External elastic membrane
Media
Internal elastic membrane
Lamina propria
Endothelium
Lumen

Adventitia
Enlarged media (smooth muscle)
Small lumen

Normal Blood Vessel

Vascular Hypertrophy

A fatty buildup, also called *plaque*, develops in the damaged arterial wall, clogging the flow of blood throughout the artery (*atherosclerosis*). Blood clots may form and block smaller blood vessels further down the circulation if dislodged.

Small lumen
Blood clot
Aneurysm

Atherosclerosis

Under increasing blood pressure, a weakening of the artery wall may balloon out (*aneurysm*) and even rupture, causing blood loss, tissue damage, and even death.

Blood Flow in the Heart

The right side of the heart receives blood from the veins of the body and delivers this unoxygenated blood to the lungs. The left side of the heart receives oxygen-rich blood from the lungs and pumps it through the arteries to all organs and tissues of the body.

Normal Heart

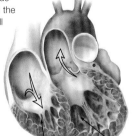

Aorta
Right ventricle   Left ventricle

Left Ventricular Hypertrophy

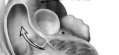

What Is Blood Pressure?

- *Blood pressure* is a measure of the force of blood against the walls of the arteries.
- It is dependent upon the action of the heart, the elasticity of the artery walls, and the volume and thickness of the blood.

- Blood pressure readings are a ratio of the maximum or systolic pressure (as the heart pushes the blood into the arteries) written over the minimum or diastolic pressure (as the heart relaxes).

$$\frac{\text{Systolic pressure}}{\text{Diastolic pressure}}$$

An example of an optimal blood pressure is: $\frac{120}{80}$

Effects in the Brain

- Hypertension is the major cause of stroke.
- The harmful effects of hypertension in the brain may be caused by blood clots blocking blood flow to parts of the brain.
- Aneurysms may burst under increasing pressure causing hemorrhage and damage to brain tissue.

Effects in the Eye

Hypertension can damage the inner lining of the back of the eye, the retina. This can serve as a marker that a patient has hypertension, and can also affect vision.

Effects in the Kidneys

- Many kidney diseases *cause* hypertension.
- The kidneys are often damaged by chronic hypertension.
- Increased blood pressure disrupts the ability of the kidneys to regulate salt and water balance in the body, which can make hypertension worse.

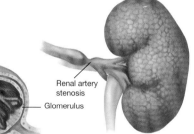

Renal artery stenosis
Glomerulus

Healthy Lifestyle Changes

Decrease your blood pressure by:
- Reducing body weight if overweight
- Restricting dietary salt
- Not smoking
- Avoiding excess alcohol
- Exercising regularly
- Developing relaxation techniques

It is very important to follow your health care provider's instructions and to take any medications as prescribed.

Effects in the Heart

- Hypertension can cause serious damage to this vital organ.
- Increased resistance in the arteries and narrowing of the vessels cause the left heart to work harder; the heart muscle thickens (termed *hypertrophy*) and becomes stiff, which can cause shortness of breath.
- The left ventricle may also become enlarged over time, with weakened contraction, resulting in heart failure. In addition, the heart muscle may suffer from decreased blood flow due to atherosclerosis of the small arteries of the heart.

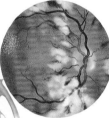

Drug Treatment	What it Does
Angiotensin-converting enzyme (ACE) inhibitors	• Relaxes blood vessels • Lowers blood pressure • Prevents diabetes-related kidney damage
Angiotensin II receptor blockers (ARBs)	• Relaxes blood vessels
Thiazide diuretics	• Increases urine production to eliminate excess sodium and fluid retention
Beta-blockers	• Slows heart rate • Decreases blood pressure
Antihypertensive drugs	• Lowers blood pressure
Calcium channel blockers	• Relaxes blood vessels • Some can slow heart rate
Vasodilators	• Works on muscles on the walls of the arteries to prevent tightening and narrowing

Understanding High Blood Pressure

Complications of High Blood Pressure

High blood pressure that is not controlled can cause long-term damage to your blood vessels, brain, heart, kidneys, and eyes. Learning about your blood pressure can help reduce your risk of having a stroke or heart attack. Ask your health care provider to check your blood pressure today.

BRAIN

Stroke—Blood vessels in the brain that are damaged, weakened, and narrowed by HBP may bulge out (aneurysm) and burst causing blood to seep into the brain tissue (hemorrhage). Or blood clots may form in the arteries leading to the brain, blocking blood flow.
Transient Ischemic Attack—TIA (mini stroke) is a brief, temporary disruption of blood supply to the brain. It's often caused by atherosclerosis or a blood clot—both of which can be a result of HBP.

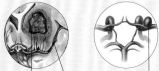

Hemorrhage   Blood clot   Aneurysm at junction of main arteries of the brain

EYES

Thickened, narrowed, or torn blood vessels in the eyes may result in vision loss.

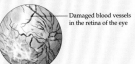

Damaged blood vessels in the retina of the eye

BLOOD VESSELS

High blood pressure can damage the inner walls of arteries causing them to thicken and harden, a condition called **arteriosclerosis**. Cholesterol and other substances (plaque) in the blood can collect on the damaged walls of the arteries, a condition called **atherosclerosis**, and may block blood flow causing problems such as chest pain (angina), heart attack, heart failure, kidney failure, stroke, blocked arteries in your legs or arms (peripheral arterial disease), eye damage, and aneurysms.

Thickened artery walls   Plaque buildup on walls of artery
Arteriosclerosis   Atherosclerosis

ANEURYSM

Over time, the constant pressure of blood moving through a weakened artery can cause a section of its wall to enlarge and form a bulge (aneurysm). An aneurysm can burst and cause internal bleeding. Aneurysms can form in any artery in the body, but they're most common in the aorta, the body's largest artery.

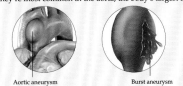

Aortic aneurysm   Burst aneurysm

HEART

Coronary Artery Disease (CAD)—Affects the arteries that supply blood to the heart. Thickened and narrowed coronary arteries prevent blood from flowing freely to the heart, causing chest pain (angina), heart attack or irregular heart rhythms (arrhythmias).
Left Ventricular Hypertrophy (LVH)—HBP forces the heart to work harder to pump blood to the rest of the body. This causes the heart's left pumping chamber (the left ventricle) to thicken or stiffen limiting the ventricle's ability to pump blood, increasing the risk of heart attack, heart failure, and sudden cardiac death.
Heart failure—Over time, the strain on the heart from HBP can cause the heart to weaken and work less efficiently, eventually failing to meet the body's demand for blood.

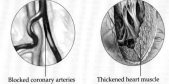

Blocked coronary arteries   Thickened heart muscle
Angina   Left Ventricular Hypertrophy

KIDNEYS

High blood pressure is one of the most common causes of kidney failure. It can damage both the large arteries leading to the kidneys and the tiny blood vessels within the kidneys. Damage to either prevents the kidneys from effectively filtering waste from the blood, allowing dangerous levels of fluid and waste to accumulate.

Glomerulus—filters waste from blood

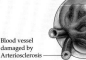

Blood vessel damaged by Arteriosclerosis

Prevention and Management

High blood pressure can be prevented and managed best by adjusting your lifestyle. Decrease your blood pressure by the following measures:

- Reduce body weight if overweight.
- Maintain a healthy weight.
- Eat healthy foods.
- Decrease salt in your diet.
- Decrease fat in your diet.
- Increase fiber in your diet.
- Do not smoke.
- Avoid excessive alcohol intake.
- Exercise regularly.
- Manage stress.
- Follow your physician's instructions and take any medications as prescribed.

What Is High Blood Pressure?

When the heart beats, it pumps blood out to all parts of the body through the arteries creating force or pressure against the walls of the arteries. Like air in a tire, blood fills arteries to a certain capacity. But just as too much air pressure can damage a tire, high blood pressure can damage healthy arteries. When blood pressure is high, the heart must work harder to pump the same amount of blood through the arteries. Blood pressure rises and falls during the day, but when blood pressure stays high over time, it is called high blood pressure (HBP) or hypertension. The wear and tear caused by untreated HBP can cause damage to the heart, kidneys, and eyes, and increases the risk for heart attack, stroke, kidney failure, CAD, and other serious health problems.

Signs and Symptoms of High Blood Pressure

Most of the time, HBP does not cause any symptoms. It is often diagnosed when a patient visits his or her physician for a routine checkup. Many people do not realize they have HBP until it has caused damage to their body. In rare cases, headaches can result from extremely HBP.

How Is Blood Pressure Measured?

Blood pressure is measured with a simple test using a blood pressure cuff. The cuff is wrapped around your upper arm and inflated enough to stop the blood flow in your artery for a few seconds. When the cuff is released or deflated, the first sound heard by your health care provider through the stethoscope is the whooshing sound of your heart pushing blood into your arteries. This is called the "systolic" blood pressure. The "diastolic" blood pressure is when this noise disappears, indicating the heart is relaxed. The systolic blood pressure number is always stated first followed by the diastolic number. For example, your blood pressure may be read as "117 over 76," or written "117/76."

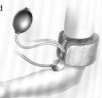

Two numbers are used to describe blood pressure:

Systolic (top number) The top number called "systolic blood pressure" measures blood pressure when the heart pumps blood forward through the arteries to the rest of your body. This force creates pressure on the arteries. Blood pressure is highest when the heart beats, pumping the blood. A normal healthy number is around 117.

117 / 76 **mm Hg**

mm Hg is a measurement of pressure

Diastolic (bottom number) The second number is lower than the systolic pressure and measures blood pressure when the heart relaxes between beats. This is called "diastolic blood pressure." A normal healthy number is around 76. Your blood pressure normally changes throughout the day. It rises when you are active and lowers when you are resting.

Healthy and Unhealthy Blood Pressure Levels

Blood Pressure Category	Systolic mm Hg (upper #)		Diastolic mm Hg (lower #)
Normal	**<120**	and	**<80**
Prehypertension	**120-139**	or	**80-89**
High Blood Pressure (Hypertension) Stage 1	**140-159**	or	**90-99**
High Blood Pressure (Hypertension) Stage 2	**160** or higher	or	**100** or higher
Hypertensive Crisis (Emergency care needed)	Higher than **180**	or	Higher than **110**

http://www.heart.org/HEARTORG/   *Your doctor should evaluate unusually low blood pressure readings.

Types and Causes of High Blood Pressure (Hypertension)

Primary or essential hypertension is the most common type of HBP. In most cases the exact causes are unknown; however, there are several factors that increase or contribute to your chances of developing HBP:
- Obesity or being overweight
- Lack of physical activity
- Poor diet, especially one that includes too much salt and too little potassium
- Genetics and family medical history
- Age and gender
- High levels of alcohol consumption
- Ethnic background
- Stress
- Smoking and secondhand smoke

Secondary hypertension may result from a known cause such as:
- Chronic kidney disease
- Adrenal and thyroid problems or tumors
- Diabetes
- Pregnancy
- Some neurologic disorders

High Blood Pressure in Children

Teens, children, and even babies can have HBP. Although HBP is far more common among adults, the rate among kids is on the rise, a trend that experts link to the increase in childhood obesity. Early diagnosis and treatment can reduce or prevent the harmful complications of HBP. The American Heart Association recommends that all children have their blood pressure measured yearly. Children have the same test for HBP as do adults; however, interpreting the numbers is more difficult. Your child's physician will use charts based on your child's gender, height, age, and blood pressure numbers to determine whether or not your child has HBP.

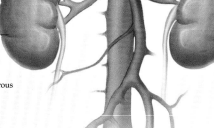

© 2014   Wolters Kluwer   Published by Anatomical Chart Company | Developed in consultation with Dr. Douglas S. Moodie.

Heart Failure

What Is Heart Failure?

- Heart failure is when the heart is unable to pump enough blood to meet the body's needs.
- Fatigue, shortness of breath, and swelling from fluid retention are symptoms.
- Most frequently diagnosed in hospitalized patients older than age 65.

What Causes Heart Failure?

Heart failure can result from almost any type of heart disease, including a heart attack, high blood pressure, congenital heart defects, valve problems, or abnormalities of heart muscle.

What Are the Types of Heart Failure?

The two main groups of heart failure are divided by the way the left ventricle, the main pumping chamber, is impaired:

- **Systolic Heart Failure** is due to the thinning of the heart muscle. Causes may include:
  - ♦ Prior heart attacks
  - ♦ Leaky heart valves
  - ♦ Diseases of the heart muscle

- **Diastolic Heart Failure** is due to a thickening of the heart muscle that prevents the ventricle from filling normally. Causes may include:
  - ♦ Long-standing high blood pressure
  - ♦ Diabetes

Symptoms and Signs

Common heart failure symptoms include:

- Fatigue
- Weakness
- Shortness of breath even at rest

Abnormal findings include:

- Weight gain from fluid buildup
- Increased pulse and breathing rates
- Bulging of the veins on the sides of the neck

- Difficulty breathing when lying flat and at rest
- Cough

- Swelling of the legs
- Enlargement of the liver and belly

With proper treatment these symptoms and signs improve.

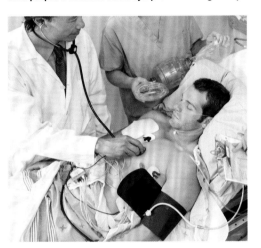

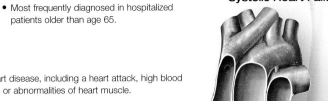

Systolic Heart Failure

Stretched and thin chambers

Heart can't pump

Left ventricle

Diastolic Heart Failure

Stiff and thick chambers

Heart can't fill

Left ventricle

Conditions that Worsen Symptoms of Heart Failure

Factors that place additional strain on the heart and can worsen heart failure symptoms include:

- Infections such as pneumonia
- Fever
- Rapid heart rhythms
- Low blood count (anemia)
- Uncontrolled high blood pressure

- An overactive thyroid gland
- Too much salt in the diet
- Drinking too many alcoholic beverages
- Taking certain medications, including some over-the-counter anti-inflammatory medications

Diagnosis

Patient's symptoms and findings by a health care provider on physical examination include:

- Fluid in the lungs
- Abnormal heart sounds
- Prominence of the veins in the neck

- Enlarged liver
- Swelling in the legs

Tests

- A chest x-ray may show fluid buildup in the lungs and/or an enlarged heart size.
- An ultrasound of the heart ("echocardiogram") can demonstrate which type of heart failure is present (systolic or diastolic).

Advanced Therapies

For patients with severe heart failure who do not respond to medication, advanced therapies include:

- Implanting a special pacemaker to improve the coordination of the heart's contraction.
- An implanted defibrillator to monitor and automatically treat life-threatening abnormal heart rhythms that can occur.

- A single implanted device can provide both of these functions if needed.

For the most severely affected, and carefully selected patients:

- Internal or external mechanical pumps can be placed (including "ventricular assist devices" and totally artificial hearts) to take over for the heart's poor function.
- Cardiac transplantation can be considered.

Staging

Doctors describe how advanced a patient's heart failure symptoms are using this classification:

Class 1	• The patient has no current symptoms	
Class 2	• There is a limitation of activity	• Shortness of breath that comes on only when climbing a flight of stairs quickly
Class 3	• There is marked limitation of activity	• Shortness of breath climbing stairs slowly
Class 4	• There is severe limitation	• Shortness of breath at rest

Treatment

The goals of heart failure treatment are to improve symptoms and prolong survival. Underlying causes of the heart failure should be addressed, such as managing high blood pressure, coronary artery disease, and valve abnormalities.

	Treatment	**What they do**
Systolic Heart Failure	• Beta-blockers	• Block neurotransmitters to allow the heart rate to slow and blood vessels to relax
	• ACE inhibitors • Angiotensin receptor blockers • Aldosterone • Antagonists	• Block certain hormones and allow blood vessels to relax
	• Inotropic drugs	• Improve strength of the heart's contraction
	• Combination of angiotensin receptor antagonist and neprilysin inhibitor	• Combines two different approaches to relaxing blood vessels
Diastolic Heart Failure	• Diuretic medications	• Reduce water retention

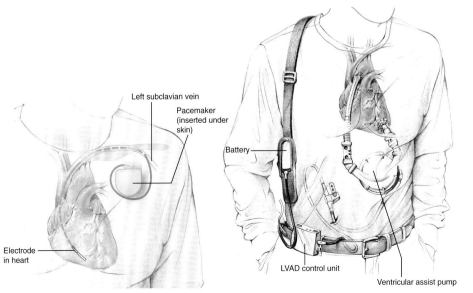

Left subclavian vein

Pacemaker (inserted under skin)

Battery

Electrode in heart

LVAD control unit

Ventricular assist pump

© 2017 Wolters Kluwer Medical illustrations by Jennifer Smith, in consultation with Leonard S. Lilly, MD, Harvard Medical School, Brigham and Women's Hospital, Boston, MA.

Peripheral Artery Disease

What Is Peripheral Artery Disease?

- **Peripheral artery disease** (PAD) refers to the narrowing of vessels in the legs and pelvis, causing insufficient blood flow and oxygen.
- PAD affects both men and women.
- PAD is most common after the age of 60.

Atherosclerosis of Peripheral Arteries

The main cause of PAD is **atherosclerosis,** also known as "hardening of the arteries." In this condition there is buildup of fatty plaque on the walls of arteries, making them narrower, reducing blood flow, and not allowing the normal, necessary increase in blood flow with physical activity.

Conditions that lead to atherosclerosis include the following:

- Cigarette smoking
- Diabetes
- High cholesterol

Symptoms and Signs of PAD of the Lower Extremities

- The most common symptom is **claudication**, a feeling of aching or cramping in the calf, thigh, or buttocks brought on by exercise, which is relieved by rest.
  - Initially, this may only occur walking up an incline, climbing a long flight of stairs, or walking quickly.
  - Later, with progressive narrowing of the arteries, symptoms occur with less exertion.
  - In severe cases, there may be severe and continuous pain in the feet and toes even at rest.
  - Pulse points are reduced or absent in affected areas of the legs.
  - In advanced PAD, the feet and lower legs have shiny, tight skin and may be pale and cool with weakened, shrunken muscles. There may be ulcerations of the skin that do not heal.

Treatments and Lifestyle Modifications

To effectively manage PAD, reducing the risk factors that lead to atherosclerosis is recommended. These include the following:

- Smoking cessation.
- Controlling blood pressure and cholesterol levels.
- Walking exercises to increase endurance and improve claudication symptoms.
- Certain medications are sometimes helpful for improving blood flow to the limbs and reducing discomfort.
- If symptoms do not improve or become more limiting, a procedure known as a balloon catheterization and the insertion of a stent may be necessary to improve blood flow.
- Extensive narrowing and blockages may require surgery to bypass the blocked arteries.

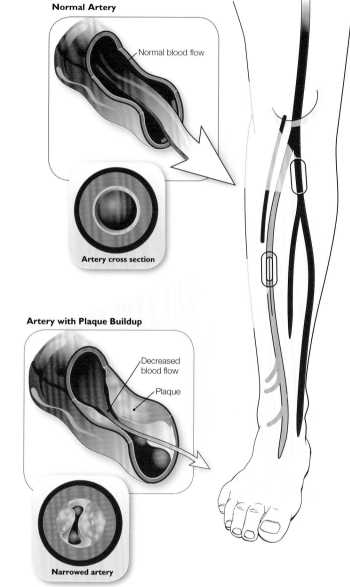

Normal Artery

Normal blood flow

Artery cross section

Artery with Plaque Buildup

Decreased blood flow

Plaque

Narrowed artery

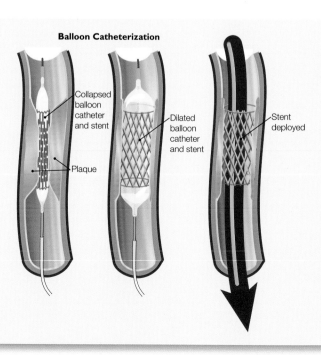

Balloon Catheterization

Collapsed balloon catheter and stent

Dilated balloon catheter and stent

Stent deployed

Plaque

©2019 Wolters Kluwer   Anatomical Chart Company, Philadelphia, PA. Medical illustrations by Jennifer Smith, in consultation with Leonard S. Lilly, MD, Harvard Medical School, Brigham and Women's Hospital, Boston, MA.

Stenosis refers to abnormal narrowing of one or more heart valves, which prevents the smooth flow of blood from one chamber to the next.

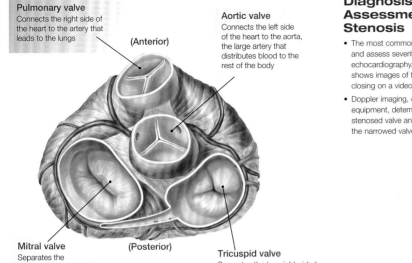

Pulmonary valve
Connects the right side of the heart to the artery that leads to the lungs

(Anterior)

Aortic valve
Connects the left side of the heart to the aorta, the large artery that distributes blood to the rest of the body

Mitral valve
Separates the two left-sided heart chambers

(Posterior)

Tricuspid valve
Separates the two right-sided heart chambers

Diagnosis and Assessment of Valve Stenosis

- The most common test to diagnose and assess severity of valve stenosis is echocardiography. This noninvasive procedure shows images of the valves opening and closing on a video screen.
- Doppler imaging, obtained with the same equipment, determines the pressure across a stenosed valve and calculates the severity of the narrowed valve.

Pulmonary Valve Stenosis

- Pulmonary valve stenosis is uncommon and is almost always a result of deformity of the valve at birth.
- When severe, it causes fatigue, light-headedness, and blood backup—symptoms similar to tricuspid stenosis.
- Doppler echocardiography confirms the diagnosis and severity.
- Catheter balloon valvuloplasty is often effective for symptomatic patients.

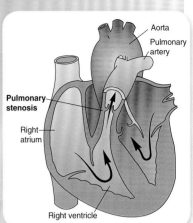

Aorta
Pulmonary artery
Pulmonary stenosis
Right atrium
Right ventricle

Aortic Valve Stenosis
Causes

- Birth deformity of the valve (bicuspid aortic valve)
- Thickening and calcium deposits on the valve observed in older individuals, especially those with high cholesterol, those with high blood pressure, and smokers
- Rheumatic fever, a condition that can follow a streptococcal throat infection

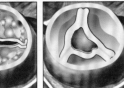

Bicuspid aortic valve   Calcific aortic stenosis   Rheumatic aortic stenosis

Signs, Symptoms, Diagnosis

- Narrowing of the valve in aortic stenosis progresses over many decades causing symptoms only when it becomes severely narrowed.
- Symptoms usually occur with exertion and include the following:
  - Chest pain
  - Shortness of breath
  - Light-headedness spells
  - Heart murmur (a turbulent noise) heard through a stethoscope
  - Weakened pulse of blood, on the sides of the neck, felt on physical examination
- Echocardiography shows thickening and calcium deposits, reduced opening, and a high pressure difference across the valve.
- Cardiac catheterization is usually performed if valve surgery is planned. This procedure looks for narrowings in the coronary arteries.

Treatment

- The usual procedure is open heart surgery with removal of the old narrowed valve and placement of a healthy artificial valve made of mechanical parts or biologic tissue.
- Aortic valve replacement can also be performed in a less invasive way (called **TAVR** or **TAVI**), in which a new artificial valve is compressed to a narrow form, placed on a tube (catheter) that is inserted into the vascular system through the skin and then threaded to the position of the diseased, narrowed valve. The new aortic valve is expanded in size and crushes the diseased one out of the way. Once the new valve is in place, the catheter is removed.

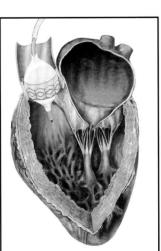

Mitral Valve Stenosis
Causes

- Mitral valve stenosis almost always results from valve damage due to rheumatic fever many years or decades earlier.
- Rheumatic fever affects the mitral valve more often than the other heart valves.

Signs, Symptoms, Diagnosis

- Symptoms include shortness of breath, initially with exertion only.
- With more severe mitral stenosis, shortness of breath can occur even at rest, and it may be difficult to lie in bed because of difficult breathing and cough.
- Patients with advanced mitral stenosis may develop a rapid, irregular heart rhythm (atrial fibrillation) that can lead to blood clots in the heart. The murmur of mitral stenosis is heard through the stethoscope placed near the tip of the heart.
- Diagnosis is confirmed by echocardiography.

Treatment

- Initial therapy may include salt restriction in the diet, diuretic medication, and drugs to slow the heart rate in order to reduce shortness of breath.
- Patients who develop atrial fibrillation need to take a blood thinner to prevent blood clots.

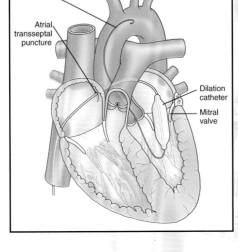

Guidewire
Atrial transseptal puncture
Dilation catheter
Mitral valve

Tricuspid Stenosis

- Tricuspid stenosis is a very rare condition that causes blood to back up into the body's veins, causing prominence of the blood vessels in the neck, enlargement of the liver, bloating of the belly, and swelling of the legs.
- Treatment of patients who are symptomatic requires mechanical opening of the valve either by balloon valvuloplasty (similar to mitral stenosis) or open heart surgery to repair or replace the valve.

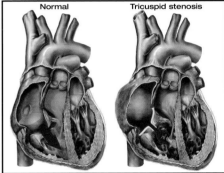

Normal   Tricuspid stenosis

Balloon Mitral Valvuloplasty

- For patients with advanced stenosis, the preferred intervention is balloon mitral valvuloplasty.
  - A catheter with a large inflatable balloon is inserted through the skin and directed through blood vessels and across the narrowed mitral valve.
  - The balloon is inflated and stretches and cracks the narrowed valve open, and then the balloon/catheter is removed.
- For patients who cannot have this procedure, heart surgery is performed to widen or replace the valve.

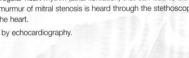
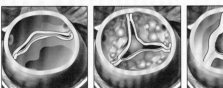

©2017 Wolters Kluwer   Medical illustrations by Jennifer Smith, Marcelo Oliver, MFA and Lik Kwong, MFA in consultation with Leonard S. Lilly, MD, Harvard Medical School, Brigham and Women's Hospital, Boston, MA.

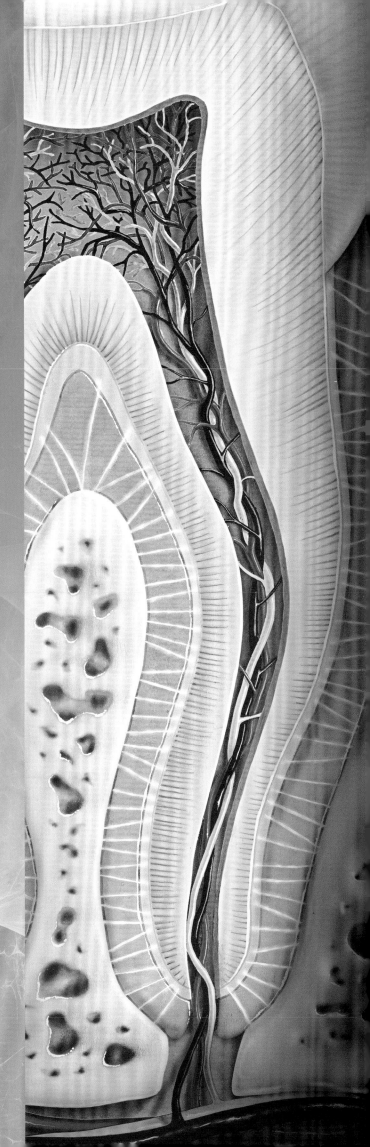

DENTAL DISEASES & DISORDERS

- Disorders of the Teeth and Jaw

- Temporomandibular Joint (TMJ)

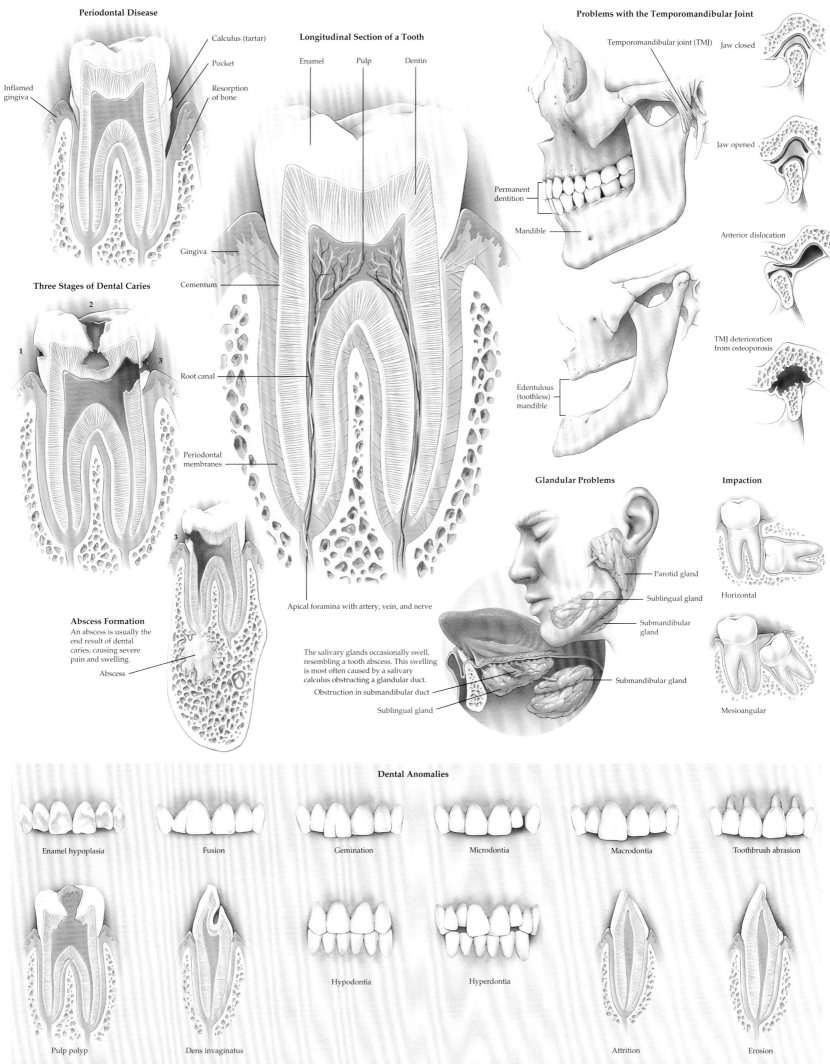

Periodontal Disease

Inflamed gingiva

Calculus (tartar)

Pocket

Resorption of bone

Longitudinal Section of a Tooth

Enamel

Pulp

Dentin

Gingiva

Cementum

Root canal

Periodontal membranes

Apical foramina with artery, vein, and nerve

Three Stages of Dental Caries

2

1

3

3

Abscess Formation

An abscess is usually the end result of dental caries, causing severe pain and swelling.

Abscess

Problems with the Temporomandibular Joint

Temporomandibular joint (TMJ)

Jaw closed

Jaw opened

Anterior dislocation

TMJ deterioration from osteoporosis

Permanent dentition

Mandible

Edentulous (toothless) mandible

Glandular Problems

The salivary glands occasionally swell, resembling a tooth abscess. This swelling is most often caused by a salivary calculus obstructing a glandular duct.

Obstruction in submandibular duct

Sublingual gland

Parotid gland

Sublingual gland

Submandibular gland

Submandibular gland

Impaction

Horizontal

Mesioangular

Dental Anomalies

Enamel hypoplasia

Fusion

Gemination

Microdontia

Macrodontia

Toothbrush abrasion

Pulp polyp

Dens invaginatus

Hypodontia

Hyperdontia

Attrition

Erosion

Key: Muscles (m.)
A. Temporalis m.
B. Temporomandibular joint
C. Masseter m.
D. Stylohyoid m.
E. Digastric m. (posterior belly)
F. Longus capitis m.
G. Levator scapulae m.
H. Trapezius m.
I. Posterior scalene m.
J. Middle scalene m.
K. Sternocleidomastoid m.
L. Inferior pharyngeal constrictor m.
M. Thyrohyoid m.
N. Sternothyroid m.
O. Omohyoid m.
P. Sternohyoid m.
Q. Hyoglossus m.
R. Mylohyoid m.
S. Digastric m. (anterior belly)

Normal Jaw (closed)

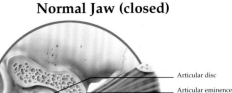

- Articular disc
- Articular eminence
- Lateral pterygoid m. (superior and inferior heads)
- Mandibular condyle

What Is TMJ Syndrome?

TMJ syndrome is a term often used to describe a disorder of the temporomandibular joints (jaw joints) and/or the muscles that control the joints and balance the head on the spinal column. It is a collection of symptoms that occur when the jaw joints and/or surrounding muscles do not work together properly. The problem also can extend down the neck and back.

Normal Jaw (open)

The purpose of the articular disc is to cushion the bones of the TMJ during opening and closing of the mouth. When the mouth opens, the mandibular condyle rotates on a horizontal axis. At the same time, the condyle and disc glide forward and downward on the articular eminence. During this entire motion, the articular disc remains attached to the condyle.

Nerves of the Temporomandibular Region

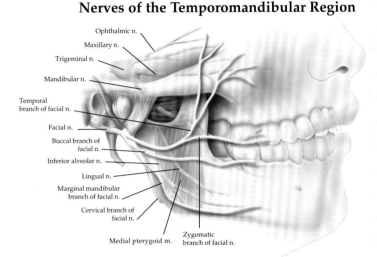

- Ophthalmic n.
- Maxillary n.
- Trigeminal n.
- Mandibular n.
- Temporal branch of facial n.
- Facial n.
- Buccal branch of facial n.
- Inferior alveolar n.
- Lingual n.
- Marginal mandibular branch of facial n.
- Cervical branch of facial n.
- Medial pterygoid m.
- Zygomatic branch of facial n.

Common TMJ Syndrome Causes and Disorders

Whiplash

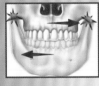

Whiplash causes the muscles of the neck to be jarred and pulled violently, often resulting in ligament tears, stretching of structures to their limits, and discal tearing. All can lead to the development of TMJ symptoms.

Malocclusion

Malocclusion is the abnormal contact of opposing teeth with respect to the temporomandibular joint that interferes with the efficient movement of the jaw during mastication. It is one of the most frequent triggers of TMJ syndrome. Malocclusion, even on a minute scale, can trigger the spasm of muscles, resulting in pain.

Bruxism/Clenching

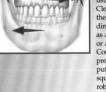

Bruxism, the grinding of teeth, usually occurs during sleep. Clenching can occur throughout the day or night. Both can be directly related to TMJ, either as a trigger for muscle spasms or as a result of malocclusion. Constant grinding also causes pressure on the TMJ. Bruxism can put pressure on the articular disc, squeezing out synovial fluid and robbing it of lubrication.

Systemic Diseases

The TMJ, like any other joint, is susceptible to any of the systemic diseases. Immune disorders such as osteoarthritis, rheumatoid arthritis, psoriatic arthritis, and systemic lupus erythematosus and electrolyte imbalances can produce inflammation and muscle cramping in the TMJ. In addition, viral infections can cause damage to the surfaces of the TMJ.

Loss of Teeth

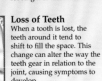

When a tooth is lost, the teeth around it tend to shift to fill the space. This change can alter the way the teeth gear in relation to the joint, causing symptoms to develop.

Disc Displacement

The jaw joint, in addition to being a ball and socket joint, glides forward and backward. When functioning correctly, the articular cartilage lies between the condyle head of the mandible and the roof of the joint. It normally follows the condylar head in its forward and backward movement. If the ligaments that hold the disc to the condylar head are injured, the disc can slip out of place and can no longer serve as a normal cushion between the lower and upper parts of the jaw. Typically, the disc is pulled forward. Mild displacements can cause a clicking or popping sound in the joint and sometimes can be painful. Permanent damage may result from the displacements.

Symptoms

Extracapsular—Outside the jaw joint
- Headaches
- Tooth pain (caused by bruxism)
- Numbness or tingling of fingers
- Dizziness
- Neck, shoulder, or back pain
- Pain behind eyes
- Earaches or ringing in ears

Intracapsular—Within the jaw joint
- Crepitus (grinding sound)
- Clicking or popping
- Locking or limited range of motion
- Pain in and around jaw joints

Disorders Sometimes Mistaken for TMJ Syndrome
- Migraine headache
- Chemical allergies
- Temporal tendinitis
- Psychosomatic headache
- Ernest syndrome
- Sinusitis
- Brain tumors
- Trauma

Treatment

Phase 1—Attempts to break the cycle of muscle spasms, thereby relieving pain and producing a physiological relationship between the maxilla and mandible. Treatments can include the following:
- Use of an intraoral orthotic or splint
- Anti-inflammatory medications
- Stress management
- Physical therapy
- Muscle relaxants
- Manipulative treatment

Phase 2—Attempts to break the cycle of pain through more permanent means of treatment. Treatments can include the following:
- Adjustment of dental occlusion
- Orthodontics
- Reconstruction of teeth
- Orthognathic surgery (surgical relocation of teeth or jaw)
- Replacement of missing teeth
- Surgery on TMJ itself (last resort)

DIGESTIVE SYSTEM DISEASES & DISORDERS

- Gastroesophageal Disorders and Digestive Anatomy
- Diseases of the Digestive System
- Understanding Ulcers
- Ulcerative Colitis and Crohn's Disease
- Understanding Irritable Bowel Syndrome (IBS)

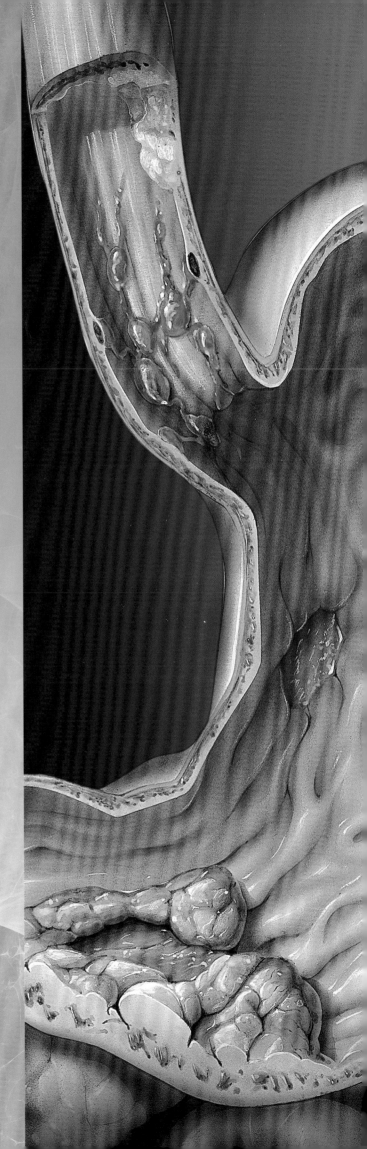

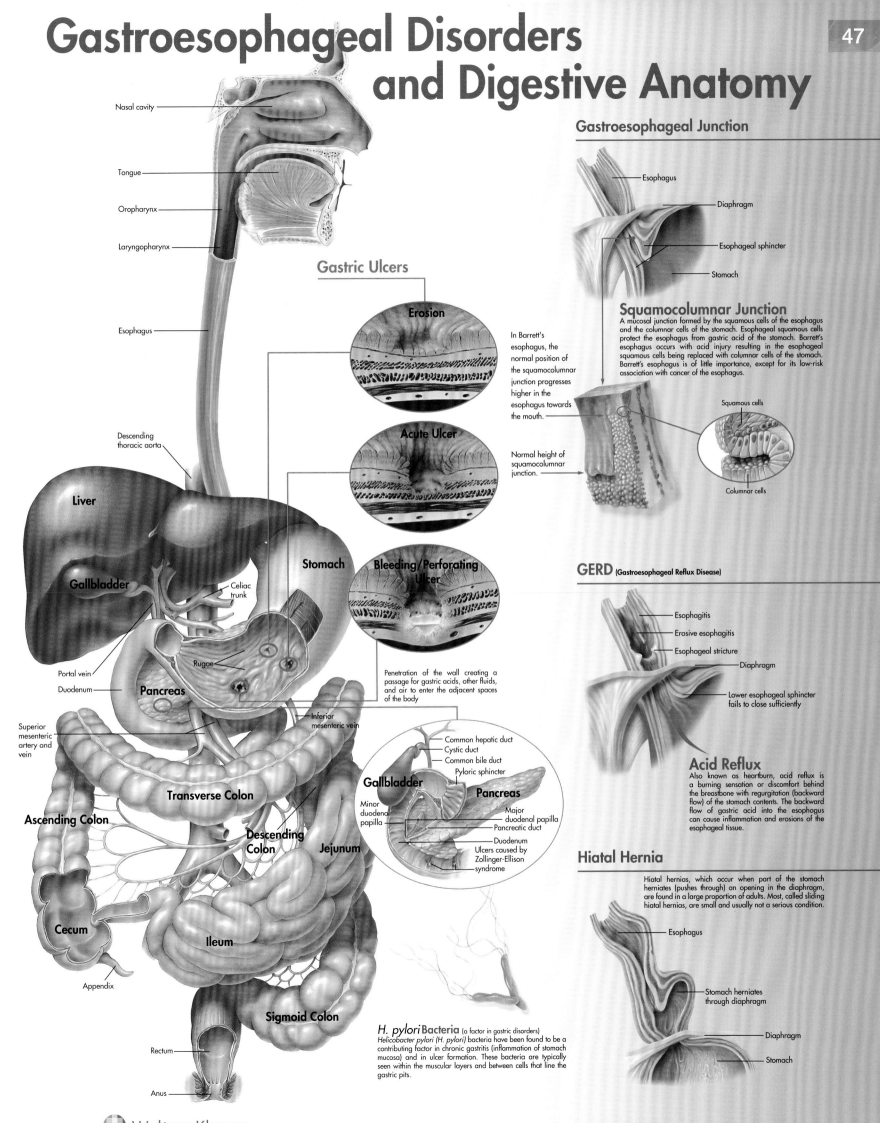

Gastroesophageal Disorders and Digestive Anatomy

Nasal cavity

Tongue

Oropharynx

Laryngopharynx

Esophagus

Descending thoracic aorta

Liver

Gallbladder

Portal vein

Duodenum

Pancreas

Celiac trunk

Rugae

Stomach

Superior mesenteric artery and vein

Ascending Colon

Transverse Colon

Descending Colon

Jejunum

Cecum

Ileum

Appendix

Sigmoid Colon

Rectum

Anus

Inferior mesenteric vein

Gastric Ulcers

Erosion

Acute Ulcer

Bleeding/Perforating Ulcer

Penetration of the wall creating a passage for gastric acids, other fluids, and air to enter the adjacent spaces of the body

In Barrett's esophagus, the normal position of the squamocolumnar junction progresses higher in the esophagus towards the mouth.

Normal height of squamocolumnar junction.

Common hepatic duct
Cystic duct
Common bile duct
Pyloric sphincter

Gallbladder

Minor duodenal papilla

Pancreas

Major duodenal papilla
Pancreatic duct
Duodenum
Ulcers caused by Zollinger-Ellison syndrome

H. pylori Bacteria (a factor in gastric disorders)
Helicobacter pylori (H. pylori) bacteria have been found to be a contributing factor in chronic gastritis (inflammation of stomach mucosa) and in ulcer formation. These bacteria are typically seen within the muscular layers and between cells that line the gastric pits.

Gastroesophageal Junction

Esophagus

Diaphragm

Esophageal sphincter

Stomach

Squamocolumnar Junction
A mucosal junction formed by the squamous cells of the esophagus and the columnar cells of the stomach. Esophageal squamous cells protect the esophagus from gastric acid of the stomach. Barrett's esophagus occurs with acid injury resulting in the esophageal squamous cells being replaced with columnar cells of the stomach. Barrett's esophagus is of little importance, except for its low-risk association with cancer of the esophagus.

Squamous cells

Columnar cells

GERD (Gastroesophageal Reflux Disease)

Esophagitis

Erosive esophagitis

Esophageal stricture

Diaphragm

Lower esophageal sphincter fails to close sufficiently

Acid Reflux
Also known as heartburn, acid reflux is a burning sensation or discomfort behind the breastbone with regurgitation (backward flow) of the stomach contents. The backward flow of gastric acid into the esophagus can cause inflammation and erosions of the esophageal tissue.

Hiatal Hernia

Hiatal hernias, which occur when part of the stomach herniates (pushes through) an opening in the diaphragm, are found in a large proportion of adults. Most, called sliding hiatal hernias, are small and usually not a serious condition.

Esophagus

Stomach herniates through diaphragm

Diaphragm

Stomach

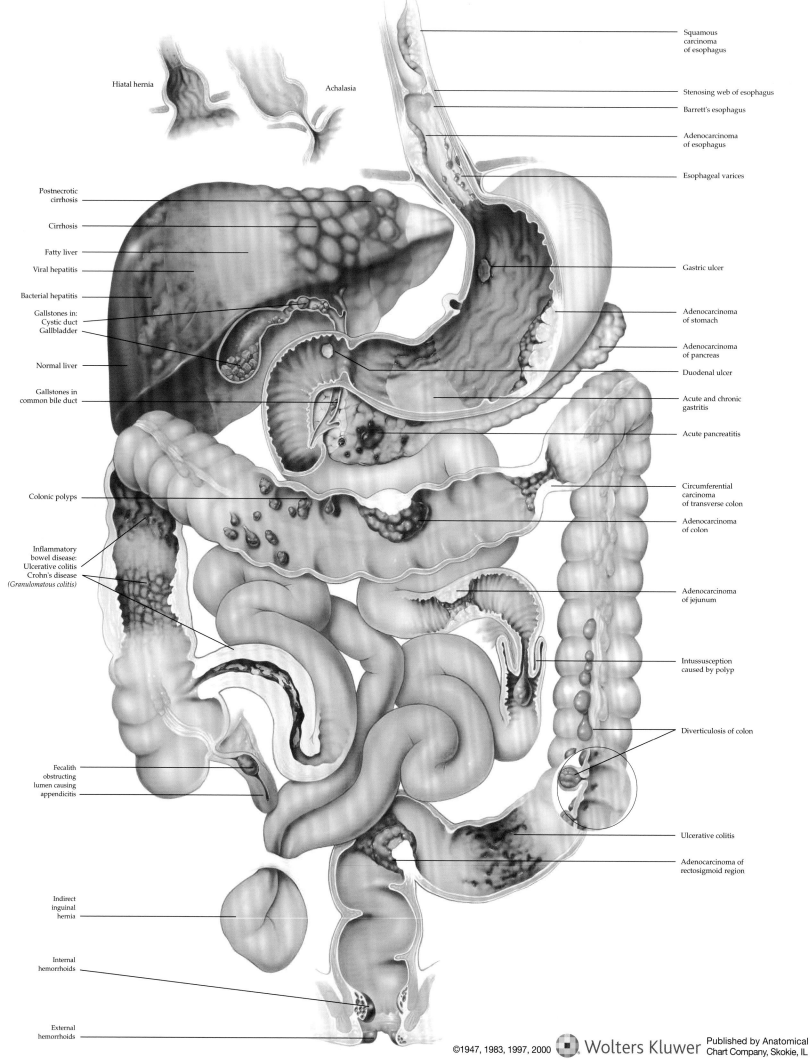

Hiatal hernia

Achalasia

Squamous carcinoma of esophagus

Stenosing web of esophagus

Barrett's esophagus

Adenocarcinoma of esophagus

Esophageal varices

Postnecrotic cirrhosis

Cirrhosis

Fatty liver

Viral hepatitis

Bacterial hepatitis

Gallstones in: Cystic duct Gallbladder

Normal liver

Gallstones in common bile duct

Gastric ulcer

Adenocarcinoma of stomach

Adenocarcinoma of pancreas

Duodenal ulcer

Acute and chronic gastritis

Acute pancreatitis

Colonic polyps

Circumferential carcinoma of transverse colon

Adenocarcinoma of colon

Inflammatory bowel disease: Ulcerative colitis Crohn's disease (Granulomatous colitis)

Adenocarcinoma of jejunum

Intussusception caused by polyp

Diverticulosis of colon

Fecalith obstructing lumen causing appendicitis

Ulcerative colitis

Adenocarcinoma of rectosigmoid region

Indirect inguinal hernia

Internal hemorrhoids

External hemorrhoids

Wolters Kluwer   Published by Anatomical Chart Company, Skokie, IL

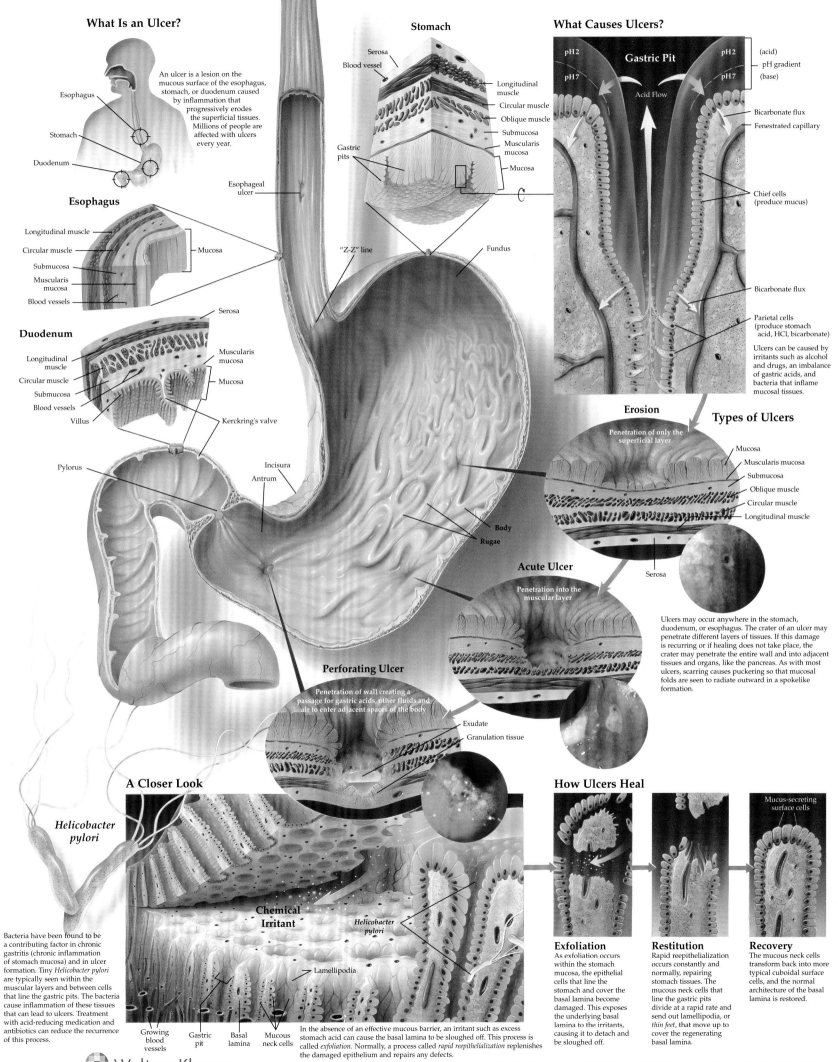

What Is an Ulcer?

Esophagus
Stomach
Duodenum

An ulcer is a lesion on the mucous surface of the esophagus, stomach, or duodenum caused by inflammation that progressively erodes the superficial tissues. Millions of people are affected with ulcers every year.

Esophagus

Longitudinal muscle
Circular muscle
Submucosa
Muscularis mucosa
Blood vessels
Mucosa

Duodenum

Longitudinal muscle
Circular muscle
Submucosa
Blood vessels
Villus
Serosa
Muscularis mucosa
Mucosa
Kerckring's valve

Pylorus
Incisura
Antrum
Body
Rugae

Stomach

Serosa
Blood vessel
Gastric pits
Longitudinal muscle
Circular muscle
Oblique muscle
Submucosa
Muscularis mucosa
Mucosa

Esophageal ulcer
"Z-Z" line
Fundus

What Causes Ulcers?

pH 2
pH 7
Gastric Pit
Acid Flow
pH 2
pH 7

(acid)
pH gradient
(base)

Bicarbonate flux
Fenestrated capillary

Chief cells (produce mucus)

Bicarbonate flux

Parietal cells (produce stomach acid, HCl, bicarbonate)

Ulcers can be caused by irritants such as alcohol and drugs, an imbalance of gastric acids, and bacteria that inflame mucosal tissues.

Types of Ulcers

Erosion

Penetration of only the superficial layer

Mucosa
Muscularis mucosa
Submucosa
Oblique muscle
Circular muscle
Longitudinal muscle
Serosa

Acute Ulcer

Penetration into the muscular layer

Ulcers may occur anywhere in the stomach, duodenum, or esophagus. The crater of an ulcer may penetrate different layers of tissues. If this damage is recurring or if healing does not take place, the crater may penetrate the entire wall and into adjacent tissues and organs, like the pancreas. As with most ulcers, scarring causes puckering so that mucosal folds are seen to radiate outward in a spokelike formation.

Perforating Ulcer

Penetration of wall creating a passage for gastric acids, other fluids and air to enter adjacent spaces of the body

Exudate
Granulation tissue

A Closer Look

Helicobacter pylori

Chemical Irritant
Helicobacter pylori

Bacteria have been found to be a contributing factor in chronic gastritis (chronic inflammation of stomach mucosa) and in ulcer formation. Tiny *Helicobacter pylori* are typically seen within the muscular layers and between cells that line the gastric pits. The bacteria cause inflammation of these tissues that can lead to ulcers. Treatment with acid-reducing medication and antibiotics can reduce the recurrence of this process.

Lamellipodia

Growing blood vessels
Gastric pit
Basal lamina
Mucous neck cells

In the absence of an effective mucous barrier, an irritant such as excess stomach acid can cause the basal lamina to be sloughed off. This process is called *exfoliation*. Normally, a process called *rapid reepithelialization* replenishes the damaged epithelium and repairs any defects.

How Ulcers Heal

Mucus-secreting surface cells

Exfoliation

As exfoliation occurs within the stomach mucosa, the epithelial cells that line the stomach and cover the basal lamina become damaged. This exposes the underlying basal lamina to the irritants, causing it to detach and be sloughed off.

Restitution

Rapid reepithelialization occurs constantly and normally, repairing stomach tissues. The mucous neck cells that line the gastric pits divide at a rapid rate and send out lamellipodia, or *thin feet*, that move up to cover the regenerating basal lamina.

Recovery

The mucous neck cells transform back into more typical cuboidal surface cells, and the normal architecture of the basal lamina is restored.

Ulcerative Colitis and Crohn's Disease

Ulcerative colitis (UC) and Crohn's disease (CD) are the two most common forms of inflammatory bowel disease (IBD)

Who Gets Crohn's Disease?
CD affects about 780,000 Americans. CD is more common in young people between 15 and 35 years of age.

Who Gets Ulcerative Colitis?
UC affects about 900,000 Americans, both men and women, at any age. Most people are diagnosed in their mid-30s, but the disease develops in some after age 60.

Similar, But Different

SIMILARITIES

- Age: usually before 30 years, but can occur at any age
- Ethnicity: whites and people of Ashkenazi Jewish descent have highest risk
- Family history: risk higher if you have a close relative with the disease
- Symptoms: mild to severe and include abdominal pain and cramping, diarrhea, blood, mucus, or pus in stool, weight loss, fatigue and fever, possible nausea and vomiting
- Complications: can be life-threatening
- Remission: symptom-free periods can last months to years between flare-ups

DIFFERENCES

Crohn's disease (CD)	Ulcerative colitis (UC)
Location	
• Anywhere in GI tract, from mouth to anus; most common at end of small intestine (ileum) and beginning of large intestine	• Affects only the colon (large bowel) and rectum
Risk Factors	
• Cigarette smoking increases risk of developing CD and of more severe disease	• Nicotine may play a role in UC prevention... but causes a host of other problems
	• Use of isotretinoin for acne may increase risk of IBD, particularly UC
• Living in a developed country, urban area, or northern climate increases risk of developing CD	
Symptoms	
• Possible mouth sores	• Half of patients with UC have mild symptoms
• Tears in lining of anus or a fistula in severe CD	
Surgery	
• Up to 75% of patients with CD will eventually require surgery	• About 23%-45% of patients with UC will eventually require surgery
• Surgery can relieve symptoms not responding to other treatments, but it is not a cure.	• Removal of the colon and rectum is a cure, but complications may be severe, and quality of life is reduced.

Your Doctor's Toolkit
Currently there are no tests for the diagnosis of CD or UC. Your doctor may use these tools to diagnose, assess, and monitor your IBD.

Blood and fecal tests—to check for anemia, infection, inflammation, parasites, or blood in the stool

Endoscopic procedures are painless and easily accomplished during an outpatient visit:

- **Colonoscopy**—to examine the entire colon using a thin, flexible lighted tube. During colonoscopy, small samples of tissue (biopsy) may be taken for laboratory analysis.
- **Chromoendoscopy**—to detect slight changes in the lining of your intestine, blue dye is sprayed during a colonoscopy. You may have blue bowel movements for a short time after this procedure!
- **Flexible sigmoidoscopy**—similar to colonoscopy, except specifically examines the last section of your colon, called the sigmoid.
- **Capsule endoscopy (CE)**—to examine the small bowel when the results of other techniques are uncertain, and your doctor suspects CD. You swallow a tiny camera that takes hundreds of photographs while moving naturally with intestinal movements. The capsule painlessly exits in your stool.
- **Balloon endoscopy**—to assess areas of the small bowel where other endoscopes cannot reach, using a longer scope. Also useful if the diagnosis is still uncertain after CE.
- **Upper gastrointestinal endoscopy:** to examine the upper GI tract in patients with CD accompanied by vomiting and indigestion.

Imaging procedures—computed tomography (CT scan), magnetic resonance imaging (MRI), x-rays, ultrasound.

Enterography—to view part of the small bowel that cannot easily be seen by other methods. You drink a contrast material that helps produce high-resolution images via CT scan or MRI.

Treatment and Management
Your doctor will discuss various therapeutic options with you before making recommendations. Options include anti-inflammatories, corticosteroids, biologic therapy (anti-TNF drugs), and surgery. The ideal therapy for you is based on many factors, including disease symptoms, location, and severity.

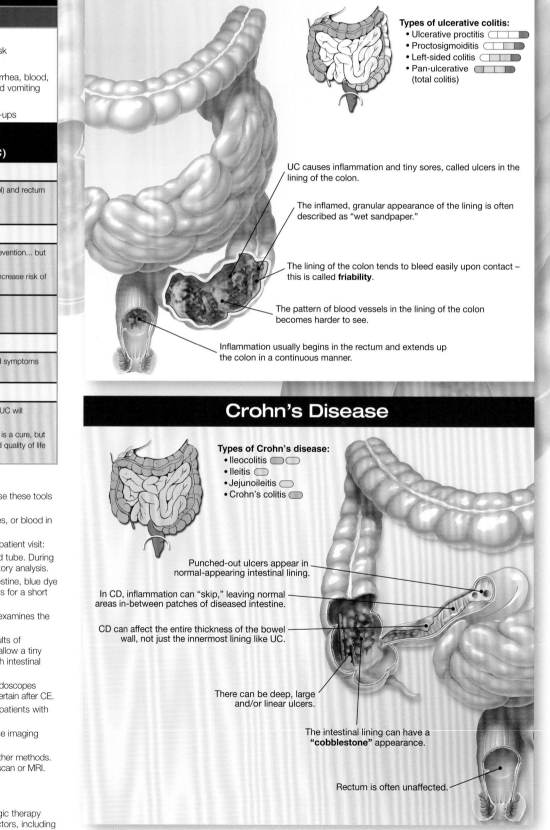

Ulcerative Colitis

Types of ulcerative colitis:
- Ulcerative proctitis
- Proctosigmoiditis
- Left-sided colitis
- Pan-ulcerative (total colitis)

UC causes inflammation and tiny sores, called ulcers in the lining of the colon.

The inflamed, granular appearance of the lining is often described as "wet sandpaper."

The lining of the colon tends to bleed easily upon contact – this is called **friability**.

The pattern of blood vessels in the lining of the colon becomes harder to see.

Inflammation usually begins in the rectum and extends up the colon in a continuous manner.

Crohn's Disease

Types of Crohn's disease:
- Ileocolitis
- Ileitis
- Jejunoileitis
- Crohn's colitis

Punched-out ulcers appear in normal-appearing intestinal lining.

In CD, inflammation can "skip," leaving normal areas in-between patches of diseased intestine.

CD can affect the entire thickness of the bowel wall, not just the innermost lining like UC.

There can be deep, large and/or linear ulcers.

The intestinal lining can have a "cobblestone" appearance.

Rectum is often unaffected.

Causes

Researchers have yet to discover any one specific cause for IBS; however, some theories include the following:

- People who suffer from IBS have a colon (or large intestine) that is particularly sensitive and reactive to factors that would not otherwise bother most people, such as stress, large meals, gas, medicines, caffeine, and alcohol.
- Colon motility (movement). In IBS, food may move through the intestines too quickly, resulting in gas, bloating, diarrhea, and strong muscle contractions, called spasms. For other people, the movement is too slow, causing constipation.
- Serotonin, a neurotransmitter, delivers messages from one part of your body to another. Ninety-five percent of the serotonin in your body is located in the gastrointestinal (GI) tract, and the other five percent is in your brain. People with IBS have abnormal levels of serotonin and more sensitive pain receptors in their GI tract. As a result, they experience problems with bowel movement, motility (movement), and sensation.
- Researchers indicate that IBS may be caused by a bacterial infection in the GI tract. People who have had gastroenteritis sometimes develop IBS, otherwise called postinfectious IBS.

Signs and Symptoms

Abdominal pain or discomfort at least 3 days per month in the last 3 months associated with 2 or more of the following:

- Improvement with defecation
- Onset associated with a change in frequency of stool
- Onset associated with a change in form (appearance) of stool

Certain symptoms may also be present, such as:

- A change in frequency of bowel movements
- A change in appearance of bowel movements
- Feelings of uncontrollable urgency to have a bowel movement
- Difficulty or inability to pass stool
- Mucus in the stool
- Bloating

Bleeding, fever, weight loss, and persistent severe pain are alarm symptoms and not symptoms of IBS and may indicate other problems such as inflammation, or rarely cancer.

The following have been associated with a worsening of IBS symptoms:

- Gassy foods such as beans, cabbage, cauliflower, and broccoli
- Milk/dairy products
- Alcohol or drinks with caffeine, such as coffee, tea, or carbonated beverages such as colas
- Sugar-free sweeteners such as sorbitol or mannitol
- Stress, conflict or emotional upsets; lack of exercise or adequate sleep

Researchers have found that women with IBS may have more symptoms during their menstrual periods, suggesting that reproductive hormones can worsen IBS.

In addition, people with IBS frequently suffer from depression and anxiety, which can worsen symptoms.

Risk Factors

- Age—Symptoms begins before the age of 35 for 50% of IBS sufferers.
- Female—Overall, about twice as many women as men have the condition.
- Family History of IBS—Studies have shown that people who have a first-degree relative—such as a parent or sibling—with IBS are at increased risk of the condition.

Diagnosis

There is no specific test for IBS. If you fit IBS criteria and don't have any alarm symptoms, your doctor may suggest a course of treatment without any testing. However, if you don't respond to treatment, diagnostic tests can be performed to rule out other problems. These tests may include the following:

- Colonoscopy—allows the doctor to examine the entire length of the colon.
- CT Scan—takes x-ray images of internal organs.
- Blood Tests—celiac disease is sensitivity to wheat protein that may cause signs and symptoms like those of IBS.
- Lactose Intolerance Tests.

Treatment and Management

No one medication or combination of medications will work for everyone with IBS. Patients need to work with a doctor to find the best combination of medicine, diet, counseling, and support to control their symptoms.

Mild IBS can be controlled by making dietary changes and learning to manage stress.

- Eat a healthy diet and avoid foods that trigger an increase in your symptoms.
- Small meals during the day (instead of 3 large meals) may be beneficial.

However, if your symptoms are moderate or severe, your doctor may recommend the following:

- Fiber supplements
- Eliminating gassy foods
- Antidiarrhea medications
- Anticholinergic medications to relieve painful bowel spasms
- Antidepressant medications if your symptoms include pain or depression
- Antibiotics (rarely)

Stress management is an important part of treatment for IBS because the colon has many nerves that connect it to the brain. Feeling mentally or emotionally tense, troubled, angry, or overwhelmed can stimulate colon spasms in people with IBS.

- Learn relaxation techniques such as meditation.
- Obtain counseling and support.
- Exercise regularly: walking or yoga.
- Change the stressful situations in your life.
- Get adequate sleep.

Understanding Irritable Bowel Syndrome (IBS)

Irritable bowel syndrome (IBS) is a common disorder that affects the large intestine (colon) and is characterized by cramping, abdominal pain, bloating, constipation, and diarrhea. IBS can cause a great deal of discomfort and distress, but it does not permanently damage your colon, nor does it lead to a more serious disease. Most people can control IBS with diet, stress management, and medications. Rarely, for others, the disorder makes it difficult to work, attend social events, or even travel short distances.

As many as 20% of the adult population, or one in five Americans, have symptoms of IBS, making it one of the most common disorders diagnosed by doctors.

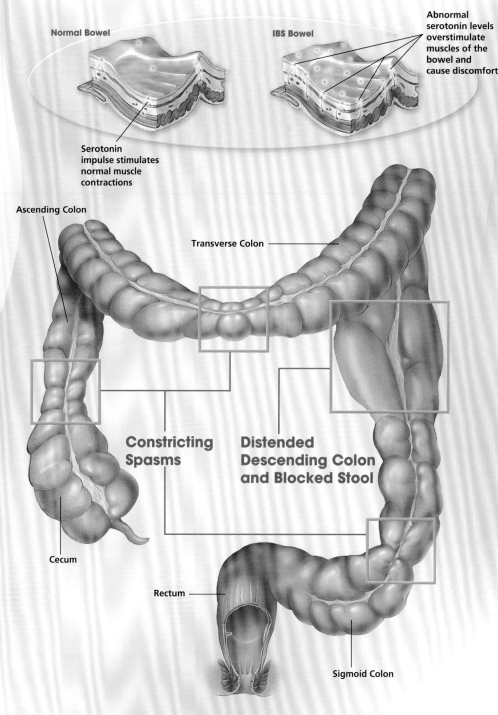

Normal Bowel

IBS Bowel

Abnormal serotonin levels overstimulate muscles of the bowel and cause discomfort

Serotonin impulse stimulates normal muscle contractions

Ascending Colon

Transverse Colon

Constricting Spasms

Distended Descending Colon and Blocked Stool

Cecum

Rectum

Sigmoid Colon

ENDOCRINE SYSTEM DISEASES & DISORDERS

What Is Diabetes?

Diabetes mellitus or diabetes is a group of diseases that affect the body cells' ability to convert and use sugar (glucose) from food for energy. The result is too much sugar (glucose) in the blood. Hyperglycemia (high blood sugar) can damage organs such as the eyes, kidneys, nerves, heart, and blood vessels, increasing risk of stroke and heart attacks.

Patients with hypertension, high cholesterol, heart disease, and a family history of diabetes and those who are overweight or Hispanic or African American should be screened for diabetes beginning at age 45. Early diagnosis can slow the progression of the disease and lessen the risk of long-term complications.

Blood tests are used to diagnose diabetes. All diabetes blood tests involve drawing blood and sending it to a lab for analysis. Your health care provider may perform the following to test for diabetes:

- **A1C blood test** shows the average blood glucose levels over the past 3 months, and is reported as a percentage; the higher the percentage, the higher your blood glucose levels have been. An A1C test of >6.5% is considered abnormal.
- **Fasting plasma glucose test** measures blood glucose after fasting for at least 8 hours. Fasting glucose levels above 126 mg/dL are considered abnormal.
- **2-Hour oral glucose test** measures blood glucose levels before and 2 hours after drinking a special sweet liquid. Two-hour postmeal glucose levels >200 mg/dL are considered abnormal.

Types of Diabetes

Type 1 Diabetes Mellitus (T1DM) People with T1DM do not produce insulin because their immune system (the body's system for fighting infection) attacks and destroys the insulin-producing beta cells in the pancreas, leaving little or no insulin. Without insulin, sugar builds up in the blood instead of being transferred to the cells.
The cause of T1DM is not known, but it is thought to be a combination of genetic and environmental factors (exposure to certain viruses). T1DM accounts for about 5% of diagnosed diabetes in the United States. It can appear at any age, but develops most often in children and young adults.

Type 2 Diabetes Mellitus (T2DM) is when the pancreas does not produce enough insulin, or the body cannot use insulin properly (a condition called insulin resistance). T2DM is the most common form of diabetes, and genetics play a part in its development. The following factors play an important role in causing **high blood sugar and insulin resistance** in individuals genetically prone to type 2 diabetes:

- Beta cells in the pancreas slowly stop producing insulin.
- Alpha cells in the pancreas produce too much of a hormone called glucagon that stimulates the liver to make sugar, which the body can't use, and it's released into the blood.
- The liver fails to store sugar as an energy source.
- The kidney overproduces glucose and INCREASES absorption of glucose into the blood.
- Low insulin levels cause the fat cells to break down and release "free fatty acids" (FFAs). FFAs cause the liver to make more sugar, destroy the insulin-producing beta cells in the pancreas, and block the muscles from using glucose for energy.
- Muscle cells are unable to absorb and use glucose for energy. Unused glucose stays in the blood, increasing sugar levels.
- Eating releases hormones that tell the pancreas to produce/release insulin, prevent the liver from making sugar, slow the passage of food through the stomach, and send the brain a message to "feel full." In T2DM, these hormones are impaired resulting in weight gain and reduced insulin levels.
- As one gains weight, appetite is increased causing more weight gain and adding to insulin resistance.

Prediabetes is when the blood sugar level is higher than normal, but is still low enough not to be considered diabetes. Ninety-two million Americans have prediabetes which is defined as having fasting blood sugar levels of 100-125 mg/dL, 2-hour postmeal blood sugar levels of 140-199 mg/dL, or an A1C of 5.7%-6.4%. People with prediabetes are at high risk for some diabetes-related complications, especially heart disease. Weight loss and exercise can reverse prediabetes. Eleven percent of patients with prediabetes convert to clinical diabetes each year.

Gestational diabetes is a condition that women can get when they are pregnant. The exact cause is unknown, but it is believed that pregnancy hormones make your cells more resistant to insulin resulting in high blood sugar. Gestational diabetes usually disappears after the baby is born, but women who have had it are at higher risk of developing T2DM later.

What Happens in Diabetes

Brain

Lung

Heart

Liver

Kidney

Pancreas

Large intestine

Small intestine

Pancreas

1 Food is broken down into glucose. Glucose is a form of sugar in the blood and is the main source of energy for the body.

2 Glucose needs the help of a hormone called **insulin** to enter the cells. A hormone is a chemical substance made in one part of the body that travels to other parts of the body to help cells and organs do their jobs.

3 **Insulin** is made by special cells in the pancreas called beta cells. Insulin makes it possible for glucose to enter the cells. The insulin opens a door in the cell that allows glucose to enter.

4 In diabetes, your pancreas doesn't make enough insulin, or your cells don't respond properly to the insulin produced, or a combination of both.

5 Without the help of insulin, glucose builds up in your blood causing your blood sugar levels to rise.

Normal beta cells secrete insulin, which drives glucose into muscle, liver and fat cells maintaining blood sugar levels in the normal range

Diabetic beta cells During prediabetes, up to 80% of beta cell function is lost, insulin levels drop, and glucose levels rise while fasting and after eating.

Insulin

Insulin cannot attach to cell

Glucose moves into the blood

Cell door is closed, glucose is not able to enter and moves into the blood

Red blood cells

Increased blood sugar (glucose) level

Insulin from pancreas attaches to cell

Glucose from food

Cell "door" is opened allowing glucose (sugar) to enter the cell

Glucose converted to energy

Energy deprived cell

Insulin attaches to cell and opens a "door" allowing glucose to enter

Normal Body Cell
Insulin acts as a "key" to open a door in the cell that lets glucose enter, where it will be converted to energy.

Diabetic Body Cell
Cells develop a resistance to insulin, the insulin does not work correctly, or not enough insulin is made by the pancreas. Cells do not get the fuel they need for energy, and sugar builds up in the blood.

Symptoms of Diabetes

Patients with type 1 diabetes usually report rapidly developing symptoms. With type 2 diabetes, symptoms usually develop gradually and may not appear until many years after the onset of the disease.

- Weight loss even when eating properly
- Frequent urination
- Excessive thirst
- Extreme hunger
- Fatigue
- Blurred vision
- Dry, itchy skin
- More infections than usual
- Numbness in feet and/or hands
- Slow-healing cuts or sores
- No symptoms

Risk Factors

Type 2 Diabetes and Prediabetes
- Overweight or obesity.
- Physical inactivity/lack of exercise.
- Family history of diabetes.
- Certain racial and ethnic groups (African Americans, Hispanic/Latino Americans, Asian Americans, Pacific Islanders, Native Americans, and Alaska Natives).
- Older age—but onset is increasing dramatically among children, adolescents, and younger adults.
- History of gestational diabetes or delivery of a baby weighing 9 lb or more at birth.
- High blood pressure, low HDL (good) cholesterol, and/or high triglyceride levels.
- Polycystic ovary syndrome.

Type 1 Diabetes
- Parent or sibling who has T1DM.
- Environmental factors (exposure to a virus or toxin).
- Race—T1DM is more common in whites than in other races.
- Geography—certain countries, such as Finland and Sweden, have higher rates of T1DM.

Diabetes in Youth

Diabetes is one of the most common chronic diseases in children and adolescents. About 1 in 400 people younger than 20 years has type 1 or type 2 diabetes. Although type 1 diabetes is more prevalent among children nationwide, type 2 diabetes is becoming more common in U.S. kids and teens, especially if they are overweight. There is no known way to prevent type 1 diabetes, but experts agree that healthy eating and an active lifestyle can help to prevent type 2 diabetes in youth.

Diabetes Management

People with type 1 diabetes require insulin to manage their diabetes. Insulin pens and insulin pumps are safe, effective, and accurate ways to take insulin. Treatment for type 1 diabetes is a lifelong commitment to blood sugar monitoring, taking insulin, healthy eating, exercise, and regular visits to your health care provider.

Type 2 diabetes may be treated with a variety of different antidiabetic medications determined by blood sugar levels and symptoms. Patients may also be prescribed medicine to control cholesterol and blood pressure.

People with diabetes can prevent or delay problems by keeping blood sugar levels as close to normal as possible, keeping blood pressure and cholesterol under control, and getting regular medical care. Although diabetes is a common disease, each individual needs professional care. Consulting with a diabetes health care team will help you to maintain the correct balance between medication, blood sugar monitoring, diet, and exercise.

5 Tips for Successful Diabetes Self-Management

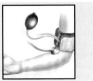

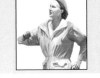

1 Know your metabolic targets: blood sugar levels (A1C), blood pressure, and cholesterol.

2 Practice living a healthy lifestyle: exercise, lose weight if overweight, and make healthy food choices.

3 Stop smoking.

4 Take your medication as prescribed.

5 Follow up frequently with health care providers who are knowledgeable about diabetes.

© 2015 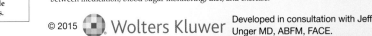 Wolters Kluwer   Developed in consultation with Jeff Unger MD, ABFM, FACE.

What Is Type 1 Diabetes?

Diabetes mellitus type 1 or type 1 diabetes (T1DM), once known as insulin-dependent or juvenile diabetes, is a chronic metabolic disorder that prevents the body from making energy from food. Most people develop T1DM when they are children or young adults, but it can occur at any age.

People with T1DM cannot produce the hormone insulin, because their immune system (the body's system for fighting infection) attacks or destroys the insulin-producing beta cells in the pancreas. Without the beta cells, the body can no longer produce the insulin needed to help sugar (glucose) enter the cell to be used for energy, and the sugar (glucose) builds up in the blood. High blood sugar levels can lead to many long-term health problems.

Although the exact cause of type 1 diabetes is not known, it is thought that the destruction of the pancreatic beta cells by the immune system is triggered in genetically susceptible individuals after exposure to a series of viral illnesses.

What Happens in Type 1 Diabetes?

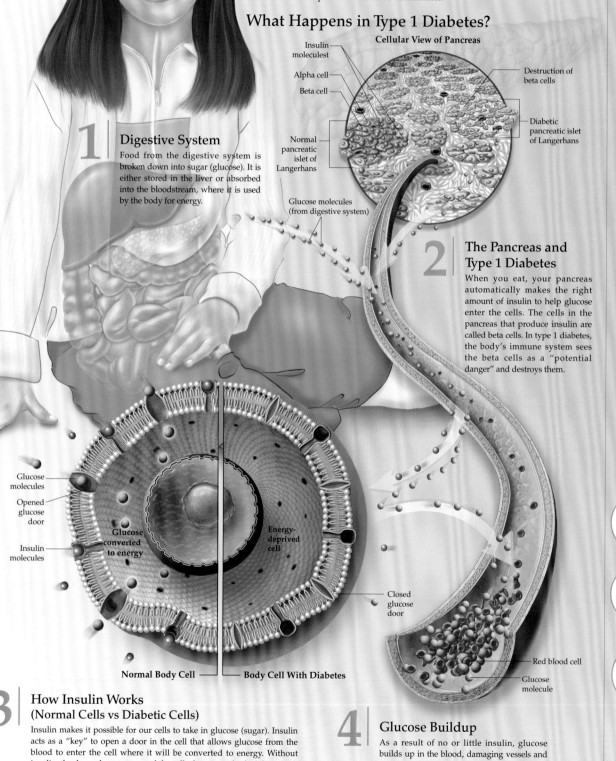

Cellular View of Pancreas

Insulin moleculest
Alpha cell
Beta cell
Normal pancreatic islet of Langerhans
Glucose molecules (from digestive system)
Destruction of beta cells
Diabetic pancreatic islet of Langerhans

1 Digestive System

Food from the digestive system is broken down into sugar (glucose). It is either stored in the liver or absorbed into the bloodstream, where it is used by the body for energy.

2 The Pancreas and Type 1 Diabetes

When you eat, your pancreas automatically makes the right amount of insulin to help glucose enter the cells. The cells in the pancreas that produce insulin are called beta cells. In type 1 diabetes, the body's immune system sees the beta cells as a "potential danger" and destroys them.

Glucose molecules
Opened glucose door
Insulin molecules
Glucose converted to energy
Energy-deprived cell
Closed glucose door
Normal Body Cell — Body Cell With Diabetes
Red blood cell
Glucose molecule

3 How Insulin Works (Normal Cells vs Diabetic Cells)

Insulin makes it possible for our cells to take in glucose (sugar). Insulin acts as a "key" to open a door in the cell that allows glucose from the blood to enter the cell where it will be converted to energy. Without insulin, the doors do not open and the cells do not get the fuel they need.

4 Glucose Buildup

As a result of no or little insulin, glucose builds up in the blood, damaging vessels and vital organs.

Managing Type 1 Diabetes

At this time, there is no cure or prevention for type 1 diabetes. Patients with type 1 diabetes require insulin to manage their diabetes. Insulin pens and insulin pumps are safe, effective, and accurate ways to take insulin. Managing this disease requires individualized care from a diabetes health care team to help maintain the correct balance between medication, blood sugar monitoring, diet, and exercise.

- Know your prescribed metabolic targets (blood sugar (A1C), blood pressure, cholesterol).
- Exercise 5 days each week for 30-45 minutes per session.
- Eat healthy meals; see a certified diabetic educator or a registered dietician for assistance in meal planning.

- Never stop taking your insulin or prescription medicines without the consent of your health care provider.
- Stop smoking and minimize your alcohol consumption.
- Make sure that your health care provider is well trained in managing patients with type 1 diabetes.

Complications
SHORT-TERM

Hypoglycemia (low blood sugar)

Hypoglycemia is when blood sugar falls below 70 mg/dL. This is also known as an insulin reaction. Low blood sugar can be caused by eating too little, not eating often enough, too much physical activity without eating, or too much insulin. Hypoglycemia can develop quickly in people with diabetes.

Symptoms include the following:
- Weakness/dizziness
- Sweating
- Headache
- Loss of coordination
- Seizure
- Hunger
- Loss of consciousness
- Inability to concentrate
- Blurred vision
- Fatigue
- Tremor
- Irritability
- Slurred speech
- Awakening from sleep
- Falling out of bed
- Facial tingling

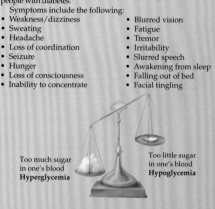

Too much sugar in one's blood
Hyperglycemia

Too little sugar in one's blood
Hypoglycemia

Hyperglycemia (high blood sugar)

Hyperglycemia is when blood sugar increases and stays above the normal level (>120 mg/dL before meals and >180 mg/dL after meals). Symptoms can develop slowly, sometimes over a period of days, so it is important to monitor blood sugar levels. High blood sugar for an extended time can result in damage to various parts of the body.

Symptoms include the following:
- Frequent urination
- Fatigue
- Increased thirst
- Blurred vision

Ketoacidosis

When the body cannot make enough insulin to help glucose enter cells for energy, the body begins to break down fat. When fat is used for energy, chemicals called ketones are released into the blood. Some of the ketones are passed out of the body through the urine, but ketones can build up to a poisonous level in the blood causing **diabetic ketoacidosis (DKA)**.

This condition can develop slowly and can lead to a diabetic coma or even death.

Symptoms include the following:
- Thirst
- Fatigue
- Nausea and vomiting
- Stomach pain
- Possible infection
- Loss of consciousness

LONG-TERM

Heart Disease and Stroke

Poor blood sugar (glucose) control, high blood pressure, and high cholesterol can damage arteries increasing risk for heart attack or stroke.

Kidney Disease (Nephropathy)

High levels of blood glucose can damage the glomeruli (the filtering units of the kidney), which can reduce the kidney's ability to remove waste and retain important nutrients such as protein.

Eye Problems

- Diabetic retinopathy occurs when one of the arteries that supplies blood to the retina becomes blocked causing diminished blood flow to the retina and can lead to blindness.
- Diabetic macular edema (DME) results in vision loss due to the effects of chronic inflammation from exposure to high blood sugar levels.

Nerve Damage (Neuropathy)

High blood sugar levels can damage nerves resulting in pain and loss of function. Sensory neuropathy results in tingling and burning sensation in the feet while at rest. If sensation to the feet is lost completely, patients risk developing ulcers, infections, and foot deformities that may require an amputation. Sleep and balance may be disrupted.

Other examples of diabetic neuropathy include the following:
- Rapid heart rate
- Dizziness when standing upright
- Inability to completely empty the bladder or urinary incontinence
- Fullness in the abdomen after eating a few bites
- Diarrhea and/or constipation
- Erectile dysfunction/vaginal dryness
- Loss of ability to sweat
- Excessive sweating while eating
- Charcot foot and ankle

What Is Type 2 Diabetes?

Type 2 diabetes or T2DM, once known as non-insulin-dependent or adult-onset diabetes, is a progressive metabolic disorder that affects how your body uses sugar (glucose) from food. Glucose is an important source of energy for the cells of your body and organs. If you have diabetes, it means you have too much glucose (sugar) in your blood, which can lead to serious health problems.

T2DM is a complex disease with multiple factors linked to its cause and development, but is mainly characterized by a reduction in insulin secretion from the pancreas along with the body's inability to use insulin properly (a condition called insulin resistance) to keep blood glucose (blood sugar) levels normal. Insulin is the hormone that is needed to transport glucose (sugar) from the food you eat to your cells.

Type 2 diabetes is the most common and increasingly widespread form of diabetes, and it is believed that genetic and environmental factors play a role in its development. Being overweight is strongly linked to the development of T2DM, but not everyone with T2DM is overweight. It is most often associated with older age, but is a growing problem among U.S. children and adolescents. Type 2 diabetes in youth can have a devastating effect on one's kidneys and heart at a young age.

Symptoms

(Many patients may have no symptoms)
- Increased thirst
- Initial weight gain followed by weight loss
- Fatigue
- Frequent urination
- Dry skin
- Blurred vision
- Tingling in hands and feet
- Erectile dysfunction, vaginal dryness

Risk Factors

High-risk patients without symptoms should be screened every 3 years beginning at age 45. Patients with symptoms should be screened as soon as possible.

T2DM risk factors include the following:
- Obesity or overweight
- Lack of physical activity
- Parent or sibling with T2DM
- High-risk ethnicity: African American, Latino, Native American, Asian American, Pacific Islander
- Women who had gestational diabetes (high blood sugar during pregnancy) or who have had a baby weighing 9 lb or more at birth
- History of prediabetes; prediabetes is blood sugar levels higher than normal, but not yet high enough to be diagnosed as diabetes
- History of high blood pressure (hypertension) and/or cardiovascular disease
- Abnormal cholesterol
- Exposure to secondhand smoke
- Abnormal sleep patterns
- History of mental illness
- Women with a history of polycystic ovarian syndrome

Managing Type 2 Diabetes

People with T2DM can prevent or delay problems by keeping the level of glucose (sugar) in the blood as close to normal as possible (85-130 mg/dL), keeping blood pressure and cholesterol under control, and getting regular medical care. Although diabetes is a common disease, every individual needs personalized care. T2DM may be treated with a variety of different medications determined by blood sugar levels and symptoms. Patients may be prescribed medicine to control cholesterol and blood pressure. Your diabetes health care provider will help you to maintain the correct balance between medications, blood sugar monitoring, diet, and exercise.

The 5 Keys to Successful Diabetes Management

1. Know your metabolic target levels for glucose, blood pressure, and cholesterol.
2. Incorporate healthy lifestyle practices into your life: exercise, lose weight if you are overweight, and make healthy food choices.
3. Stop smoking.
4. Take your prescribed medicines.
5. Follow up frequently with health care providers who are knowledgeable in diabetes.

What Happens in Type 2 Diabetes

Much of the food you eat is broken down into glucose. Glucose is the form of sugar in the blood and is the main source of energy for the body. Glucose needs the help of a hormone called insulin to enter the body cells. Normally the pancreas releases the right amount of insulin needed to transfer glucose from your blood to your cells. In Type 2 diabetes, problems occur when the insulin that is produced in the pancreas doesn't work correctly, not enough insulin is made, or the body's cells resist insulin.

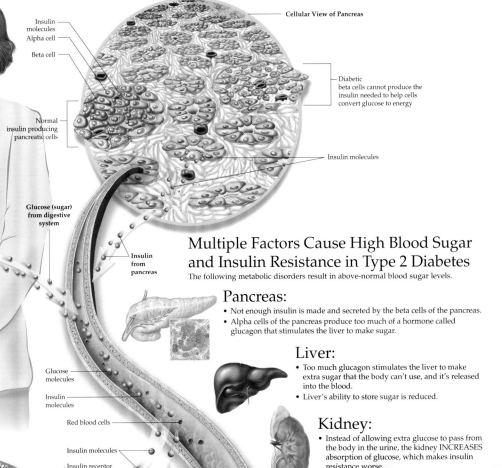

Cellular View of Pancreas

Insulin molecules
Alpha cell
Beta cell
Normal insulin producing pancreatic cells

Diabetic beta cells cannot produce the insulin needed to help cells convert glucose to energy

Insulin molecules

Glucose (sugar) from digestive system

Heart
Liver
Stomach
Pancreas
Large intestine
Small intestine

Insulin from pancreas

Glucose molecules
Insulin molecules
Red blood cells
Insulin molecules
Insulin receptor

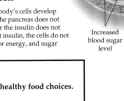

Glucose molecules
Cell "door" is opened allowing glucose (sugar) to enter the cell
Insulin attaches to cell and opens a "door"
Glucose converted to energy
Energy-deprived cell

Cell door is closed, glucose is not able to enter and moves into the blood.
Glucose moves into the blood

Increased blood sugar level

Normal Body Cell | **Diabetic Body Cell**

The insulin acts as a "key" to open a door in the cell that lets glucose enter the cell where it will be converted to energy.

In Type 2 diabetes, the body's cells develop a resistance to insulin, the pancreas does not make enough insulin, or the insulin does not work correctly. Without insulin, the cells do not get the fuel they need for energy, and sugar builds up in the blood.

Multiple Factors Cause High Blood Sugar and Insulin Resistance in Type 2 Diabetes

The following metabolic disorders result in above-normal blood sugar levels.

Pancreas:
- Not enough insulin is made and secreted by the beta cells of the pancreas.
- Alpha cells of the pancreas produce too much of a hormone called glucagon that stimulates the liver to make sugar.

Liver:
- Too much glucagon stimulates the liver to make extra sugar that the body can't use, and it's released into the blood.
- Liver's ability to store sugar is reduced.

Kidney:
- Instead of allowing extra glucose to pass from the body in the urine, the kidney INCREASES absorption of glucose, which makes insulin resistance worse.
- The kidney itself increases the amount of glucose it makes.

Brain:
- As one gains weight, appetite is increased.
- Obese people have a high risk of developing diabetes because they have difficulty controlling their appetite.

Skeletal Muscles:
- Muscle cells are unable to absorb and use glucose for energy.
- Unused glucose stays in the blood, increasing sugar levels, adding to insulin resistance.

Fat Cells:
- Low insulin levels cause the fat cells to break down and release "free fatty acids" (FFAs).
- FFAs cause the liver to make more sugar, destroy the insulin producing beta cells in the pancreas, and block the muscles from using glucose for energy.

Alimentary Canal or Gut:
- When you eat, your gut releases hormones that tell the pancreas to produce/release insulin, prevent the liver from making sugar, slow the passage of food through the stomach, and send the brain a message to "feel full."
- In T2DM, these hormones are impaired, which stops the pancreas from making insulin, stimulates the liver to make more sugar, and causes the stomach to empty faster.
- The brain does not feel full after eating resulting in weight gain and increased blood sugar levels.

Complications

Long-term diabetes can damage many parts of the body. See your health care provider at least once a year to find and treat any problems early.

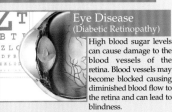

Eye Disease (Diabetic Retinopathy)
High blood sugar levels can cause damage to the blood vessels of the retina. Blood vessels may become blocked causing diminished blood flow to the retina and can lead to blindness.

Heart Disease and Stroke
Poor blood sugar control, high blood pressure, and high cholesterol can damage arteries and increase risk of heart attack or stroke.

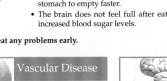

Kidney Disease (Nephropathy)
High levels of blood sugar can damage the small blood vessels in the filtering units of the kidney (the glomeruli), and may cause them to leak or lose their filtering ability leading to CKD (chronic kidney disease), and possible kidney failure.

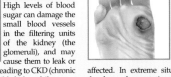

Vascular Disease
Poor diabetes control can cause circulation problems in the blood vessels of the legs and feet. Healing of wounds and infections may also be affected. In extreme situations, gangrene can develop and amputations may be necessary.

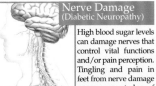

Nerve Damage (Diabetic Neuropathy)
High blood sugar levels can damage nerves that control vital functions and/or pain perception. Tingling and pain in feet from nerve damage may progress to loss of feeling. Neuropathy can also affect balance, sleep, and sexual function and can cause urinary tract incontinence.

Developed in consultation with Jeff Unger MD, ABFP, FACE.

Metabolic Syndrome

What Is Metabolic Syndrome?

■ **Metabolic syndrome** describes a common condition in which **obesity, high blood glucose ("blood sugar"), high blood pressure,** and an **abnormal cholesterol profile (dyslipidemia)** cluster together in one person.
■ When these risk factors occur together, the chance of developing **coronary heart disease, stroke,** and **diabetes** is much greater than when these risk factors develop independently.

■ According to the American Heart Association, almost 25% of Americans are affected by metabolic syndrome.

Metabolic Syndrome Risk Factors

To be diagnosed with metabolic syndrome, patients need to have at least three of the following risk factors:

Obesity

■ **Obesity** is defined as having too much body fat.
■ A person is considered obese when his/her weight is 20% or more above ideal weight.
■ Obesity promotes insulin resistance, an inability to respond normally to insulin.

■ People with fat situated mainly around the stomach (abdomen) are considered **"apple shaped"** and have a higher risk of many of the serious conditions associated with metabolic syndrome.
■ Ask your health care provider what your ideal weight should be.

Apple-shaped: Excess fat mostly around the abdomen

Metabolic Syndrome Risk Factor:
Waist measurement >35 in (women) or 40 in (men)

High Blood Glucose

■ Sugar (glucose) is what supplies the body with energy.
■ Normally, this sugar (glucose) is rapidly cleared from the blood and stored as energy, but if sugar stays in the blood it causes an unhealthy buildup called **high blood glucose**.

■ Glucose in the blood reaches all of the body's organs and systems, including the heart, arteries and veins, kidneys, and nervous system.
■ This constant "sugar attack" has the same effect as eating too much candy and not brushing your teeth—it causes organ system decay or degeneration.
■ People with high blood glucose are at risk for many diseases, including heart attack, stroke, blindness, and amputation. High blood glucose levels (or prediabetes) often lead to the development of type 2 diabetes.

Metabolic Syndrome Risk Factor:
Glucose of at least 110 mg/dL or greater

High Blood Pressure

■ Blood pressure is the force that helps the blood flow through the blood vessels.
■ Blood vessels that are subjected to high blood pressure for an extended period of time thicken and become less flexible, causing arteriosclerosis affecting the supply of blood to the heart.

■ Blood pressure is measured using two numbers:
1. Systolic pressure is measured just after the heart contracts and the pressure is greatest.
2. Diastolic pressure is measured when the heart relaxes and the pressure is lowest.
■ Normal blood pressure is about 110/75 mm Hg. High blood pressure alone causes no symptoms, but it does increase the risk of heart attack, stroke, and kidney failure.

Metabolic Syndrome Risk Factor:
Blood pressure >130/85 mm Hg

Abnormal Cholesterol Profile (Dyslipidemia)

■ **Cholesterol** is a type of fat in your blood.
■ Cholesterol either comes from the foods you eat or is made by your liver and is found in all of the body's cells.

■ Triglycerides and LDL are considered bad cholesterol.
■ HDL is a good cholesterol.
■ Too much bad cholesterol and not enough good cholesterol increase the risk for coronary heart disease and is an important indicator of metabolic syndrome.

Triglycerides

High triglyceride levels in the blood can help clog the arteries with fatty deposits called plaque (atherosclerosis), making it difficult for oxygen-rich blood to reach the heart. High triglyceride levels increase your risk of having a heart attack.

Metabolic Syndrome Risk Factor:
Triglyceride level >150 mg/dL

HDL Cholesterol

HDL cholesterol (the "good cholesterol") helps remove deposits from within the blood vessels and it stops the blood vessels from becoming blocked. The more the HDL in your blood, the better it is for your heart. When HDL cholesterol levels are low, there is a greater risk of developing a heart attack or stroke.

Metabolic Syndrome Risk Factor:
HDL cholesterol level <50 mg/dL (women) and <40 mg/dL (men)

High blood glucose: sugar (glucose) builds up in bloodstream

High blood pressure, if not treated, causes damage to the lining of the arteries

Fibrous plaque (atherosclerosis)

Medical Conditions Associated With Metabolic Syndrome

People with untreated metabolic syndrome are at a higher risk of cardiovascular disease (such as coronary heart disease and stroke) and type 2 diabetes.

A **Stroke**—The term stroke refers to the sudden death of brain tissue caused by a lack of oxygen to the brain. In ischemic stroke, blood flow to an area of the brain is either blocked or reduced. This blockage may result from atherosclerosis and blood clot formation.

B **Coronary Heart Disease**—Narrowing of the arteries in the heart usually causes coronary heart disease, which can lead to heart attacks. The buildup of plaque in the lining of the arteries (atherosclerosis) can cause this narrowing. All of the metabolic syndrome risk factors can result in atherosclerosis. Heart attacks occur when blood cannot flow through the clogged arteries.

As a result, the heart does not get enough oxygen and stops working.

C **Type 2 Diabetes**—Type 2 diabetes is a disease in which the pancreas produces little or no insulin and/or the body loses the ability to respond normally to insulin (insulin resistance). Insulin is needed to transport glucose into the cells for use as energy. Without insulin, body tissues have less access to essential nutrients for energy and storage. Without proper management, diabetes can lead to complications that affect the eyes, mouth, cardiovascular system, kidneys, nerves, and extremities.

How Is Metabolic Syndrome Treated?

Metabolic syndrome is a disease that requires long-term management of each of the risk factors. Poor nutrition and lack of exercise are underlying causes of these risk factors. It has been shown that with lifestyle changes and treatment, including medications, people with metabolic syndrome can greatly decrease their chances of developing serious complications. Regular monitoring of blood pressure, cholesterol, and glucose is important to detect the syndrome.

Treatment options usually include the following:

■ **Weight loss**—If you are obese, a weight loss of 5%-10% of your body weight can help your body regain its ability to recognize insulin.
■ **Exercise**—Increased activity reverses insulin resistance. It also helps lower blood pressure, lower "bad" cholesterol levels, raise "good" cholesterol levels, and reduce the risk of developing type 2 diabetes.

■ **Eat a heart-healthy diet**—Reduce saturated fat, processed foods, salt, white flour, potatoes, and rice. Include two servings of fruit per day. Increase greens, vegetables, fat-free dairy, lean protein, and whole grains.

© 2019 Wolters Kluwer · Anatomical Chart Company, Philadelphia, PA. Medical illustrations by Jennifer Smith, in consultation with Jessica Shank Coviello, DNP, APRN, ANP-BC.

What Is the Thyroid?

The thyroid is a small gland that is wrapped around the windpipe (trachea), just below the thyroid cartilage. The thyroid plays an important role in health and affects every organ, tissue, and cell in the body. It makes hormones that maintain the normal function of many organ systems and regulate metabolism (how the body uses and stores energy from foods eaten).

When the thyroid is not working properly (called thyroid disorder), it can affect the following:

- Body weight
- Energy level
- Sleeping patterns
- Skin and hair
- Fertility and menstruation
- Memory and concentration
- Bone strength
- Cholesterol level

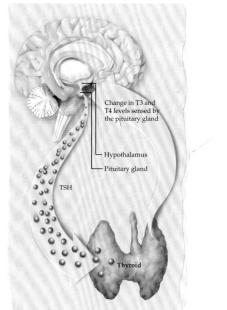

Change in T3 and T4 levels sensed by the pituitary gland

Hypothalamus

Pituitary gland

TSH

Thyroid

Normal Hormone Production

The thyroid gland is controlled by the pituitary gland. When the level of thyroid hormones (T3 and T4) drops too low, the pituitary gland responds by producing thyroid-stimulating hormone (TSH). TSH is a good marker of thyroid hormone balance: when the thyroid gland is underactive, TSH is high; when overactive, TSH is low.

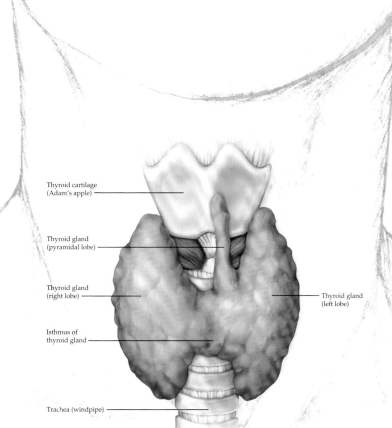

Thyroid cartilage (Adam's apple)

Thyroid gland (pyramidal lobe)

Thyroid gland (right lobe)

Thyroid gland (left lobe)

Isthmus of thyroid gland

Trachea (windpipe)

How to Check Your Thyroid

As a first step in identifying an underlying thyroid problem, you should do a simple thyroid self-examination.

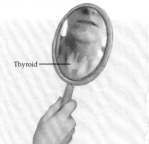

Thyroid

1. While holding a mirror, look at the area of your neck just below the Adam's apple. This is where you will find your thyroid.

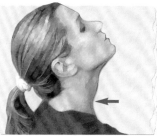

2. Tip your head back, while focusing on the thyroid area in the mirror.

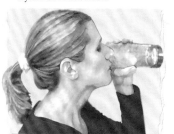

3. Take a drink of water. Look at your neck and check for any lumps in this area while you swallow.

Overactive Thyroid

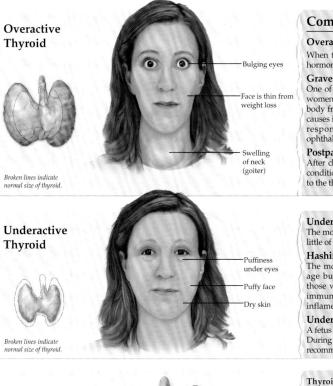

Bulging eyes

Face is thin from weight loss

Swelling of neck (goiter)

Broken lines indicate normal size of thyroid.

Common Thyroid Disorders

Overactive thyroid (hyperthyroidism):
When the thyroid gland is overactive, it makes too much of the thyroid hormone. This condition affects women more than men.

Graves' disease:
One of the most common causes of overactive thyroid, especially among women. It occurs when the immune system, which normally protects the body from bacteria and viruses, mistakenly attacks the thyroid gland and causes it to overproduce the thyroid hormone thyroxine. This autoimmune response can also affect the tissue behind the eyes (Graves' ophthalmopathy) and the skin on the shins (Graves' dermopathy).

Postpartum thyroiditis:
After childbirth, a woman's thyroid can become larger or inflamed. This condition usually goes away within 6 months, with no permanent damage to the thyroid.

Symptoms

- Sudden weight loss, even when appetite and food intake remain normal or increase
- Rapid or irregular heartbeat or pounding of the heart
- Nervousness, irritability, tremor
- Sweating
- Changes in menstrual patterns
- Increased sensitivity to heat
- Changes in bowel patterns, especially more frequent bowel movements
- Enlarged thyroid (goiter), which may appear as a swelling at the base of the neck
- Fatigue, muscle weakness
- Difficulty sleeping
- Pain or discomfort in the neck

Underactive Thyroid

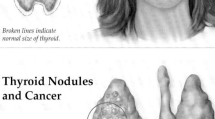

Puffiness under eyes

Puffy face

Dry skin

Broken lines indicate normal size of thyroid.

Underactive thyroid (hypothyroidism):
The most common type of thyroid disorder, where the thyroid makes too little of the thyroid hormone.

Hashimoto's disease:
The most often cause of underactive thyroid, which can occur at any age but is most common in middle-aged and older women and in those who have a family history of this problem. It occurs when the immune system reacts against the thyroid gland, causing it to become inflamed (chronic thyroiditis).

Underactive thyroid and pregnancy:
A fetus depends on its mother's thyroid hormone for normal development. During pregnancy, women need more thyroid hormone, so thyroid testing is recommended every few weeks to ensure that the levels remain in balance.

- Increased sensitivity to cold
- Constipation
- Rough, cold, and dry skin
- Puffy face
- Hoarse voice
- Poor concentration
- Heavier-than-normal menstrual periods
- Depression
- Tingling sensations in legs and arms
- Sleepiness
- Unexplained weight gain
Note: There may be no symptoms.

Thyroid Nodules and Cancer

Nodules

Cancer

Thyroid nodules are extremely common, and the vast majority are benign (not cancerous). Most commonly, nodules are discovered when a lump is noticed in the neck, or during an examination for another condition. Endocrinologists (thyroid specialists) often check to see if the nodule is not cancerous, and if surgery is recommended.

If thyroid cancer is found, it is usually highly treatable with an excellent prognosis. Surgical removal is usually the first step in treatment of thyroid cancer, sometimes followed by treatment with radioactive iodine.

- Lump in the front of the neck, on either side of the windpipe just below the Adam's apple
- Tight feeling in the throat
- Coughing
- Hoarseness
- Swollen lymph nodes, especially in the neck
- Pain in the throat or neck, sometimes spreading up to the ears

Other symptoms may occur depending on the cause of the lump(s).

EYE AND EAR DISEASES & DISORDERS

- Middle Ear Conditions
- Disorders of the Eye
- Understanding Glaucoma
- Age-Related Macular Degeneration

Middle Ear Conditions

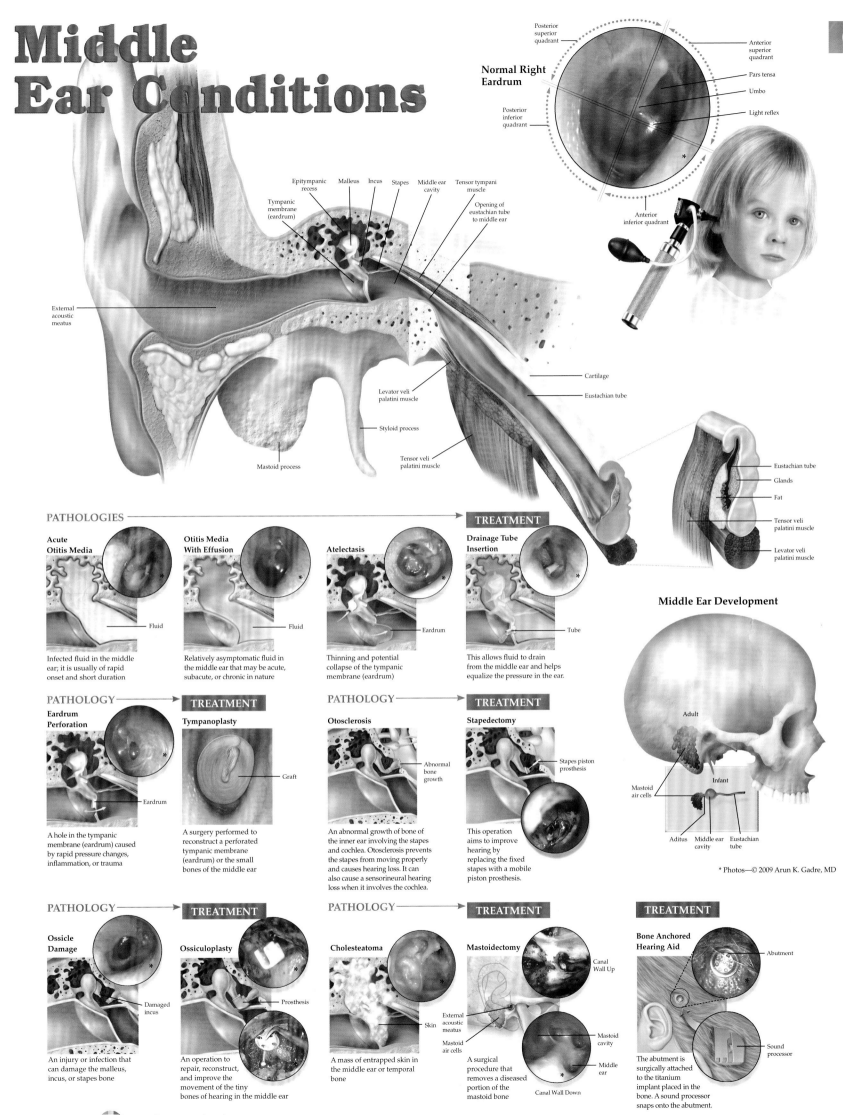

Normal Right Eardrum

Posterior superior quadrant · Posterior inferior quadrant · Anterior inferior quadrant · Anterior superior quadrant · Pars tensa · Umbo · Light reflex

Epitympanic recess · Malleus · Incus · Stapes · Middle ear cavity · Tensor tympani muscle · Opening of eustachian tube to middle ear

Tympanic membrane (eardrum) · External acoustic meatus · Levator veli palatini muscle · Mastoid process · Styloid process · Tensor veli palatini muscle · Cartilage · Eustachian tube

Eustachian tube · Glands · Fat · Tensor veli palatini muscle · Levator veli palatini muscle

Middle Ear Development

Adult · Mastoid air cells · Infant · Aditus · Middle ear cavity · Eustachian tube

* Photos—© 2009 Arun K. Gadre, MD

PATHOLOGIES — TREATMENT

Acute Otitis Media
Fluid
Infected fluid in the middle ear; it is usually of rapid onset and short duration

Otitis Media With Effusion
Fluid
Relatively asymptomatic fluid in the middle ear that may be acute, subacute, or chronic in nature

Atelectasis
Eardrum
Thinning and potential collapse of the tympanic membrane (eardrum)

TREATMENT — Drainage Tube Insertion
Tube
This allows fluid to drain from the middle ear and helps equalize the pressure in the ear.

PATHOLOGY — TREATMENT

Eardrum Perforation
Eardrum
A hole in the tympanic membrane (eardrum) caused by rapid pressure changes, inflammation, or trauma

Tympanoplasty
Graft
A surgery performed to reconstruct a perforated tympanic membrane (eardrum) or the small bones of the middle ear

PATHOLOGY — TREATMENT

Otosclerosis
Abnormal bone growth
An abnormal growth of bone of the inner ear involving the stapes and cochlea. Otosclerosis prevents the stapes from moving properly and causes hearing loss. It can also cause a sensorineural hearing loss when it involves the cochlea.

Stapedectomy
Stapes piston prosthesis
This operation aims to improve hearing by replacing the fixed stapes with a mobile piston prosthesis.

PATHOLOGY — TREATMENT

Ossicle Damage
Damaged incus
An injury or infection that can damage the malleus, incus, or stapes bone

Ossiculoplasty
Prosthesis
An operation to repair, reconstruct, and improve the movement of the tiny bones of hearing in the middle ear

PATHOLOGY — TREATMENT

Cholesteatoma
Skin
A mass of entrapped skin in the middle ear or temporal bone

Mastoidectomy
Canal Wall Up · External acoustic meatus · Mastoid air cells · Mastoid cavity · Middle ear · Canal Wall Down
A surgical procedure that removes a diseased portion of the mastoid bone

TREATMENT

Bone Anchored Hearing Aid
Abutment · Sound processor
The abutment is surgically attached to the titanium implant placed in the bone. A sound processor snaps onto the abutment.

©1999, 2000, 2009 Wolters Kluwer Published by Anatomical Chart Company in consultation with Arun K. Gadre, MD, Heuser Hearing Institute Professor of Otology & Neurotology, University of Louisville.

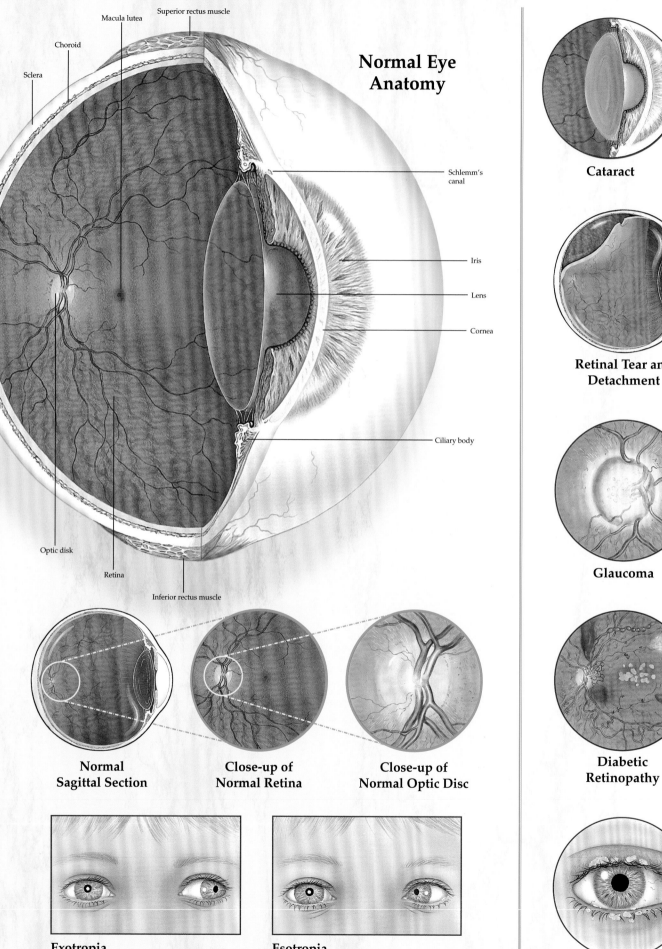

Normal Eye Anatomy

Superior rectus muscle

Macula lutea

Choroid

Sclera

Schlemm's canal

Iris

Lens

Cornea

Ciliary body

Optic disk

Retina

Inferior rectus muscle

Normal Sagittal Section

Close-up of Normal Retina

Close-up of Normal Optic Disc

Exotropia
A deviation of the visual axis of one eye away from the other eye.

Esotropia
A deviation of the visual axis of one eye toward that of the other eye

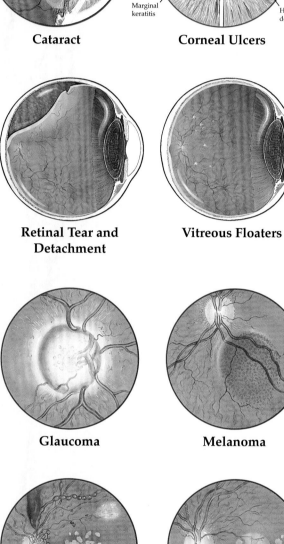

Hypopyon ulcer

Marginal keratitis

Herpes dendrite

Cataract   **Corneal Ulcers**

Retinal Tear and Detachment   **Vitreous Floaters**

Glaucoma   **Melanoma**

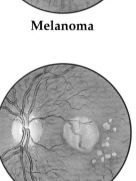

Diabetic Retinopathy   **Macular Degeneration**

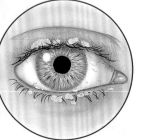

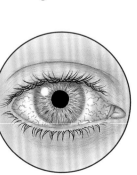

Blepharitis   **Conjunctivitis**

Normal External Anatomy of the Left Eye

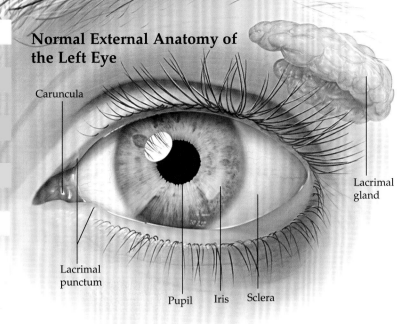

Caruncula

Lacrimal gland

Lacrimal punctum

Pupil Iris Sclera

Understanding Glaucoma

Glaucoma is a group of eye diseases that gradually steals sight without warning and often without symptoms. It is a condition in which normal fluid pressure inside the eyes (intraocular pressure, or IOP) slowly rises when the aqueous humor that normally flows in and out of the eye cannot drain properly. Instead, the fluid collects and causes pressure damage to the optic nerve (a bundle of more than 1 million nerve fibers that connect the retina with the brain) with subsequent loss of vision. There are subtypes of primary glaucoma: open angle, narrow angle, and congenital.

Narrow-Angle Glaucoma

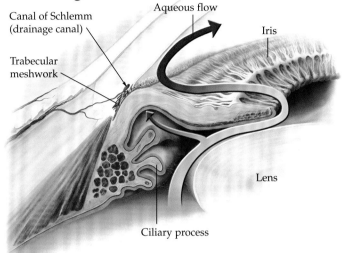

Aqueous flow

Canal of Schlemm (drainage canal)

Iris

Trabecular meshwork

Lens

Ciliary process

Narrow-angle glaucoma, also known as closed-angle glaucoma, is much more rare and different from open-angle glaucoma. Eye pressure usually goes up very fast. This happens when the drainage canal gets blocked or covered. The angle between the iris and the cornea is not as wide and open as it should be. Outer edges of the iris bunch up over the drainage canal when the pupil enlarges too much or too quickly.

Open-Angle (Chronic) Glaucoma

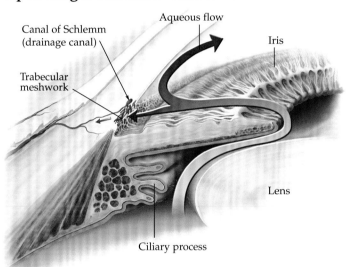

Aqueous flow

Canal of Schlemm (drainage canal)

Iris

Trabecular meshwork

Lens

Ciliary process

Open-angle (chronic) glaucoma is the most common form of glaucoma. This happens when the aqueous fluid drainage canals (canal of Schlemm) become constricted or obstructed over time. The inner eye pressure (intraocular pressure or IOP) rises because the correct amount of fluid cannot drain out of the eye. With open-angle glaucoma, the entrances to the drainage canals are clear and should be working correctly. The obstruction occurs inside the drainage canals.

Congenital Glaucoma

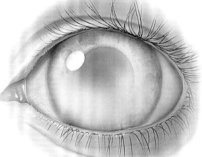

Congenital glaucoma is a rare form of glaucoma that occurs in babies and young children. This condition can be inherited. It is usually the result of incorrect or incomplete development of the eye's drainage canals during the prenatal period.

Sagittal View of the Eye

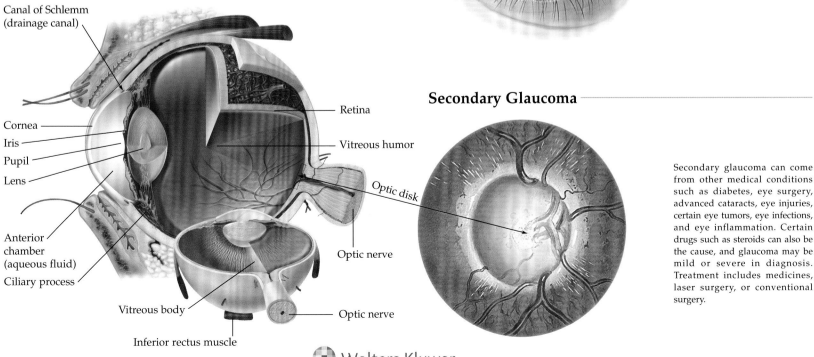

Canal of Schlemm (drainage canal)

Cornea
Iris
Pupil
Lens

Anterior chamber (aqueous fluid)
Ciliary process

Vitreous body

Inferior rectus muscle

Retina

Vitreous humor

Optic disk

Optic nerve

Optic nerve

Secondary Glaucoma

Secondary glaucoma can come from other medical conditions such as diabetes, eye surgery, advanced cataracts, eye injuries, certain eye tumors, eye infections, and eye inflammation. Certain drugs such as steroids can also be the cause, and glaucoma may be mild or severe in diagnosis. Treatment includes medicines, laser surgery, or conventional surgery.

Age-Related Macular Degeneration

What Is Macular Degeneration?

- Age-related macular degeneration (AMD) is a degenerative condition of the macula.
- The macula is the part of the retina responsible for sharp central vision needed for driving, reading, watching TV, and facial recognition.
- AMD is the leading cause of permanent vision loss in those aged 50 or older in developed countries.

Signs and Symptoms

- Dim or blurred central vision
- Distorted central vision
- Diminished or altered color vision

Screening

- Dilated eye examination
- Scanning laser ophthalmoscopy
- Angiography or fluorescein angiography, an examination of the blood vessels by x-ray after a radiopaque dye is injected for better viewing
- Fundus autofluorescence or noninvasive retinal imaging

AMD Types

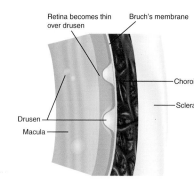

Macula with Dry AMD

Retina becomes thin over drusen
Bruch's membrane
Choroid
Sclera
Drusen
Macula

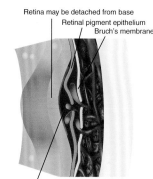

Macula with Wet AMD

Retina may be detached from base
Retinal pigment epithelium
Bruch's membrane

Blood vessels break through Bruch's membrane and retinal epithelium leaking fluid and blood

- In the early stages of macular degeneration, scattered deposits on the retina called drusen and atrophy of the retina in certain areas in more advanced AMD.
- Drusen can interfere with vision, causing blurriness or dimness.
- Advanced cases of dry AMD cause further vision loss.

- When fluid, swelling, and abnormal blood vessels are present in more advanced stages of AMD, it is categorized as "wet."
- As the new blood vessels and swelling displace the retina, more acute vision loss and distortion of vision may occur.

Lifestyle Modifications

Steps that can slow the progression of AMD:

- Smoking cessation.
- Proper management of blood pressure and cholesterol.
- Proper weight management.
- Specially formulated vitamins.
- Proper diet: Choose foods rich in omega-3 fatty acids and antioxidants, as well as leafy green vegetables with high zinc content.

Ora serrata
Conjunctiva
Canal of Schlemm
Scleral spur
Cornea
Iris
Pupil
Anterior chamber
Lens
Nucleus
Cortex
Posterior chamber
Sclera
Optic disk
Retina
Macula

Treatment

- There is no cure for AMD.
- Dry AMD—No treatment is currently available, but there are a number of clinical trials under way.
- Wet AMD—There are a number of treatments that may be used alone or in combination in the management of wet AMD.

Wet AMD Treatments	
Laser Photocoagulation	• New or abnormal blood vessels are cauterized using laser therapy. • Technique prevents further leakage and vision loss.
Photodynamic Therapy	• New or abnormal blood vessels are frozen. • Technique prevents further leakage and vision loss.
Anti-VEGF (Vascular Endothelial Growth Factor)	• VEGF is an inflammatory chemical present in patients with wet AMD. • Administration of intraocular anti-VEGF therapy prevents the growth of new blood vessels and reduces swelling and inflammation of the macula.
Steroids	• Steroids are used to reduce swelling and inflammation of the macula.

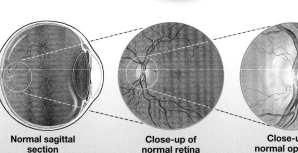

Normal sagittal section

Close-up of normal retina

Close-up of normal optic disk

© 2017 Wolters Kluwer

Medical illustrations by Jennifer Smith, in consultation with Virgil Alfaro, III, MD, Charleston, SC.

WillsEye Hospital

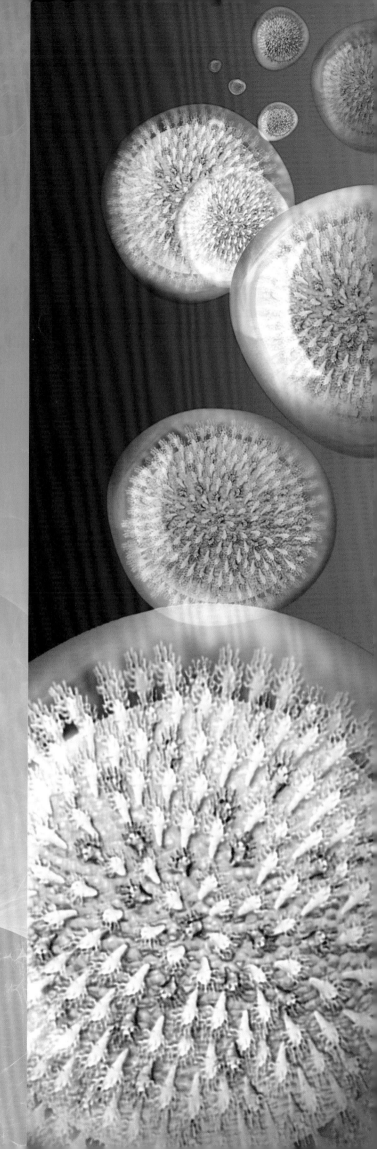

INFECTIOUS DISEASES & DISORDERS

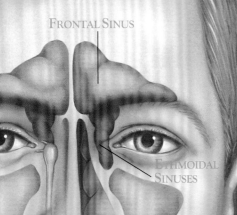

FRONTAL SINUS

ETHMOIDAL SINUSES

MAXILLARY SINUS

Understanding **The Common Cold**

COMMON COLD IS A VIRAL INFECTION OF THE UPPER RESPIRATORY TRACT (NOSE AND THROAT), WHICH CAUSES THE MUCOUS MEMBRANES OF THE HEAD AND THROAT TO BECOME INFLAMED. USUALLY COLDS LAST FROM 3 TO 7 DAYS ALTHOUGH SOME OF THE SYMPTOMS CAN LAST FOR 2 WEEKS. RARELY, A BACTERIAL INFECTION MAY COMPLICATE A COLD CAUSED BY A VIRUS.

RHINOVIRUS

HEADACHE

SINUS PAIN

RUNNY OR STUFFY NOSE

COUGHING OR SORE THROAT

CAUSES AND RISK FACTORS

Most colds are caused by the rhinovirus and are highly contagious (especially the first 2-4 days). The virus enters the body through the mouth or nose.

Colds can be caught by:

- Inhaling the droplets of the virus from someone who is sick as they cough, sneeze, or talk
- Having direct physical contact with someone who has a cold; touching objects that they have touched and then touching your own eyes, nose, or mouth can transfer the virus into your system

Risk Factors

- Age: Infants and younger children are more susceptible to colds because of their immature immune systems and their close contact with other children. As the immune system develops over time, the frequency of colds diminishes.
- Season: Children and adults are more likely to catch colds in the fall and winter (or during rainy seasons) when more time is spent indoors.
- Additionally: Fatigue, stress, and allergies that have nose or throat symptoms can increase the risk of getting a cold.

SIGNS AND SYMPTOMS

The symptoms you experience during a cold are due to inflammation. When foreign microorganisms such as viruses enter the body, your body's defenses react with an inflammatory response; this response is characterized by redness, heat, swelling, and pain. As the body attacks and breaks down the cold virus, the resulting debris is blown out from the nose or coughed up from the air passages in the lungs.

The symptoms resulting from this process can include the following:

- Runny or stuffy nose
- Sneezing
- Sore or tickly throat
- Watery eyes
- Coughing
- Headache
- Sinus pain or teeth pain (viral sinusitis can occur with a cold)
- Muscle aches
- Mild fever
- Fatigue

COMPLICATIONS OF THE COMMON COLD

When you have a cold, asthma may become worse, including wheezing.

You may also acquire bacterial infections such as:

- Sinusitis
- Bronchitis
- Ear infections (usually in children)
- Pneumonia

TREATMENT AND MANAGEMENT

There is no cure for the common cold, but there are things you can do to make yourself more comfortable, including the following:

- Drink plenty of liquids.
- Eat chicken soup.
- Rest and consider staying home while you are sick.
- Gargle with warm salt water.
- Use nasal saline or a Neti pot.
- Use a humidifier—remember to change the water daily.
- For adults and children, pain relievers such as acetaminophen or ibuprofen can help reduce muscle aches or fever.
- Always talk to your doctor before giving cold medicine to children 6 years of age and younger.

It is important to note that antibiotics are not effective against viral infections such as the common cold. Antibiotics work only against bacterial infections.

When to suspect a bacterial infection or complications from a cold and seek medical help:

- If symptoms do not improve or they worsen after 7-10 days
- If you have difficulty breathing
- If you have persistent fever

TO PREVENT GETTING THE COLD VIRUS...

Keep your hands away from your face and eyes.

Wash your hands frequently with soap and water for 15-30 seconds. If a sink is not available, alcohol-based rubs can be used as an alternative.

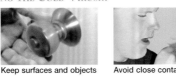
Keep surfaces and objects (countertops, door knobs, toys, etc.) that can be exposed to the virus clean.

Avoid close contact with people who have a cold.

TO PREVENT SPREADING THE COLD VIRUS...

Avoid close contact with others, and don't share utensils or drinking glasses.

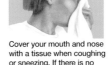
Cover your mouth and nose with a tissue when coughing or sneezing. If there is no tissue available, cough or sneeze into your elbow rather than your hands.

UNDERSTANDING HEPATITIS

What Is Viral Hepatitis?

Viral hepatitis is a fairly common disease leading to the destruction of liver cells. It is caused by one or more of five different hepatic viruses (hepatitis A, B, C, D, and E) some singly, some in combination. The disease progresses from the preicteric (before the onset of jaundice) period, through the icteric period, and finally to the posticteric period. While most people are asymptomatic and recover completely, others develop chronic hepatitis. People at increased risk for hepatitis include intravenous drug users, health care workers, infants born to infected mothers, hemodialysis patients, recipients of plasma-derived products, travelers from areas where hepatitis is endemic, and people who have multiple sexual partners.

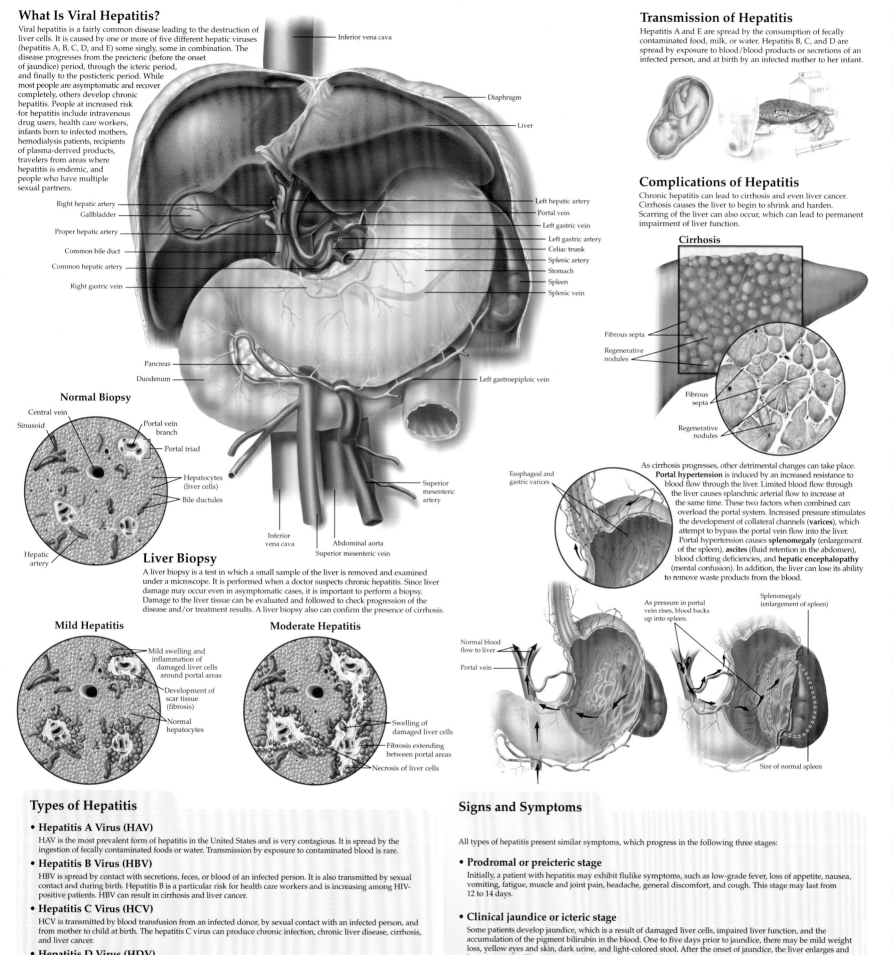

Labels (center illustration): Inferior vena cava; Diaphragm; Liver; Left hepatic artery; Portal vein; Left gastric vein; Left gastric artery; Celiac trunk; Splenic artery; Stomach; Spleen; Splenic vein; Left gastroepiploic vein; Right hepatic artery; Gallbladder; Proper hepatic artery; Common bile duct; Common hepatic artery; Right gastric vein; Pancreas; Duodenum; Superior mesenteric artery; Inferior vena cava; Abdominal aorta; Superior mesenteric vein

Normal Biopsy

Labels: Central vein; Sinusoid; Portal vein branch; Portal triad; Hepatocytes (liver cells); Bile ductules; Hepatic artery

Liver Biopsy

A liver biopsy is a test in which a small sample of the liver is removed and examined under a microscope. It is performed when a doctor suspects chronic hepatitis. Since liver damage may occur even in asymptomatic cases, it is important to perform a biopsy. Damage to the liver tissue can be evaluated and followed to check progression of the disease and/or treatment results. A liver biopsy also can confirm the presence of cirrhosis.

Mild Hepatitis

Labels: Mild swelling and inflammation of damaged liver cells around portal areas; Development of scar tissue (fibrosis); Normal hepatocytes

Moderate Hepatitis

Labels: Swelling of damaged liver cells; Fibrosis extending between portal areas; Necrosis of liver cells

Transmission of Hepatitis

Hepatitis A and E are spread by the consumption of fecally contaminated food, milk, or water. Hepatitis B, C, and D are spread by exposure to blood/blood products or secretions of an infected person, and at birth by an infected mother to her infant.

Complications of Hepatitis

Chronic hepatitis can lead to cirrhosis and even liver cancer. Cirrhosis causes the liver to begin to shrink and harden. Scarring of the liver can also occur, which can lead to permanent impairment of liver function.

Cirrhosis

Labels: Fibrous septa; Regenerative nodules; Fibrous septa; Regenerative nodules

As cirrhosis progresses, other detrimental changes can take place. **Portal hypertension** is induced by an increased resistance to blood flow through the liver. Limited blood flow through the liver causes splanchnic arterial flow to increase at the same time. These two factors when combined can overload the portal system. Increased pressure stimulates the development of collateral channels (**varices**), which attempt to bypass the portal vein flow into the liver. Portal hypertension causes **splenomegaly** (enlargement of the spleen), **ascites** (fluid retention in the abdomen), blood clotting deficiencies, and **hepatic encephalopathy** (mental confusion). In addition, the liver can lose its ability to remove waste products from the blood.

Labels: Esophageal and gastric varices; Normal blood flow to liver; Portal vein; As pressure in portal vein rises, blood backs up into spleen; Splenomegaly (enlargement of spleen); Size of normal spleen

Types of Hepatitis

- **Hepatitis A Virus (HAV)**

  HAV is the most prevalent form of hepatitis in the United States and is very contagious. It is spread by the ingestion of fecally contaminated foods or water. Transmission by exposure to contaminated blood is rare.

- **Hepatitis B Virus (HBV)**

  HBV is spread by contact with secretions, feces, or blood of an infected person. It is also transmitted by sexual contact and during birth. Hepatitis B is a particular risk for health care workers and is increasing among HIV-positive patients. HBV can result in cirrhosis and liver cancer.

- **Hepatitis C Virus (HCV)**

  HCV is transmitted by blood transfusion from an infected donor, by sexual contact with an infected person, and from mother to child at birth. The hepatitis C virus can produce chronic infection, chronic liver disease, cirrhosis, and liver cancer.

- **Hepatitis D Virus (HDV)**

  HDV occurs only in those infected with the hepatitis B virus. It causes cirrhosis as well as sudden, severe illness that can be fatal. It is usually transmitted by contact with contaminated blood.

- **Hepatitis E Virus (HEV)**

  HEV occurs primarily in those who have traveled to developing countries. It is transmitted by the consumption of fecally contaminated food or water.

- **Hepatitis G Virus (HGV) and Transfusion Transmitted Virus (TTV)**

  HGV and TTV are recently discovered viruses. So far, these viruses do not appear to be associated with clinical hepatitis or any liver injury. Research is being conducted to provide more information about these viruses.

Signs and Symptoms

All types of hepatitis present similar symptoms, which progress in the following three stages:

- **Prodromal or preicteric stage**

  Initially, a patient with hepatitis may exhibit flulike symptoms, such as low-grade fever, loss of appetite, nausea, vomiting, fatigue, muscle and joint pain, headache, general discomfort, and cough. This stage may last from 12 to 14 days.

- **Clinical jaundice or icteric stage**

  Some patients develop jaundice, which is a result of damaged liver cells, impaired liver function, and the accumulation of the pigment bilirubin in the blood. One to five days prior to jaundice, there may be mild weight loss, yellow eyes and skin, dark urine, and light-colored stool. After the onset of jaundice, the liver enlarges and becomes tender. The spleen may also become enlarged. This stage lasts from 1 to 2 weeks.

- **Recovery or posticteric stage**

  Most symptoms abate or disappear. There is also a decrease in the size of the liver. This stage lasts from 2 to 12 weeks, often longer in patients with hepatitis B, C, or E.

Anatomical Chart Company, Skokie, IL. Medical illustrations by Liana Bauman, MAMS, in consultation with Hari Conjeevaram, MD.

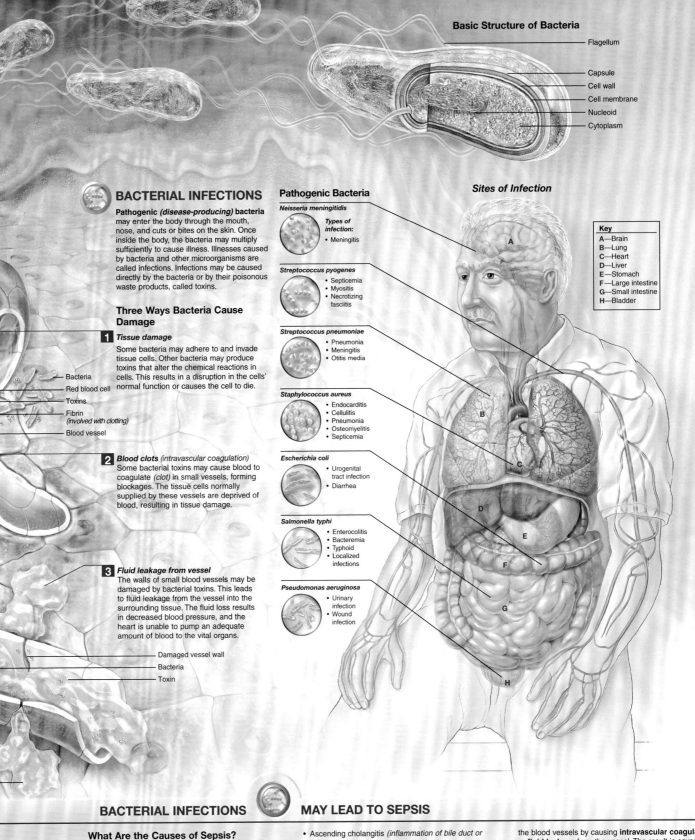

Basic Structure of Bacteria

- Flagellum
- Capsule
- Cell wall
- Cell membrane
- Nucleoid
- Cytoplasm

BACTERIAL INFECTIONS

Pathogenic *(disease-producing)* bacteria may enter the body through the mouth, nose, and cuts or bites on the skin. Once inside the body, the bacteria may multiply sufficiently to cause illness. Illnesses caused by bacteria and other microorganisms are called infections. Infections may be caused directly by the bacteria or by their poisonous waste products, called toxins.

Three Ways Bacteria Cause Damage

1 *Tissue damage*

Some bacteria may adhere to and invade tissue cells. Other bacteria may produce toxins that alter the chemical reactions in cells. This results in a disruption in the cells' normal function or causes the cell to die.

- Toxins
- Bacteria
- Damaged tissue

- Bacteria
- Red blood cell
- Toxins
- Fibrin *(involved with clotting)*
- Blood vessel

2 *Blood clots (intravascular coagulation)*

Some bacterial toxins may cause blood to coagulate *(clot)* in small vessels, forming blockages. The tissue cells normally supplied by these vessels are deprived of blood, resulting in tissue damage.

3 *Fluid leakage from vessel*

The walls of small blood vessels may be damaged by bacterial toxins. This leads to fluid leakage from the vessel into the surrounding tissue. The fluid loss results in decreased blood pressure, and the heart is unable to pump an adequate amount of blood to the vital organs.

- Damaged vessel wall
- Bacteria
- Toxin

- Fluid leakage

Pathogenic Bacteria

Neisseria meningitidis

Types of infection:
- Meningitis

Streptococcus pyogenes
- Septicemia
- Myositis
- Necrotizing fasciitis

Streptococcus pneumoniae
- Pneumonia
- Meningitis
- Otitis media

Staphylococcus aureus
- Endocarditis
- Cellulitis
- Pneumonia
- Osteomyelitis
- Septicemia

Escherichia coli
- Urogenital tract infection
- Diarrhea

Salmonella typhi
- Enterocolitis
- Bacteremia
- Typhoid
- Localized infections

Pseudomonas aeruginosa
- Urinary infection
- Wound infection

Sites of Infection

Key
A—Brain
B—Lung
C—Heart
D—Liver
E—Stomach
F—Large intestine
G—Small intestine
H—Bladder

BACTERIAL INFECTIONS ⬤ MAY LEAD TO SEPSIS

What Is Sepsis?

Sepsis is a systemic inflammatory response syndrome resulting from a **bacterial infection**. In sepsis, bacteria from the infected site, or the toxins they produce, enter the bloodstream and spread throughout the body. This sets off a chain of chemical reactions that lead to excessive systemic inflammation and intravascular coagulation. Without proper treatment, this may lead to organ dysfunction, multiple organ failure, and eventually death.

What Are the Risk Factors?

People with inefficient immune systems or blood disorders are at particular risk for sepsis. The risk factors associated with sepsis include the following:

- Major surgery
- Chemotherapy
- Immunosuppressive medications
- Therapy with antibiotics
- Indwelling catheters/tubes
- An endoscopic procedure
- A cardiovascular procedure

What Are the Causes of Sepsis?

Sepsis is a result of a bacterial infection that can originate anywhere in the body. **Sites of infection** may include the lungs, digestive tract, kidneys, bladder, joints, skin, or the coverings around the brain.
Infections that can cause sepsis include the following:

- Meningitis *(inflammation of the brain membrane)*
- Bacterial pneumonia *(inflammation of the lungs)*
- Bacterial peritonitis *(inflammation of the peritoneum)*
- Osteomyelitis *(infection of the cortical bone)*
- Septic arthritis *(inflammation of synovial membrane of joints)*
- Cellulitis *(inflammation of subcutaneous, connective tissue)*
- Endocarditis *(infection of the valves of the heart)*
- Bacterial enterocolitis *(infection of the small and large intestines)*
- Cholecystitis *(inflammation of the gallbladder)*
- Ascending cholangitis *(inflammation of bile duct or biliary tree)*
- Pyelonephritis *(inflammation of the kidney)*
- Cystitis *(inflammation of the urinary bladder)*

What Are the Symptoms?

Symptoms of sepsis include the following:
- High fever
- Low body temperature
- Chills with body shaking
- Confusion or changes in mental status
- Hyperventilation *(rapid breathing)*
- Tachycardia *(rapid heartbeat)*
- Low urine production

What Are the Complications?

When an infection worsens, bacteria may enter the bloodstream. Toxins produced by the bacteria can affect the blood vessels by causing **intravascular coagulation** or **fluid leakage** from the vessel. The result is severe hypotension *(low blood pressure)*, which is known as *septic shock*. Impaired blood flow can result in damage to vital organs such as the brain, heart, and kidneys.

What Is the Treatment?

Hospitalization is necessary to treat sepsis successfully. Blood culture tests are performed to identify the causative **pathogenic bacteria**. While the test results are pending, intravenous antibiotic therapy is administered to the patient. This consists of a broad-spectrum *(kills a variety of bacteria)* antibiotic or multiple antibiotics. When the test results become available, the treatment can then be tailored to combat the causative pathogenic bacteria. Further testing may be done to identify the source or originating **site of the infection**. Supportive therapy with oxygen, intravenous fluids, and medications to restore normal blood pressure, is also important for a complete recovery.

UNDERSTANDING HIV AND AIDS

HIV virion (virus particle)

HIV
Life Cycle

① HIV binds to the T cell.

② Viral RNA is released into the host cell.

③ Reverse transcriptase converts viral RNA into viral DNA.

④ Viral DNA enters the T cell's nucleus and inserts itself into the T cell's DNA.

⑤ The T cell begins to make copies of the HIV components.

⑥ Protease (an enzyme) helps create new virus particles.

⑦ The new HIV virion (virus particle) is released from the T cell.

Viral RNA

Reverse transcriptase

Viral DNA

T cell

Viral RNA

HIV proteins

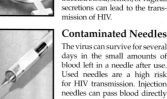

New HIV virion (virus particle)

What Are HIV and AIDS?

Since it was first reported in 1981, HIV/AIDS has become a major worldwide epidemic. AIDS (acquired immunodeficiency syndrome) is a chronic, life-threatening condition caused by the human immunodeficiency virus (HIV). HIV damages or destroys certain cells of the immune system, particularly T cells, weakening the body's response to infections and certain types of cancers. The virus and the infection are known as HIV, while the term "AIDS" refers to the later stages of HIV infection.

How Is HIV Transmitted?

Sexual Activity

Having unprotected sexual contact with an infected partner is the most common method of spreading HIV. Contact with infected blood, semen, or vaginal secretions can lead to the transmission of HIV.

Contaminated Needles

The virus can survive for several days in the small amounts of blood left in a needle after use. Used needles are a high risk for HIV transmission. Injection needles can pass blood directly from one person's bloodstream to another.

HIV Testing

HIV tests tell patients if they are infected with HIV. The tests look for the presence of antibodies (proteins made by the immune system to fight a specific disease) to HIV antigens or HIV RNA. The most common type of HIV test is a blood test known as an enzyme-linked immunosorbent assay (ELISA) screening. It searches for antibodies to HIV in the blood. A positive result should always be confirmed with a second test. Another blood test is called the Western blot analysis, which looks for antibodies to several HIV proteins.

Pregnancy

A woman can transmit the virus to her unborn infant during pregnancy, delivery, or after birth when she is breast-feeding. Babies born to infected mothers have a 15%-25% chance of becoming infected.

Blood or Blood Products

Infected blood is where HIV is found in the highest concentrations. Since 1985, the HIV antibody test has been used to screen blood donations for the virus. Now it is rare to become infected by receiving blood or blood products through transfusion.

HIV is **not** transmitted by insect bites; casual contact; sharing dishes or food; swimming pools and hot tubs; pets; contact with saliva, tears, or sweat; contact with toilets; or donating blood.

Risk Factors

Anyone of any age, race, gender, or sexual orientation can become infected with HIV, but a person is at greatest risk if he or she:

• Has unprotected sex with multiple partners

• Has unprotected sex with a partner who is HIV positive

• Has another sexually transmitted infection such as syphilis, herpes, or gonorrhea

• Shares needles during intravenous drug use

• Is a hemophiliac who received blood products before April 1985

• Received a blood transfusion or blood products before 1985

Newborns or nursing infants whose mothers are HIV positive are also at high risk. Anyone at risk should be tested for HIV infection.

AIDS-Related Illnesses

Opportunistic infections (OIs) occur only when the immune system is severely damaged. These infections cause life-threatening illnesses in people with AIDS. Below is a partial list of some of the infections/cancers associated with AIDS, along with some of their symptoms.

Nervous system:

• **Toxoplasmosis**—fever, headache, partial loss of vision, seizures, paralysis on one side of the body, confusion

• **Cryptococcosis**—confusion, fever, headache, seizures

• **Non-Hodgkin lymphoma**—one or more painless swellings in neck, armpits, or groin; fever, sweats

• **Herpes zoster (shingles)**—painful rash of fluid-filled blisters found on chest, abdomen, face or extremities

Respiratory system:

• *Pneumocystis carinii* **pneumonia (PCP)**—fatigue, fever, dry cough, shortness of breath

• **Tuberculosis (TB)**—persistent cough, chest pain, shortness of breath, weight loss, coughing up of blood (hemoptysis), fever

Skin:

• **Herpes simplex**—painful blisters on or around lips or genitals

• **Kaposi sarcoma**—raised, purple or pinkish-brown lesions on skin

Digestive system:

• **Cryptosporidiosis**—watery diarrhea, abdominal pain, fever, vomiting

• **Candidiasis**—white plaques in mouth and/or throat, pain with swallowing or eating

• **Cytomegalovirus (CMV)**—diarrhea, nonitchy rash, fever, abdominal pain, visual changes, yellowing of skin and whites of eyes (very rare)

• **Isosporiasis**—watery diarrhea, abdominal pain, weight loss, fever

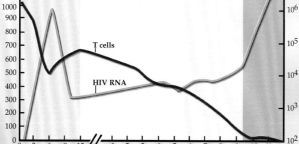

Stages of HIV Infection

1. Acute Stage

Occurs about 1-2 weeks after initial infection. During this stage, the virus undergoes massive replication. Patients may be asymptomatic or have a flulike syndrome.

2. Asymptomatic HIV

During this stage, chronic signs or symptoms are not present. T-cell count may be used to monitor progression of the disease. With the patient's own resistance and drug therapy, this stage can last for 10-12 years or longer.

3. Symptomatic HIV

This stage has two phases: early and late. When the T-cell count falls below 200 cells per cubic millimeter of blood, it is the late phase. This stage of HIV is defined mainly by the emergence of opportunistic infections and cancers to which the immune system normally helps maintain resistance.

4. Advanced HIV

A T-cell count of 50 cells per cubic millimeter or less represents advanced HIV. With the onset of this stage, patients are at the highest risk for opportunistic infections and malignancies.

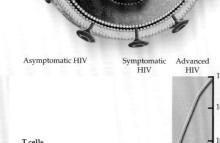

Acute stage | Asymptomatic HIV | Symptomatic HIV | Advanced HIV

T-cells (CD4)/mm³ — 1200, 1100, 1000, 900, 800, 700, 600, 500, 400, 300, 200, 100

HIV RNA Copies per mL Plasma — 10^7, 10^6, 10^5, 10^4, 10^3, 10^2

T cells

HIV RNA

Weeks — 0 3 6 9 12

Years — 1 2 3 4 5 6 7 8 9 10 11

Signs and Symptoms of HIV Infection

Depending on the stage of infection, the symptoms of HIV vary. Symptoms can include the following:

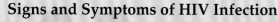

• Short-term memory loss
• Persistent headaches
• High fever
• Confusion and forgetfulness
• Seizures and lack of coordination

• Persistent or frequent oral infections
• Difficult or painful swallowing
• Loss of appetite
• Heavy night sweats
• Cough and shortness of breath

• Swollen lymph nodes in neck, armpits, and groin
• Persistent skin rashes or flaky skin
• Severe weight loss
• Chronic diarrhea
• Lack of energy and muscle weakness

Treatment

HIV and AIDS are not curable, but early detection and treatment can increase life expectancy. There are no vaccines available, but medications can slow the progression of HIV and the development of AIDS. Other medications are available to protect against and treat the variety of illnesses that may develop. Consult with a physician who specializes in caring for HIV-infected individuals. It is critical that all prescribed medication be taken as directed.

Wolters Kluwer Anatomical Chart Company, Skokie, IL. Medical illustrations by Liana Bauman, MAMS, in consultation with Michele Till, MD.

What Is Influenza?

Influenza, also known as the flu, is caused by the influenza virus. It is a contagious infection of the nose, throat, and lungs.

Influenza virus spreads in the little drops that spray out of an infected person's mouth and nose when he/she sneezes, coughs, laughs, or even talks.

When someone else breathes in these drops or gets them on the hands and then touches his or her own mouth or nose, the virus can enter his or her body.

Flu Symptoms

Headache	Almost always
Fever	Usually high, 102°F-104°F or 38.9°C-40°C
Fatigue, weakness	Can last up to 2-3 weeks
Runny or stuffy nose	Sometimes
Sneezing	Sometimes
Sore throat	Sometimes
Cough	Can become severe
Chest discomfort	Common
General aches, pains	Usually, often severe

Bronchitis

Prevention

Ways to Help Prevent Influenza

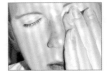

Avoid touching your eyes, nose, and mouth.

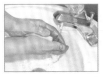

Wash your hands with soap and water frequently.

Get a vaccination (flu shot) every year before the start of the flu season. *Note: The vaccine does not cause the flu.*

Ways to Help Prevent the Spread of Influenza

Stay home when you are sick.

Avoid close contact with others.

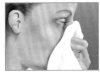

Cover your mouth and nose with a tissue when coughing or sneezing.

Special Risk Factors

Certain people have an increased risk of serious complications from influenza:

- People aged 65 years and older
- People of any age with chronic medical conditions
- Pregnant women
- Children between 6 and 23 months of age

Flu Vaccination (Flu Shot)

Because the influenza virus is different every year, you should protect yourself by getting a flu shot every year. If you are at high risk for major complications from the flu, it is especially important to get the shot before the flu season. The influenza vaccine may also lessen the severity of symptoms related to other forms of influenza that the vaccine is unable to prevent. The flu shot will not protect you from the common cold.

Complications

The complications caused by influenza include the following:
- Bacterial pneumonia.
- Dehydration.
- Worsening of chronic medical conditions, such as congestive heart failure, asthma, or diabetes.
- Children may develop sinus problems or ear infections.

Most people who get influenza recover in 1-2 weeks, but some people develop life-threatening complications (such as pneumonia) as a result of the flu. If your flu symptoms are unusually severe, you should seek medical help immediately.

Bronchitis, or inflammation of the bronchi, is another complication of influenza. In most cases, it involves the large and medium-sized bronchi. In children, older people, and those with lung disease, the infection may spread and inflame the bronchioles or lung tissue.

What to Do If You Get Sick

If you develop an influenza infection, you should:

- Get plenty of rest
- Drink plenty of liquids
- Avoid using alcohol and tobacco

You can also take medications to relieve flu symptoms, but never give aspirin to children or teenagers who have cold or flu symptoms without first speaking to your health care provider. Antiviral medications such as Oseltamivir have been approved for treatment of influenza but must be prescribed by a doctor. There is no cure for the flu. The antiviral medications can help reduce the severity and the duration of the symptoms.

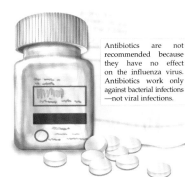

Antibiotics are not recommended because they have no effect on the influenza virus. Antibiotics work only against bacterial infections —not viral infections.

Questions & Answers

Q: How can you tell the difference between a common cold and influenza?

A: Although flu and cold symptoms can be similar, the intensity and duration are different. The symptoms of a cold may come on gradually and are milder than the symptoms of the flu. Flu symptoms are more severe and tend to come on immediately and take longer to recover.

Q: Is the stomach flu the same type of flu as influenza (flu)?

A: No. Some people use the term "stomach flu" to describe certain common illnesses that can cause nausea, vomiting, or diarrhea. Although these symptoms can sometimes be related to the flu (more commonly in children), these problems are rarely symptoms of influenza.

Q: Can the symptoms of influenza (flu) be different in children?

A: Yes. Although flu symptoms for children and adults might be similar, children might have other symptoms such as nausea, vomiting and/or diarrhea. Children are at a higher risk of complications from the flu. If a child's symptoms worsen, call your doctor.

Anatomical Chart Company, Skokie, IL. Medical illustrations by Dawn Scheuerman, MAMS, in consultation with David J. Yu, MD and William E. Burkel, PhD, University of Michigan Medical School.

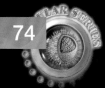

C Viral Entry Sites

Skin

Respiratory tract

Intestinal tract

Urogenital tract

Key
a—Brain
b—Lung
c—Heart
d—Liver
e—Stomach
f—Large intestine
g—Small intestine
h—Bladder

B How Viruses Infect Cells

A virus is unable to process nutrients or replicate without a host cell.

1 To invade a cell, the surface proteins on the virus attach to specific receptor sites on the host cell's outer membrane.

2 After attaching to the membrane, part or all of the virus penetrates into the host cell.

3 Depending on the specific virus, the nucleic acid of the virus is released into the host cell's cytoplasm or nucleus. Then the viral genes direct the production of proteins and nucleic acids, the components of new virus particles.

4 The host cells may burst, releasing the viruses to infect other cells. However, not all viruses destroy the cell as they leave. Some viruses form buds from the host cell's membrane and are released.

A General Structure of a Virus

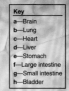

Double lipid layer

Nucleic acid (Composed of DNA or RNA)

Protein shell

Surface protein (Antigen)

D Viral Spread via the Blood

Viremia is the presence of a virus in the bloodstream. Blood-borne viruses either circulate freely in the plasma or are cell associated. Cell-associated viremia means that the virus replicates in cells found in the circulation, particularly B or T lymphocytes or monocytes, or (rarely) red blood cells.

Monocyte (White blood cell)

Red blood cell

Cell-associated viremia

Plasma viremia

Blood vessel

What Is a Virus?

Viruses are subcellular organisms made up of RNA (ribonucleic acid) or DNA (deoxyribonucleic acid) covered with proteins. Viruses are obligate intracellular parasites, meaning that they are incapable of growth or reproduction apart from living cells. Instead, they invade a host cell and stimulate it to participate in the formation of additional virus particles. Viruses are classified according to their size, shape (spherical, rod-shaped, or cubic), or means of transmission (respiratory, fecal, oral, or sexual).

A General Structure of a Virus

A virus has a core of nucleic acid, composed of DNA or RNA, depending on what type of virus it is. The nucleic acid is enclosed in one or two protein shells. Surface proteins (antigens) cover the outer shell.

B How Viruses Infect Cells

Viruses invade host cells by attaching to a specific molecule on the cell surface, which acts as a receptor. Following attachment, there is a multi-step entry process that delivers the viral nucleic acid, which contains the genes, into either the cytoplasm or the nucleus of the host cell. Once released, the viral genes dictate the synthesis of viral proteins and the replication of its genome, followed by assembly and release of new virus particles. Cell destruction is required for release of some viruses but not of others, which "bud" through the plasma membrane.

What Are the Modes of Transmission?

Most infectious diseases are transmitted in one of four ways.

1. In **contact transmission**, the susceptible host comes into direct contact (as in sexually transmitted disease) or indirect contact (contaminated inanimate objects) with the source.
2. **Airborne transmission** results from inhalation of contaminated fine mist droplets, which are sometimes suspended in airborne dust particles.
3. In **enteric** (oral-fecal) **transmission**, the infecting organisms are found in feces and are ingested by susceptible hosts, either by direct contact or, in some cases, through fecally contaminated food or water.
4. **Vector-borne transmission** occurs when an intermediate carrier (vector), such as a flea or a mosquito, transfers an organism.

C Viral Entry Sites

The first step of infection is entry into the host. This can occur at the following sites:

- Conjunctiva (mucous membranes of the eye)
- Mouth/oropharynx
- Skin
- Respiratory tract
- Intestinal tract
- Urogenital tract

How Viruses Spread in the Body

Some viruses are confined to the site of initial infection and spread only locally, whereas others spread widely. In the body, viruses may spread via the blood or via the peripheral nervous system.

D Viral Spread via the Blood

Viremia is the presence of a virus in the bloodstream. The most common source of viremia is a virus that replicates in regional lymph nodes and is transported by the thoracic duct into the circulation. Blood-borne virus either circulate freely in the plasma or are cell associated. Most viremias are acute, lasting no more than 1-2 weeks. However, certain viruses are able to evade immune defenses and persist in the blood for months or years. Human immunodeficiency virus, the cause of AIDS, is an example of a persistent viremia. Blood-borne viruses can invade almost any organ or cell type.

Viral Spread via the Peripheral Nervous System

Neural spread is a process by which a virus is transmitted within the axon of peripheral nerve fibers. The neural pathway plays an essential role in the spread of some viruses, although it is less common than viremia as a mode of spread. Neurotropic viruses are usually confined to the peripheral and central nervous systems and replicate in relatively few peripheral tissues. Rabies virus is an example of a neurotropic virus.

Anatomical Chart Company, Skokie, IL. Medical illustrations by Lik Kwong, MFA, in consultation with Neal Nathanson, MD, Departments of Microbiology and Neurology, University of Pennsylvania.

MUSCULAR AND SKELETAL DISEASES & DISORDERS

- Understanding Arthritis

- Understanding Carpal Tunnel Syndrome

- Anatomy and Injuries of the Foot and Ankle

- Anatomy and Injuries of the Hand and Wrist

- Anatomy and Injuries of the Hip

- Hip and Knee Inflammations

- Knee Injuries

- Athletic Injuries of the Knee

- Anatomy and Injuries of the Shoulder

- Human Spine Disorders

- Anatomy and Injuries of the Spine

- Understanding Osteoporosis

- Anatomy and Injuries of the Head and Neck

- Whiplash Injuries of the Head and Neck

Osteoarthritis (OA)

- Most common type of arthritis
- Primarily affects cartilage, the tissue that cushions the ends of bones within the joints
- May initially affect joints asymmetrically
- Affects hands and weight-bearing joints
- Can cause joint pain and stiffness
- Usually develops slowly over many years

○ = identifies areas most affected by OA.

Rheumatoid Arthritis (RA)

- Causes redness, warmth, and swelling of joints
- Usually affects the same joint on both sides of the body
- Often causes a general feeling of sickness, fatigue, weight loss, and fever
- May develop suddenly, within weeks or months
- Most often begins between ages 25 and 50

○ = identifies areas most affected by RA.

Other Arthritic Diseases

Many people use the word *arthritis* to refer to all rheumatic diseases. However, the word literally means joint inflammation. Other types of arthritis include the following:

Fibromyalgia (Fibrositis)

- Chronic disorder that causes pain throughout the tissues that support and move the bones and joints.
- Pain, stiffness, and localized tender points occur in the muscles and tendons, particularly those of the spine, shoulders, and hips.
- Patients may also experience fatigue and sleep disturbances.

Gout

- Results from deposits of needlelike crystals of uric acid in the joints.
- The crystals cause inflammation, swelling, and pain in the affected joint, which is often the big toe.

Juvenile Rheumatoid Arthritis

- Most common form of arthritis in children
- Causes pain, stiffness, swelling, and impaired function of the joints
- May be associated with rashes or fevers; may affect various parts of the body

Systemic Lupus Erythematosus

- Also known as *lupus* or *SLE*
- Can result in inflammation of and damage to the joints, skin, kidneys, heart, lungs, blood vessels, and brain

Bursitis

- Inflammation of a bursa, a small, fluid-filled sac that absorbs shock and reduces friction around a joint
- May be caused by arthritis in the joint or by injury or infection of the bursa
- Produces pain and tenderness and may limit the movement of nearby joints

Tendinitis

- Inflammation of a tendon, a cord of fibrous tissue that attaches muscle to bone
- May be caused by overuse, injury, or a rheumatic condition
- Produces pain and tenderness and may restrict movement of nearby joints

Common Symptoms of Arthritis

- Swelling in one or more joints
- Stiffness around the joints (each episode of stiffness for RA lasts 1 hour or more, but OA lasts 30 minutes or less)
- Constant or recurring pain or tenderness in a joint
- Difficulty using or moving a joint normally
- Warmth and redness in a joint

If you have any of these symptoms for more than 2 weeks, contact your physician.

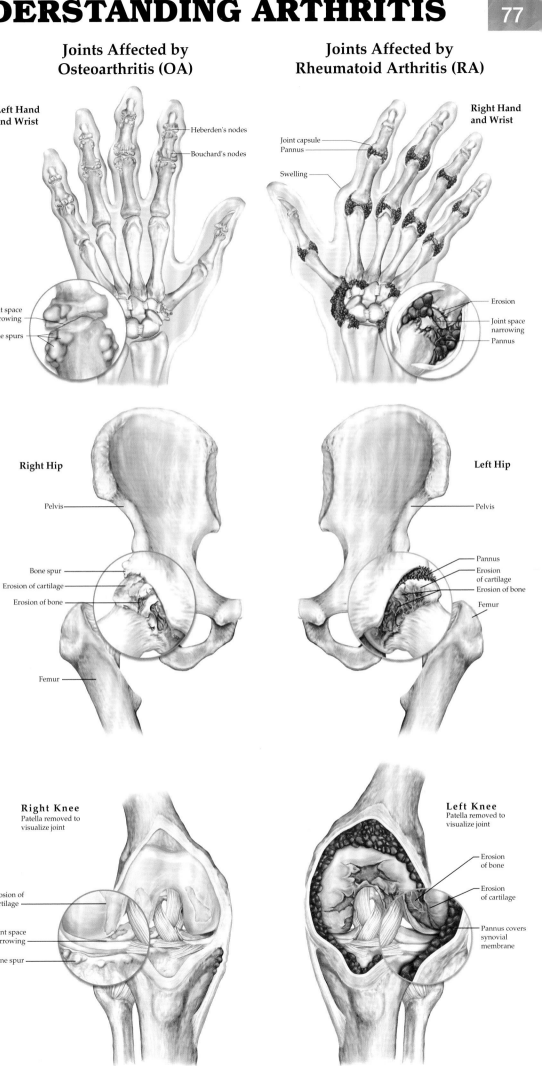

Joints Affected by Osteoarthritis (OA)

Left Hand and Wrist
Heberden's nodes
Bouchard's nodes
Joint space narrowing
Bone spurs

Joints Affected by Rheumatoid Arthritis (RA)

Right Hand and Wrist
Joint capsule
Pannus
Swelling
Erosion
Joint space narrowing
Pannus

Right Hip
Pelvis
Bone spur
Erosion of cartilage
Erosion of bone
Femur

Left Hip
Pelvis
Pannus
Erosion of cartilage
Erosion of bone
Femur

Right Knee
Patella removed to visualize joint
Erosion of cartilage
Joint space narrowing
Bone spur

Left Knee
Patella removed to visualize joint
Erosion of bone
Erosion of cartilage
Pannus covers synovial membrane

© 2004 Wolters Kluwer
Anatomical Chart Company, Skokie, IL. Medical illustrations by Dawn Scheuerman, MAMS, in consultation with Thomas J. Schnitzer, MD, PhD, Feinberg School of Medicine, Northwestern University, Chicago, IL.

UNDERSTANDING CARPAL TUNNEL SYNDROME

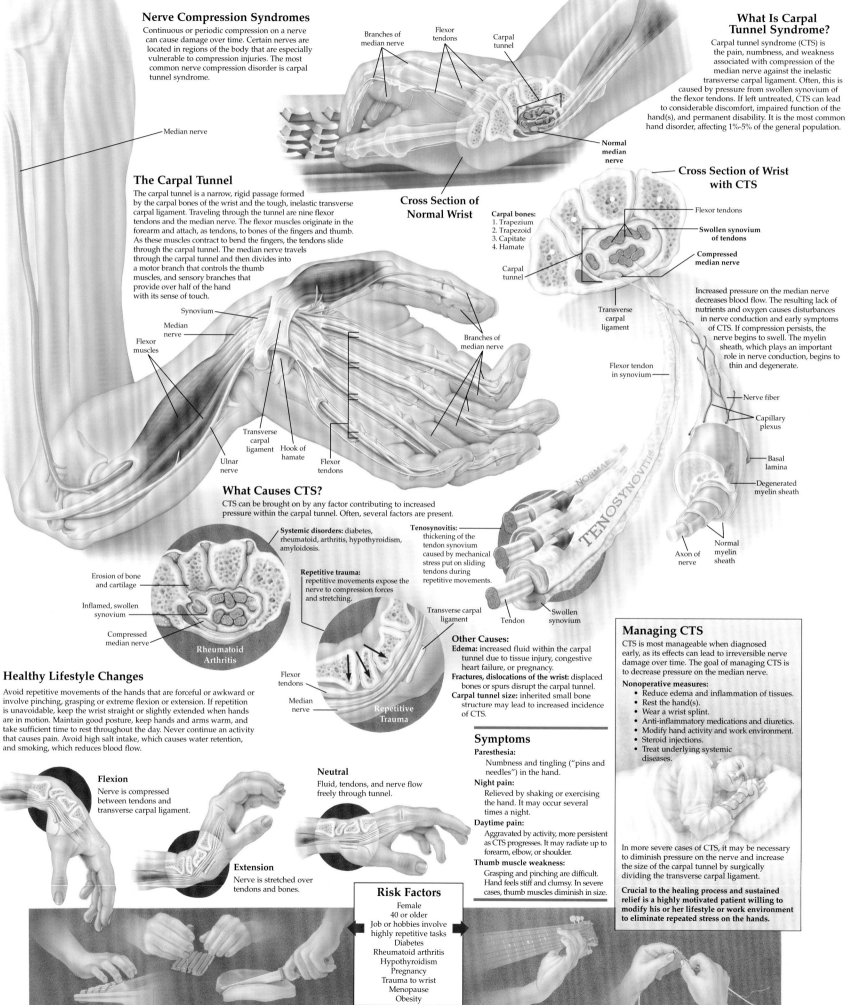

Nerve Compression Syndromes

Continuous or periodic compression on a nerve can cause damage over time. Certain nerves are located in regions of the body that are especially vulnerable to compression injuries. The most common nerve compression disorder is carpal tunnel syndrome.

Median nerve

What Is Carpal Tunnel Syndrome?

Carpal tunnel syndrome (CTS) is the pain, numbness, and weakness associated with compression of the median nerve against the inelastic transverse carpal ligament. Often, this is caused by pressure from swollen synovium of the flexor tendons. If left untreated, CTS can lead to considerable discomfort, impaired function of the hand(s), and permanent disability. It is the most common hand disorder, affecting 1%-5% of the general population.

Branches of median nerve
Flexor tendons
Carpal tunnel
Normal median nerve

The Carpal Tunnel

The carpal tunnel is a narrow, rigid passage formed by the carpal bones of the wrist and the tough, inelastic transverse carpal ligament. Traveling through the tunnel are nine flexor tendons and the median nerve. The flexor muscles originate in the forearm and attach, as tendons, to bones of the fingers and thumb. As these muscles contract to bend the fingers, the tendons slide through the carpal tunnel. The median nerve travels through the carpal tunnel and then divides into a motor branch that controls the thumb muscles, and sensory branches that provide over half of the hand with its sense of touch.

Cross Section of Normal Wrist

Carpal bones:
1. Trapezium
2. Trapezoid
3. Capitate
4. Hamate

Carpal tunnel

Cross Section of Wrist with CTS

Flexor tendons
Swollen synovium of tendons
Compressed median nerve

Transverse carpal ligament

Synovium
Median nerve
Flexor muscles
Branches of median nerve

Flexor tendon in synovium

Increased pressure on the median nerve decreases blood flow. The resulting lack of nutrients and oxygen causes disturbances in nerve conduction and early symptoms of CTS. If compression persists, the nerve begins to swell. The myelin sheath, which plays an important role in nerve conduction, begins to thin and degenerate.

Nerve fiber
Capillary plexus
Basal lamina
Degenerated myelin sheath

Transverse carpal ligament
Hook of hamate
Ulnar nerve
Flexor tendons

Axon of nerve
Normal myelin sheath

What Causes CTS?

CTS can be brought on by any factor contributing to increased pressure within the carpal tunnel. Often, several factors are present.

Systemic disorders: diabetes, rheumatoid, arthritis, hypothyroidism, amyloidosis.

Repetitive trauma: repetitive movements expose the nerve to compression forces and stretching.

Tenosynovitis: thickening of the tendon synovium caused by mechanical stress put on sliding tendons during repetitive movements.

Transverse carpal ligament
Tendon
Swollen synovium

Erosion of bone and cartilage
Inflamed, swollen synovium
Compressed median nerve

Rheumatoid Arthritis

Flexor tendons
Median nerve

Repetitive Trauma

Other Causes:
Edema: increased fluid within the carpal tunnel due to tissue injury, congestive heart failure, or pregnancy.
Fractures, dislocations of the wrist: displaced bones or spurs disrupt the carpal tunnel.
Carpal tunnel size: inherited small bone structure may lead to increased incidence of CTS.

Managing CTS

CTS is most manageable when diagnosed early, as its effects can lead to irreversible nerve damage over time. The goal of managing CTS is to decrease pressure on the median nerve.

Nonoperative measures:
- Reduce edema and inflammation of tissues.
- Rest the hand(s).
- Wear a wrist splint.
- Anti-inflammatory medications and diuretics.
- Modify hand activity and work environment.
- Steroid injections.
- Treat underlying systemic diseases.

Healthy Lifestyle Changes

Avoid repetitive movements of the hands that are forceful or awkward or involve pinching, grasping or extreme flexion or extension. If repetition is unavoidable, keep the wrist straight or slightly extended when hands are in motion. Maintain good posture, keep hands and arms warm, and take sufficient time to rest throughout the day. Never continue an activity that causes pain. Avoid high salt intake, which causes water retention, and smoking, which reduces blood flow.

Flexion
Nerve is compressed between tendons and transverse carpal ligament.

Neutral
Fluid, tendons, and nerve flow freely through tunnel.

Extension
Nerve is stretched over tendons and bones.

Symptoms

Paresthesia:
Numbness and tingling ("pins and needles") in the hand.

Night pain:
Relieved by shaking or exercising the hand. It may occur several times a night.

Daytime pain:
Aggravated by activity, more persistent as CTS progresses. It may radiate up to forearm, elbow, or shoulder.

Thumb muscle weakness:
Grasping and pinching are difficult. Hand feels stiff and clumsy. In severe cases, thumb muscles diminish in size.

In more severe cases of CTS, it may be necessary to diminish pressure on the nerve and increase the size of the carpal tunnel by surgically dividing the transverse carpal ligament.

Crucial to the healing process and sustained relief is a highly motivated patient willing to modify his or her lifestyle or work environment to eliminate repeated stress on the hands.

Risk Factors
Female
40 or older
Job or hobbies involve highly repetitive tasks
Diabetes
Rheumatoid arthritis
Hypothyroidism
Pregnancy
Trauma to wrist
Menopause
Obesity

© 1995, 2000 ◼ Wolters Kluwer   Anatomical Chart Company, Skokie, IL. Medical illustrations by Claudia M. Grosz, CMI, in consultation with Dr. Thomas Hitchcock, Marshfield Clinic, and Dr. Joseph D'Silva, D'Silva Orthopedic Center.

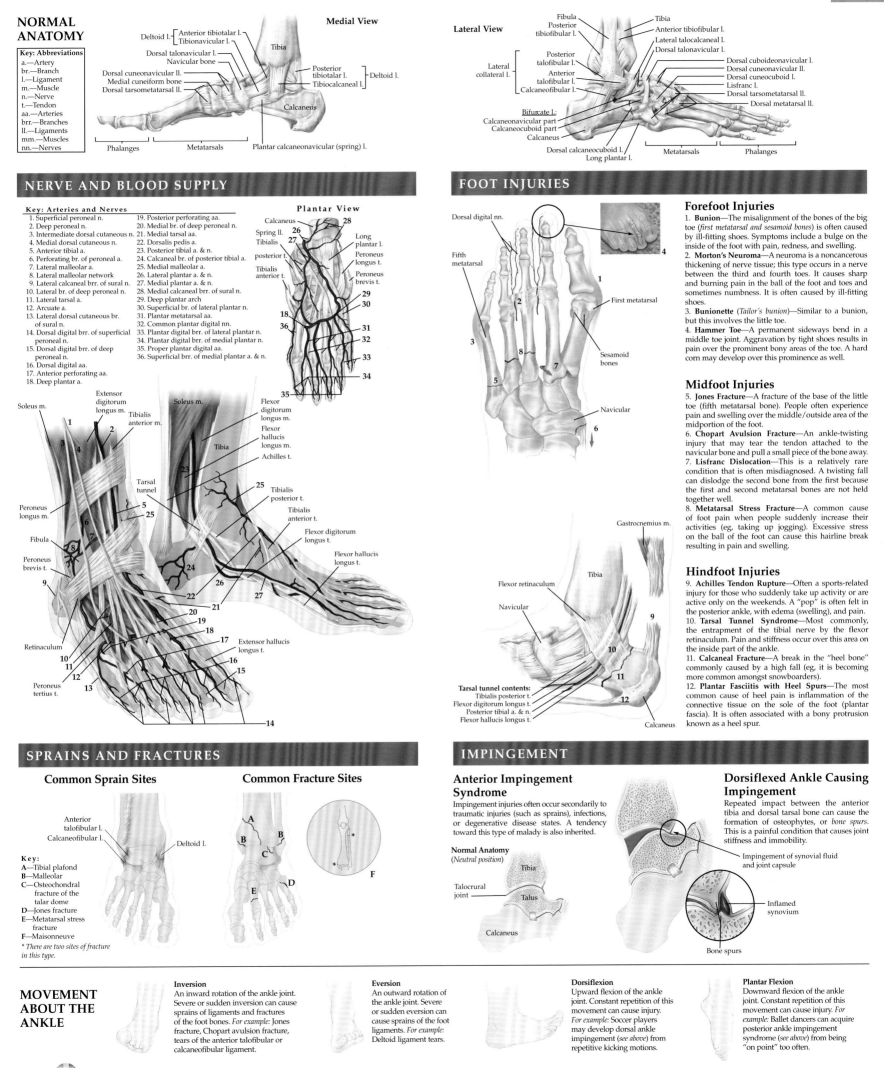

NORMAL ANATOMY

Key: Abbreviations
a.—Artery
br.—Branch
l.—Ligament
m.—Muscle
n.—Nerve
t.—Tendon
aa.—Arteries
brr.—Branches
ll.—Ligaments
mm.—Muscles
nn.—Nerves

Medial View

Deltoid l.
Anterior tibiotalar l.
Tibionavicular l.
Dorsal talonavicular l.
Navicular bone
Dorsal cuneonavicular ll.
Medial cuneiform bone
Dorsal tarsometatarsal ll.
Tibia
Posterior tibiotalar l.
Deltoid l.
Tibiocalcaneal l.
Calcaneus
Phalanges
Metatarsals
Plantar calcaneonavicular (spring) l.

Lateral View

Fibula
Posterior tibiofibular l.
Lateral collateral l.
Posterior talofibular l.
Anterior talofibular l.
Calcaneofibular l.
Bifurcate l.:
Calcaneonavicular part
Calcaneocuboid part
Calcaneus
Dorsal calcaneocuboid l.
Long plantar l.
Tibia
Anterior tibiofibular l.
Lateral talocalcaneal l.
Dorsal talonavicular l.
Dorsal cuboideonavicular ll.
Dorsal cuneonavicular ll.
Dorsal cuneocuboid l.
Lisfranc l.
Dorsal tarsometatarsal ll.
Dorsal metatarsal ll.
Metatarsals
Phalanges

NERVE AND BLOOD SUPPLY

Key: Arteries and Nerves
1. Superficial peroneal n.
2. Deep peroneal n.
3. Intermediate dorsal cutaneous n.
4. Medial dorsal cutaneous n.
5. Anterior tibial a.
6. Perforating br. of peroneal a.
7. Lateral malleolar a.
8. Lateral malleolar network
9. Lateral calcaneal brr. of sural n.
10. Lateral br. of deep peroneal n.
11. Lateral tarsal a.
12. Arcuate a.
13. Lateral dorsal cutaneous br. of sural n.
14. Dorsal digital brr. of superficial peroneal n.
15. Dorsal digital brr. of deep peroneal n.
16. Dorsal digital aa.
17. Anterior perforating aa.
18. Deep plantar a.
19. Posterior perforating aa.
20. Medial br. of deep peroneal n.
21. Medial tarsal aa.
22. Dorsalis pedis a.
23. Posterior tibial a. & n.
24. Calcaneal br. of posterior tibial a.
25. Medial malleolar a.
26. Lateral plantar a. & n.
27. Medial plantar a. & n.
28. Medial calcaneal brr. of sural n.
29. Deep plantar arch
30. Superficial br. of lateral plantar n.
31. Plantar metatarsal aa.
32. Common plantar digital nn.
33. Plantar digital brr. of lateral plantar n.
34. Plantar digital brr. of medial plantar n.
35. Proper plantar digital aa.
36. Superficial brr. of medial plantar a. & n.

Plantar View

Calcaneus 28
Spring ll. 26
Tibialis posterior t. 27
Tibialis anterior t.
Long plantar l.
Peroneus longus t.
Peroneus brevis t. 29
30
18
36
31
32
33
34
35

Soleus m.
Extensor digitorum longus m.
Tibialis anterior m.
1
2
3
4
Soleus m.
Flexor digitorum longus m.
Flexor hallucis longus m.
Achilles t.
Tibia
23
25
Tibialis posterior t.
Tibialis anterior t.
Flexor digitorum longus t.
Flexor hallucis longus t.
Tarsal tunnel
5
25
Peroneus longus m.
6
7
Fibula
8
Peroneus brevis t.
9
24
26
22
20
21
27
19
18
17
Retinaculum
10
11
12
13
Peroneus tertius t.
14
Extensor hallucis longus t.
16
15

FOOT INJURIES

Dorsal digital nn.
Fifth metatarsal
3
2
1
First metatarsal
8
5
7
Sesamoid bones
Navicular
6
4

Forefoot Injuries

1. **Bunion**—The misalignment of the bones of the big toe (*first metatarsal and sesamoid bones*) is often caused by ill-fitting shoes. Symptoms include a bulge on the inside of the foot with pain, redness, and swelling.
2. **Morton's Neuroma**—A neuroma is a noncancerous thickening of nerve tissue; this type occurs in a nerve between the third and fourth toes. It causes sharp and burning pain in the ball of the foot and toes and sometimes numbness. It is often caused by ill-fitting shoes.
3. **Bunionette** (*Tailor's bunion*)—Similar to a bunion, but this involves the little toe.
4. **Hammer Toe**—A permanent sideways bend in a middle toe joint. Aggravation by tight shoes results in pain over the prominent bony areas of the toe. A hard corn may develop over this prominence as well.

Midfoot Injuries

5. **Jones Fracture**—A fracture of the base of the little toe (fifth metatarsal bone). People often experience pain and swelling over the middle/outside area of the midportion of the foot.
6. **Chopart Avulsion Fracture**—An ankle-twisting injury that may tear the tendon attached to the navicular bone and pull a small piece of the bone away.
7. **Lisfranc Dislocation**—This is a relatively rare condition that is often misdiagnosed. A twisting fall can dislodge the second bone from the first because the first and second metatarsal bones are not held together well.
8. **Metatarsal Stress Fracture**—A common cause of foot pain when people suddenly increase their activities (eg, taking up jogging). Excessive stress on the ball of the foot can cause this hairline break resulting in pain and swelling.

Hindfoot Injuries

9. **Achilles Tendon Rupture**—Often a sports-related injury for those who suddenly take up activity or are active only on the weekends. A "pop" is often felt in the posterior ankle, with edema (swelling), and pain.
10. **Tarsal Tunnel Syndrome**—Most commonly, the entrapment of the tibial nerve by the flexor retinaculum. Pain and stiffness occur over this area on the inside part of the ankle.
11. **Calcaneal Fracture**—A break in the "heel bone" commonly caused by a high fall (eg, it is becoming more common amongst snowboarders).
12. **Plantar Fasciitis with Heel Spurs**—The most common cause of heel pain is inflammation of the connective tissue on the sole of the foot (plantar fascia). It is often associated with a bony protrusion known as a heel spur.

Gastrocnemius m.
Tibia
Flexor retinaculum
Navicular
9
10
11
12
Tarsal tunnel contents:
Tibialis posterior t.
Flexor digitorum longus t.
Posterior tibial a. & n.
Flexor hallucis longus t.
Calcaneus

SPRAINS AND FRACTURES

Common Sprain Sites

Anterior talofibular l.
Calcaneofibular l.
Deltoid l.

Key:
A—Tibial plafond
B—Malleolar
C—Osteochondral fracture of the talar dome
D—Jones fracture
E—Metatarsal stress fracture
F—Maisonneuve
* There are two sites of fracture in this type.

Common Fracture Sites

A
B
B
B
C
D
E
F
*
*

IMPINGEMENT

Anterior Impingement Syndrome

Impingement injuries often occur secondarily to traumatic injuries (such as sprains), infections, or degenerative disease states. A tendency toward this type of malady is also inherited.

Normal Anatomy
(*Neutral position*)
Talocrural joint
Tibia
Talus
Calcaneus

Dorsiflexed Ankle Causing Impingement

Repeated impact between the anterior tibia and dorsal tarsal bone can cause the formation of osteophytes, or *bone spurs*. This is a painful condition that causes joint stiffness and immobility.

Impingement of synovial fluid and joint capsule
Inflamed synovium
Bone spurs

MOVEMENT ABOUT THE ANKLE

Inversion
An inward rotation of the ankle joint. Severe or sudden inversion can cause sprains of ligaments and fractures of the foot bones. *For example:* Jones fracture, Chopart avulsion fracture, tears of the anterior talofibular or calcaneofibular ligament.

Eversion
An outward rotation of the ankle joint. Severe or sudden eversion can cause sprains of the foot ligaments. *For example:* Deltoid ligament tears.

Dorsiflexion
Upward flexion of the ankle joint. Constant repetition of this movement can cause injury. *For example:* Soccer players may develop dorsal ankle impingement (*see above*) from repetitive kicking motions.

Plantar Flexion
Downward flexion of the ankle joint. Constant repetition of this movement can cause injury. *For example:* Ballet dancers can acquire posterior ankle impingement syndrome (*see above*) from being "on point" too often.

© 2004 **Wolters Kluwer** Anatomical Chart Company, Skokie, IL. Medical illustrations by Megan E. Bluhm, MA, in consultation with Mark R. Hutchinson, MD, University of Illinois at Chicago.

NORMAL ANATOMY

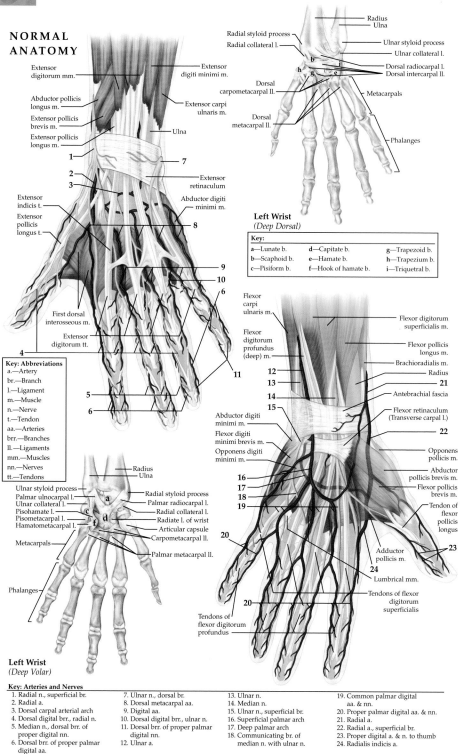

Extensor digitorum mm.
Abductor pollicis longus m.
Extensor pollicis brevis m.
Extensor pollicis longus m.
Extensor digiti minimi m.
Extensor carpi ulnaris m.
Ulna
1
2
3
Extensor indicis t.
Extensor pollicis longus t.
Extensor retinaculum
Abductor digiti minimi m.
7
8
First dorsal interosseous m.
Extensor digitorum tt.
9
10
6
11
4
5
6

Key: Abbreviations
a.—Artery
br.—Branch
l.—Ligament
m.—Muscle
n.—Nerve
t.—Tendon
aa.—Arteries
brr.—Branches
ll.—Ligaments
mm.—Muscles
nn.—Nerves
tt.—Tendons

Radius
Ulna
Radial styloid process
Radial collateral l.
Ulnar styloid process
Ulnar collateral l.
Dorsal radiocarpal l.
Dorsal intercarpal ll.
Dorsal carpometacarpal ll.
Metacarpals
Dorsal metacarpal ll.
Phalanges

Left Wrist
(Deep Dorsal)

Key:
a—Lunate b.
b—Scaphoid b.
c—Pisiform b.
d—Capitate b.
e—Hamate b.
f—Hook of hamate b.
g—Trapezoid b.
h—Trapezium b.
i—Triquetral b.

Flexor carpi ulnaris m.
Flexor digitorum profundus (deep) m.
Flexor digitorum superficialis m.
Flexor pollicis longus m.
Brachioradialis m.
12
13
14
15
Radius
21
Antebrachial fascia
Flexor retinaculum (Transverse carpal l.)
Abductor digiti minimi m.
Flexor digiti minimi brevis m.
Opponens digiti minimi m.
22
Opponens pollicis m.
Abductor pollicis brevis m.
Flexor pollicis brevis m.
Tendon of flexor pollicis longus
16
17
18
19
20
20
Adductor pollicis m.
23
24
Lumbrical mm.
Tendons of flexor digitorum superficialis
Tendons of flexor digitorum profundus

Radius
Ulna
Ulnar styloid process
Palmar ulnocarpal l.
Ulnar collateral l.
Pisohamate l.
Pisometacarpal l.
Hamatometacarpal l.
Metacarpals
Radial styloid process
Palmar radiocarpal l.
Radial collateral l.
Radiate l. of wrist
Articular capsule
Carpometacarpal ll.
Palmar metacarpal ll.
Phalanges

Left Wrist
(Deep Volar)

Key: Arteries and Nerves

1. Radial n., superficial br.
2. Radial a.
3. Dorsal carpal arterial arch
4. Dorsal digital brr., radial a.
5. Median n., dorsal brr. of proper digital nn.
6. Dorsal brr. of proper palmar digital aa.
7. Ulnar n., dorsal br.
8. Dorsal metacarpal aa.
9. Digital aa.
10. Dorsal digital brr., ulnar a.
11. Dorsal brr. of proper palmar digital nn.
12. Ulnar a.
13. Ulnar n.
14. Median n.
15. Ulnar n., superficial br.
16. Superficial palmar arch
17. Deep palmar arch
18. Communicating br. of median n. with ulnar n.
19. Common palmar digital aa. & nn.
20. Proper palmar digital aa. & nn.
21. Radial a.
22. Radial a., superficial br.
23. Proper digital a. & n. to thumb
24. Radialis indicis a.

FRACTURES

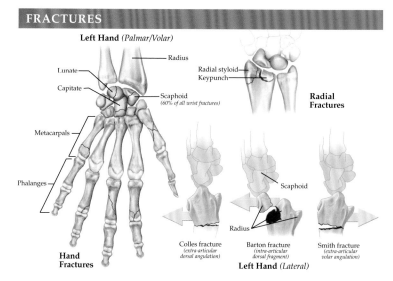

Left Hand *(Palmar/Volar)*

Radius
Lunate
Capitate
Scaphoid *(60% of all wrist fractures)*
Metacarpals
Phalanges

Radial styloid
Keypunch

Radial Fractures

Scaphoid
Radius

Hand Fractures

Colles fracture *(extra-articular dorsal angulation)*
Barton fracture *(intra-articular dorsal fragment)*
Smith fracture *(extra-articular volar angulation)*

Left Hand *(Lateral)*

HAND AND WRIST INJURIES

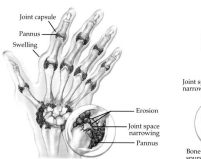

Joint capsule
Pannus
Swelling
Erosion
Joint space narrowing
Pannus

Heberden nodes
Bouchard nodes
Joint space narrowing
Bone spurs

Rheumatoid Arthritis (RA)

A chronic disease that develops over weeks or months, most often between the ages of 25 and 50, it causes a general feeling of sickness, plus fatigue, weight loss, and fever. This type of arthritis usually affects the same joint on both sides of the body with redness, warmth, and swelling. Deformity occurs in later stages of the disease.

Osteoarthritis (OA)

The most common type of arthritis, it primarily affects hyaline cartilage, the articulating surface covering the ends of the bones of the fingers and wrist. It can cause joint pain and stiffness and usually develops over many years, usually caused by trauma or simple wear and tear. Spurs and sclerosis are common findings unlike RA where erosions occur.

Carpal Tunnel Syndrome (CTS)

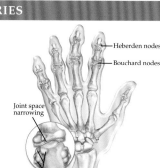

Normal Wrist Cross-Section
Median n.
Flexor retinaculum
Carpal bones
Flexor tendons

Cross Section of Affected Wrist
Compressed median n.
Inflamed tendon synovial sheaths

This common disorder causes pain, numbness, and weakness in the hand and is associated with compression of the median nerve against the inelastic transverse carpal ligament in the wrist. Continuous or periodic compression on the nerve can cause damage over time. It has a variety of causes, but it is most commonly caused by repetitive movements (eg, typing on a keyboard) that expose the nerve to compression forces and stretching.

Finger Maladies

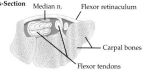

Tendon
A1 pulley
Inflamed nodule
Stuck nodule impairing extension of the finger

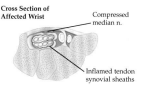

Cross section of a joint
Bursa
Bursitis
Tendon
Tendonitis
Joint capsule

Bursitis—inflammation of a bursa, the sack that separates bone from muscle near a joint.

Tendonitis—inflammation of a tendon.

Trigger Finger

A type of tenosynovitis (inflammation of the tendon and synovium), it is characterized by the inability to extend a finger after it has been flexed. An inflamed nodule in the tendon is trapped proximal to the first flexor tendon pulley.

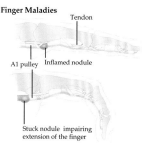

Cyst that has ballooned out from a defect in the synovial membrane of the carpometacarpal joint

Third metacarpal
Capitate
Synovial membrane

Ganglion Cyst

Occurring most often on the back of the wrist or hand, this sac is filled with the synovial fluid from a nearby joint. It is a hernia of the joint's capsule that causes the bulge. A volar wrist ganglion is less common.

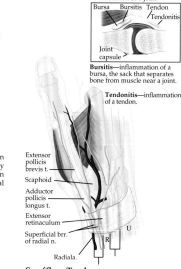

Extensor pollicis brevis t.
Scaphoid
Adductor pollicis longus t.
Extensor retinaculum
Superficial brr. of radial n.
Radial a.

Snuffbox Tenderness

The anatomical snuffbox is a superficial concavity near the radius (R) that is bound by tendons of the thumb. The radial artery passes through this space. The tendon sheaths that pass beneath the extensor retinaculum can become inflamed, causing tenderness and swelling, or de Quervain tenosynovitis. Another very common cause of pain in this region is a fracture of the scaphoid bone.

MOVEMENT ABOUT THE WRIST AND FINGERS

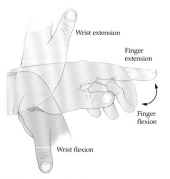

Wrist extension
Finger extension
Finger flexion
Wrist flexion

Flexion/Extension/Hyperextension

These movements occur between the forearm bones (radius and ulna) and the carpal bones of the wrist. The most common cause of wrist trauma is a fall on an extended wrist (eg, Colles, Barton, scaphoid fractures). Hyperextension of the fingers can lead to dislocation and ligament injuries on the volar aspect of the finger.

Supination/Pronation

Supination is the act of turning you palm face-up ("holds soup"), while pronation is turning your hand down facing the floor. Falls on an outstretched hand in extreme pronation have been associated with dorsal dislocations at the radioulnar (wrist) joint. A fall with the hand outstretched in a supinated position can cause a fracture of the radius (R) or volar dislocation of the radioulnar joint.

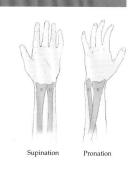

Supination
Pronation

Thumb Opposition

The ability to touch the thumb to the fifth digit (pinky finger) is the human being's unique advantage in the animal kingdom. It allows us to perform many ordinary, but essential, daily tasks, such as holding a pen or eating with a fork. Any injury to the median nerve (including carpal tunnel syndrome) inhibits our ability to use the thumb in this manner.

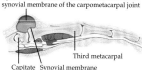

© 2005 Wolters Kluwer

Anatomical Chart Company, Skokie, IL. Medical illustrations by Megan E. Bluhm, MA in consultation with Mark R. Hutchinson, MD, University of Illinois at Chicago.

Normal Anatomy of the Hip Region

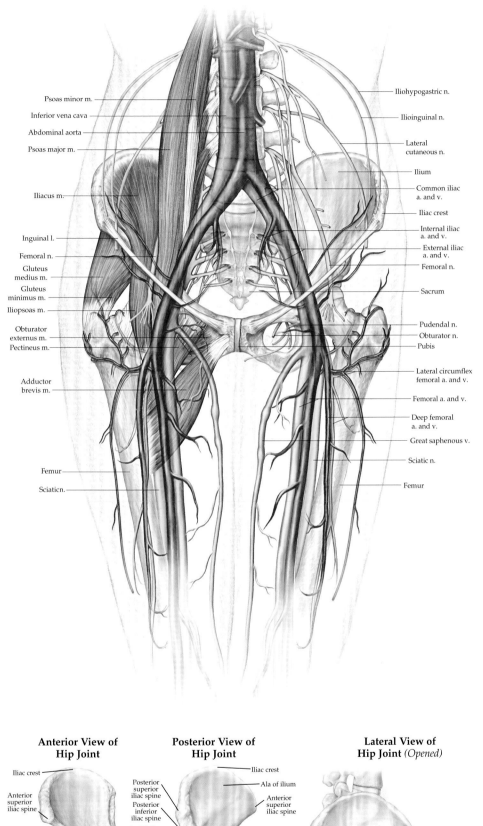

Psoas minor m.
Inferior vena cava
Abdominal aorta
Psoas major m.
Iliacus m.
Inguinal l.
Femoral n.
Gluteus medius m.
Gluteus minimus m.
Iliopsoas m.
Obturator externus m.
Pectineus m.
Adductor brevis m.
Femur
Sciaticn.

Iliohypogastric n.
Ilioinguinal n.
Lateral cutaneous n.
Ilium
Common iliac a. and v.
Iliac crest
Internal iliac a. and v.
External iliac a. and v.
Femoral n.
Sacrum
Pudendal n.
Obturator n.
Pubis
Lateral circumflex femoral a. and v.
Femoral a. and v.
Deep femoral a. and v.
Great saphenous v.
Sciatic n.
Femur

BLOOD SUPPLY AND INJURIES

Cross-section of Hip Joint Area

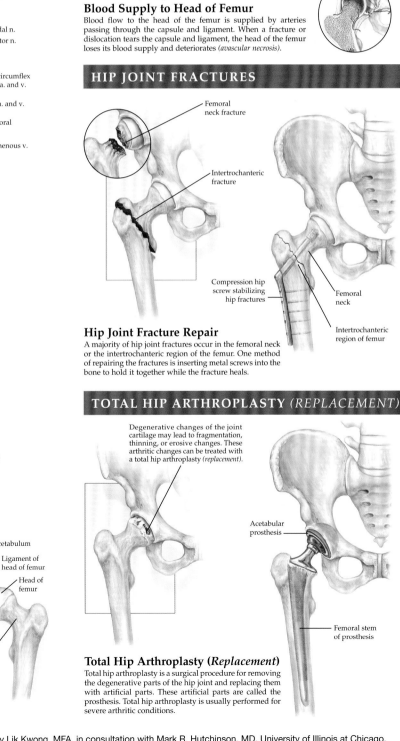

Retinacular aa.
Deep femoral a.
Lateral circumflex femoral a.:
Ascending
Transverse
Descending branches

Obturator a.
Medial circumflex femoral a.

Intertrochanteric Fracture

Head of femur
Capsule
Neck of femur

Femoral Neck Fracture

Necrosis

Dislocation

Necrosis

Blood Supply to Head of Femur

Blood flow to the head of the femur is supplied by arteries passing through the capsule and ligament. When a fracture or dislocation tears the capsule and ligament, the head of the femur loses its blood supply and deteriorates (*avascular necrosis*).

HIP JOINT FRACTURES

Femoral neck fracture

Intertrochanteric fracture

Compression hip screw stabilizing hip fractures

Femoral neck

Intertrochanteric region of femur

Hip Joint Fracture Repair

A majority of hip joint fractures occur in the femoral neck or the intertrochanteric region of the femur. One method of repairing the fractures is inserting metal screws into the bone to hold it together while the fracture heals.

TOTAL HIP ARTHROPLASTY (*REPLACEMENT*)

Degenerative changes of the joint cartilage may lead to fragmentation, thinning, or erosive changes. These arthritic changes can be treated with a total hip arthroplasty (*replacement*).

Acetabular prosthesis

Femoral stem of prosthesis

Total Hip Arthroplasty (*Replacement*)

Total hip arthroplasty is a surgical procedure for removing the degenerative parts of the hip joint and replacing them with artificial parts. These artificial parts are called the prosthesis. Total hip arthroplasty is usually performed for severe arthritic conditions.

Anterior View of Hip Joint

Iliac crest
Anterior superior iliac spine
Anterior inferior iliac spine
Iliofemoral l.
Ischium
Lesser trochanter
Pubic symphysis

Posterior View of Hip Joint

Posterior superior iliac spine
Posterior inferior iliac spine
Acetabulum
Ischial spine
Pubofemoral l.
Superior pubic ramus
Obturator foramen
Ischial tuberosity
Lesser trochanter
Femur

Iliac crest
Ala of ilium
Anterior superior iliac spine
Iliofemoral l.
Ischiofemoral l.
Greater trochanter
Zona orbicularis

Lateral View of Hip Joint (*Opened*)

Acetabulum
Ligament of head of femur
Head of femur
Neck of femur
Fat in acetabular fossa

Key: Abbreviations
Artery—a. Arteries—aa. Vein—v. Muscle—m. Ligament—l. Nerve—n.

Hip and Knee Inflammations

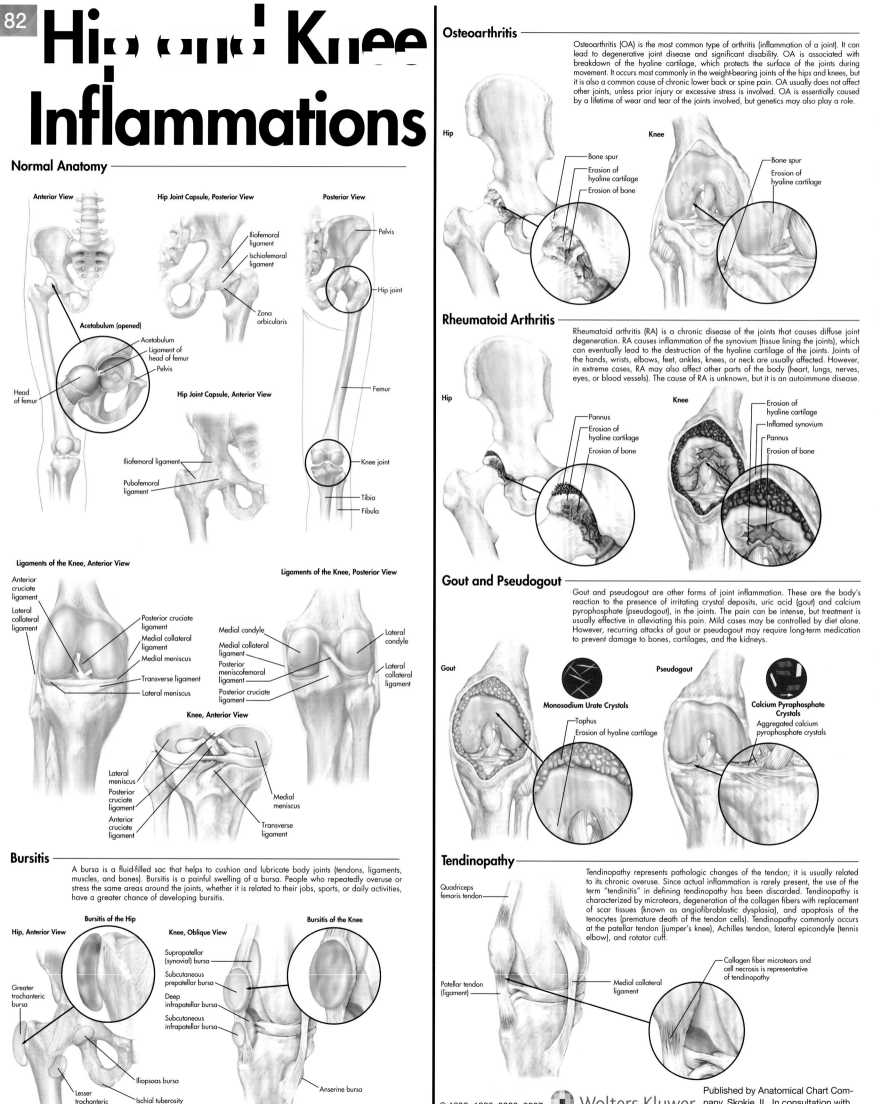

Normal Anatomy

Anterior View

Head of femur

Acetabulum (opened)
- Acetabulum
- Ligament of head of femur
- Pelvis

Hip Joint Capsule, Posterior View
- Iliofemoral ligament
- Ischiofemoral ligament
- Zona orbicularis

Hip Joint Capsule, Anterior View
- Iliofemoral ligament
- Pubofemoral ligament

Posterior View
- Pelvis
- Hip joint
- Femur
- Knee joint
- Tibia
- Fibula

Ligaments of the Knee, Anterior View
- Anterior cruciate ligament
- Lateral collateral ligament
- Posterior cruciate ligament
- Medial collateral ligament
- Medial meniscus
- Transverse ligament
- Lateral meniscus

Ligaments of the Knee, Posterior View
- Medial condyle
- Medial collateral ligament
- Posterior meniscofemoral ligament
- Posterior cruciate ligament
- Lateral condyle
- Lateral collateral ligament

Knee, Anterior View
- Lateral meniscus
- Posterior cruciate ligament
- Anterior cruciate ligament
- Medial meniscus
- Transverse ligament

Bursitis

A bursa is a fluid-filled sac that helps to cushion and lubricate body joints (tendons, ligaments, muscles, and bones). Bursitis is a painful swelling of a bursa. People who repeatedly overuse or stress the same areas around the joints, whether it is related to their jobs, sports, or daily activities, have a greater chance of developing bursitis.

Bursitis of the Hip

Hip, Anterior View
- Greater trochanteric bursa
- Lesser trochanteric bursa
- Iliopsoas bursa
- Ischial tuberosity bursa

Knee, Oblique View
- Suprapatellar (synovial) bursa
- Subcutaneous prepatellar bursa
- Deep infrapatellar bursa
- Subcutaneous infrapatellar bursa
- Anserine bursa

Bursitis of the Knee

Osteoarthritis

Osteoarthritis (OA) is the most common type of arthritis (inflammation of a joint). It can lead to degenerative joint disease and significant disability. OA is associated with breakdown of the hyaline cartilage, which protects the surface of the joints during movement. It occurs most commonly in the weight-bearing joints of the hips and knees, but it is also a common cause of chronic lower back or spine pain. OA usually does not affect other joints, unless prior injury or excessive stress is involved. OA is essentially caused by a lifetime of wear and tear of the joints involved, but genetics may also play a role.

Hip
- Bone spur
- Erosion of hyaline cartilage
- Erosion of bone

Knee
- Bone spur
- Erosion of hyaline cartilage

Rheumatoid Arthritis

Rheumatoid arthritis (RA) is a chronic disease of the joints that causes diffuse joint degeneration. RA causes inflammation of the synovium (tissue lining the joints), which can eventually lead to the destruction of the hyaline cartilage of the joints. Joints of the hands, wrists, elbows, feet, ankles, knees, or neck are usually affected. However, in extreme cases, RA may also affect other parts of the body (heart, lungs, nerves, eyes, or blood vessels). The cause of RA is unknown, but it is an autoimmune disease.

Hip
- Pannus
- Erosion of hyaline cartilage
- Erosion of bone

Knee
- Erosion of hyaline cartilage
- Inflamed synovium
- Pannus
- Erosion of bone

Gout and Pseudogout

Gout and pseudogout are other forms of joint inflammation. These are the body's reaction to the presence of irritating crystal deposits, uric acid (gout) and calcium pyrophosphate (pseudogout), in the joints. The pain can be intense, but treatment is usually effective in alleviating this pain. Mild cases may be controlled by diet alone. However, recurring attacks of gout or pseudogout may require long-term medication to prevent damage to bones, cartilages, and the kidneys.

Gout
- Tophus
- Erosion of hyaline cartilage

Monosodium Urate Crystals

Pseudogout

Calcium Pyrophosphate Crystals
- Aggregated calcium pyrophosphate crystals

Tendinopathy

Tendinopathy represents pathologic changes of the tendon; it is usually related to its chronic overuse. Since actual inflammation is rarely present, the use of the term "tendinitis" in defining tendinopathy has been discarded. Tendinopathy is characterized by microtears, degeneration of the collagen fibers with replacement of scar tissues (known as angiofibroblastic dysplasia), and apoptosis of the tenocytes (premature death of the tendon cells). Tendinopathy commonly occurs at the patellar tendon (jumper's knee), Achilles tendon, lateral epicondyle (tennis elbow), and rotator cuff.

- Quadriceps femoris tendon
- Patellar tendon (ligament)
- Medial collateral ligament
- Collagen fiber microtears and cell necrosis is representative of tendinopathy

Wolters Kluwer — Published by Anatomical Chart Company, Skokie, IL. In consultation with Mark R. Hutchinson, MD.

KNEE INJURIES

Anterior View of Normal Knee
(Patella removed)

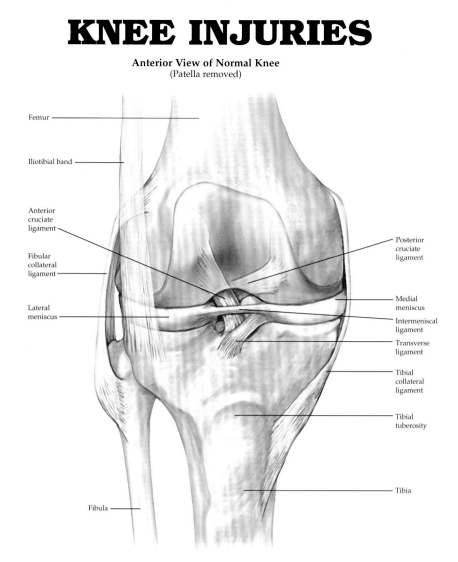

- Femur
- Iliotibial band
- Anterior cruciate ligament
- Fibular collateral ligament
- Lateral meniscus
- Fibula
- Posterior cruciate ligament
- Medial meniscus
- Intermeniscal ligament
- Transverse ligament
- Tibial collateral ligament
- Tibial tuberosity
- Tibia

Oblique View

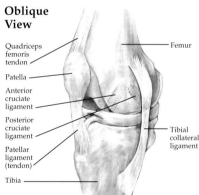

- Quadriceps femoris tendon
- Patella
- Anterior cruciate ligament
- Posterior cruciate ligament
- Patellar ligament (tendon)
- Tibia
- Femur
- Tibial collateral ligament

Posterior View

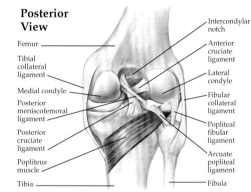

- Femur
- Tibial collateral ligament
- Medial condyle
- Posterior meniscofemoral ligament
- Posterior cruciate ligament
- Popliteus muscle
- Tibia
- Intercondylar notch
- Anterior cruciate ligament
- Lateral condyle
- Fibular collateral ligament
- Popliteal fibular ligament
- Arcuate popliteal ligament
- Fibula

Traumatic Knee Injuries

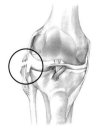

Ligament tear   Bone avulsion   Ligament sprain   Patellar dislocation

Sports-Related Ligament Injuries

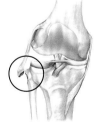

Sudden posterior movement of the tibia while the knee is flexed at 90 degrees may damage the posterior cruciate ligament.

Hyperextension of the knee joint can damage the anterior cruciate and tibial collateral ligaments.

Forcible external rotation of the foot in the "whip-kick" causes the lower leg to twist at the knee, putting excessive strain on the tibial collateral ligament. It can also cause plical irritation or exacerbate patellar instability.

A lateral blow to the knees while the feet are firmly planted may cause damage to the tibial and fibular collateral ligaments.

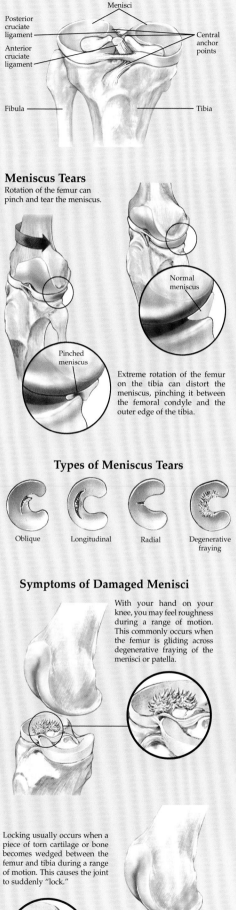

Meniscus

The meniscus is a crescent-shaped piece of cartilage that lies between the femur and tibia. Each knee has two menisci, one medial and one lateral. Together, they cushion the joint by distributing downward forces outward and away from the central anchor points of the menisci.

- Posterior cruciate ligament
- Anterior cruciate ligament
- Fibula
- Menisci
- Central anchor points
- Tibia

Meniscus Tears

Rotation of the femur can pinch and tear the meniscus.

- Pinched meniscus
- Normal meniscus

Extreme rotation of the femur on the tibia can distort the meniscus, pinching it between the femoral condyle and the outer edge of the tibia.

Types of Meniscus Tears

Oblique   Longitudinal   Radial   Degenerative fraying

Symptoms of Damaged Menisci

With your hand on your knee, you may feel roughness during a range of motion. This commonly occurs when the femur is gliding across degenerative fraying of the menisci or patella.

Locking usually occurs when a piece of torn cartilage or bone becomes wedged between the femur and tibia during a range of motion. This causes the joint to suddenly "lock."

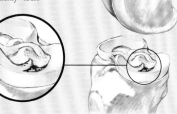

Athletic Injuries of the Knee

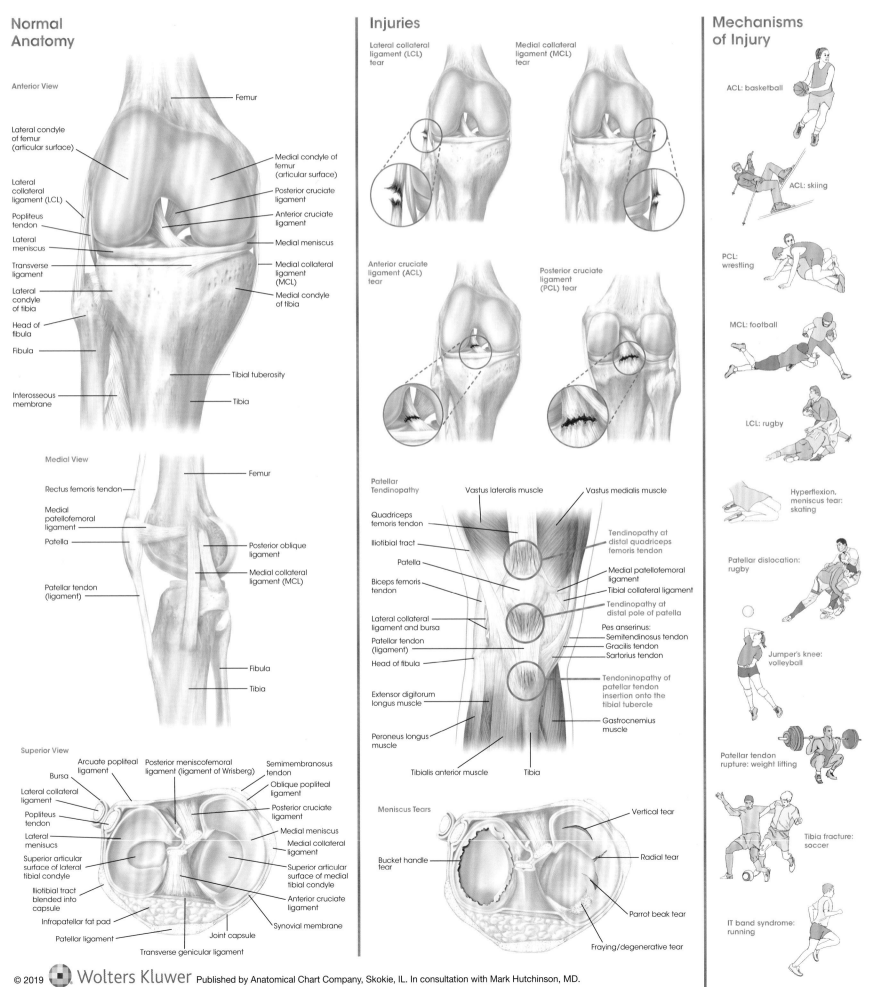

Normal Anatomy

Anterior View

- Femur
- Lateral condyle of femur (articular surface)
- Lateral collateral ligament (LCL)
- Popliteus tendon
- Lateral meniscus
- Transverse ligament
- Lateral condyle of tibia
- Head of fibula
- Fibula
- Interosseous membrane
- Medial condyle of femur (articular surface)
- Posterior cruciate ligament
- Anterior cruciate ligament
- Medial meniscus
- Medial collateral ligament (MCL)
- Medial condyle of tibia
- Tibial tuberosity
- Tibia

Medial View

- Femur
- Rectus femoris tendon
- Medial patellofemoral ligament
- Patella
- Patellar tendon (ligament)
- Posterior oblique ligament
- Medial collateral ligament (MCL)
- Fibula
- Tibia

Superior View

- Arcuate popliteal ligament
- Bursa
- Lateral collateral ligament
- Popliteus tendon
- Lateral menisucs
- Superior articular surface of lateral tibial condyle
- Iliotibial tract blended into capsule
- Infrapatellar fat pad
- Patellar ligament
- Posterior meniscofemoral ligament (ligament of Wrisberg)
- Semimembranosus tendon
- Oblique popliteal ligament
- Posterior cruciate ligament
- Medial meniscus
- Medial collateral ligament
- Superior articular surface of medial tibial condyle
- Anterior cruciate ligament
- Synovial membrane
- Transverse genicular ligament
- Joint capsule

Injuries

- Lateral collateral ligament (LCL) tear
- Medial collateral ligament (MCL) tear
- Anterior cruciate ligament (ACL) tear
- Posterior cruciate ligament (PCL) tear

Patellar Tendinopathy

- Vastus lateralis muscle
- Vastus medialis muscle
- Quadriceps femoris tendon
- Iliotibial tract
- Patella
- Biceps femoris tendon
- Lateral collateral ligament and bursa
- Patellar tendon (ligament)
- Head of fibula
- Extensor digitorum longus muscle
- Peroneus longus muscle
- Tibialis anterior muscle
- Tibia
- Tendinopathy at distal quadriceps femoris tendon
- Medial patellofemoral ligament
- Tibial collateral ligament
- Tendinopathy at distal pole of patella
- Pes anserinus: Semitendinosus tendon, Gracilis tendon, Sartorius tendon
- Tendoninopathy of patellar tendon insertion onto the tibial tubercle
- Gastrocnemius muscle

Meniscus Tears

- Bucket handle tear
- Vertical tear
- Radial tear
- Parrot beak tear
- Fraying/degenerative tear

Mechanisms of Injury

- ACL: basketball
- ACL: skiing
- PCL: wrestling
- MCL: football
- LCL: rugby
- Hyperflexion, meniscus tear: skating
- Patellar dislocation: rugby
- Jumper's knee: volleyball
- Patellar tendon rupture: weight lifting
- Tibia fracture: soccer
- IT band syndrome: running

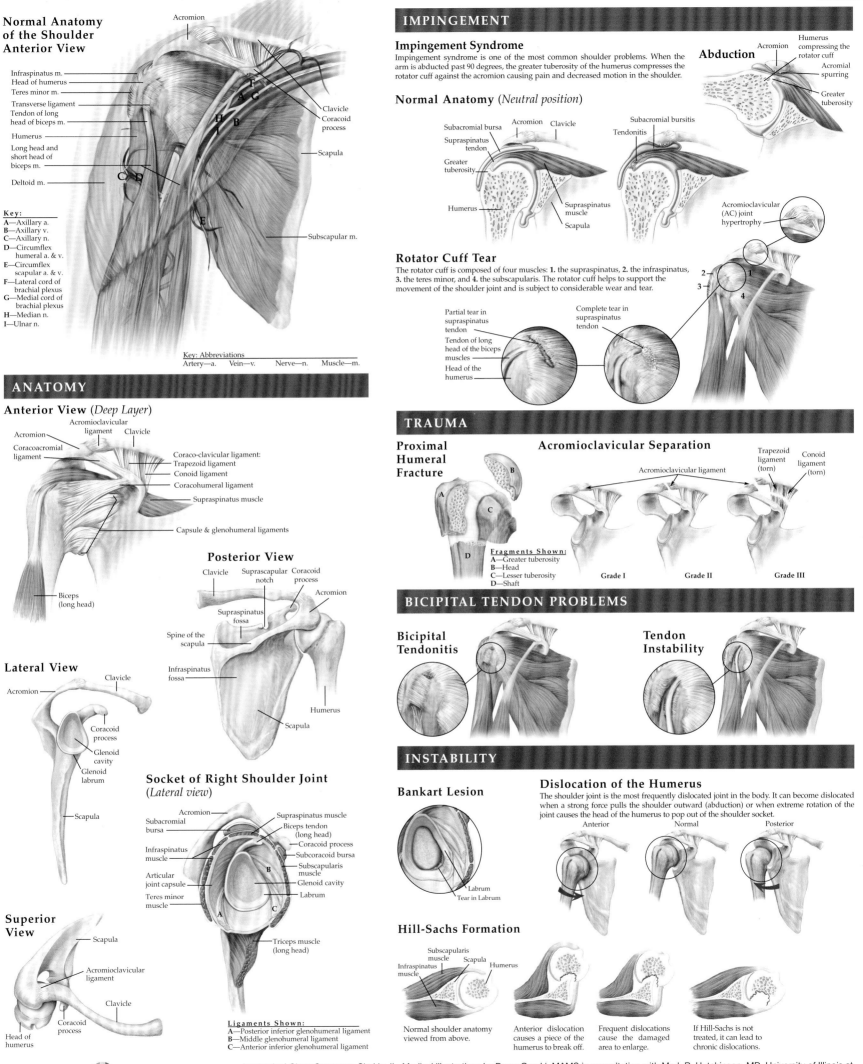

Normal Anatomy of the Shoulder Anterior View

Acromion

Infraspinatus m.
Head of humerus
Teres minor m.
Transverse ligament
Tendon of long head of biceps m.
Humerus
Long head and short head of biceps m.
Deltoid m.

Clavicle
Coracoid process
Scapula

Subscapular m.

Key:
A—Axillary a.
B—Axillary v.
C—Axillary n.
D—Circumflex humeral a. & v.
E—Circumflex scapular a. & v.
F—Lateral cord of brachial plexus
G—Medial cord of brachial plexus
H—Median n.
I—Ulnar n.

Key: Abbreviations
Artery—a.   Vein—v.   Nerve—n.   Muscle—m.

ANATOMY

Anterior View (Deep Layer)

Acromioclavicular ligament   Clavicle
Acromion
Coracoacromial ligament
Coraco-clavicular ligament:
Trapezoid ligament
Conoid ligament
Coracohumeral ligament
Supraspinatus muscle
Capsule & glenohumeral ligaments
Biceps (long head)

Posterior View

Clavicle   Suprascapular notch   Coracoid process
Acromion
Supraspinatus fossa
Spine of the scapula
Infraspinatus fossa
Humerus
Scapula

Lateral View

Clavicle
Acromion
Coracoid process
Glenoid cavity
Glenoid labrum
Scapula

Socket of Right Shoulder Joint
(Lateral view)

Acromion
Subacromial bursa
Infraspinatus muscle
Articular joint capsule
Teres minor muscle
Supraspinatus muscle
Biceps tendon (long head)
Coracoid process
Subcoracoid bursa
Subscapularis muscle
Glenoid cavity
Labrum
Triceps muscle (long head)

Ligaments Shown:
A—Posterior inferior glenohumeral ligament
B—Middle glenohumeral ligament
C—Anterior inferior glenohumeral ligament

Superior View

Scapula
Acromioclavicular ligament
Clavicle
Head of humerus
Coracoid process

IMPINGEMENT

Impingement Syndrome

Impingement syndrome is one of the most common shoulder problems. When the arm is abducted past 90 degrees, the greater tuberosity of the humerus compresses the rotator cuff against the acromion causing pain and decreased motion in the shoulder.

Normal Anatomy (Neutral position)

Subacromial bursa   Acromion   Clavicle
Supraspinatus tendon
Greater tuberosity
Humerus
Supraspinatus muscle
Scapula

Subacromial bursitis
Tendonitis

Abduction
Humerus compressing the rotator cuff
Acromion
Acromial spurring
Greater tuberosity

Acromioclavicular (AC) joint hypertrophy

Rotator Cuff Tear

The rotator cuff is composed of four muscles: **1.** the supraspinatus, **2.** the infraspinatus, **3.** the teres minor, and **4.** the subscapularis. The rotator cuff helps to support the movement of the shoulder joint and is subject to considerable wear and tear.

Partial tear in supraspinatus tendon
Tendon of long head of the biceps muscles
Head of the humerus

Complete tear in supraspinatus tendon

TRAUMA

Proximal Humeral Fracture

Fragments Shown:
A—Greater tuberosity
B—Head
C—Lesser tuberosity
D—Shaft

Acromioclavicular Separation

Acromioclavicular ligament
Trapezoid ligament (torn)
Conoid ligament (torn)

Grade I   Grade II   Grade III

BICIPITAL TENDON PROBLEMS

Bicipital Tendonitis

Tendon Instability

INSTABILITY

Bankart Lesion

Labrum
Tear in Labrum

Dislocation of the Humerus

The shoulder joint is the most frequently dislocated joint in the body. It can become dislocated when a strong force pulls the shoulder outward (abduction) or when extreme rotation of the joint causes the head of the humerus to pop out of the shoulder socket.

Anterior   Normal   Posterior

Hill-Sachs Formation

Subscapularis muscle   Scapula   Humerus
Infraspinatus muscle

Normal shoulder anatomy viewed from above.

Anterior dislocation causes a piece of the humerus to break off.

Frequent dislocations cause the damaged area to enlarge.

If Hill-Sachs is not treated, it can lead to chronic dislocations.

Anatomical Chart Company, Skokie, IL. Medical illustrations by Dawn Gorski, MAMS in consultation with Mark R. Hutchinson, MD, University of Illinois at Chicago.

HUMAN SPINE DISORDERS

The Spinal Column

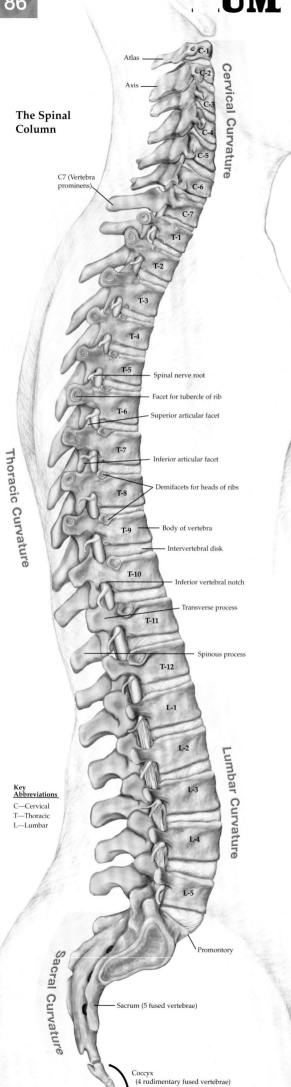

- Atlas
- Axis
- Cervical Curvature
- C-1
- C-2
- C-3
- C-4
- C-5
- C7 (Vertebra prominens)
- C-6
- C-7
- T-1
- T-2
- T-3
- T-4
- T-5 — Spinal nerve root
- — Facet for tubercle of rib
- T-6 — Superior articular facet
- T-7 — Inferior articular facet
- T-8 — Demifacets for heads of ribs
- T-9 — Body of vertebra
- — Intervertebral disk
- T-10 — Inferior vertebral notch
- — Transverse process
- T-11
- T-12 — Spinous process
- Thoracic Curvature
- L-1
- L-2 — Lumbar Curvature
- L-3
- L-4
- L-5
- Promontory
- Sacral Curvature
- Sacrum (5 fused vertebrae)
- Coccyx (4 rudimentary fused vertebrae)

Key Abbreviations
C—Cervical
T—Thoracic
L—Lumbar

Anatomy

A Typical Cervical Vertebra (Superior View)

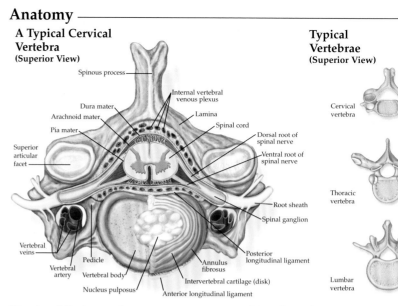

- Spinous process
- Internal vertebral venous plexus
- Dura mater
- Arachnoid mater
- Lamina
- Pia mater
- Spinal cord
- Superior articular facet
- Dorsal root of spinal nerve
- Ventral root of spinal nerve
- Root sheath
- Spinal ganglion
- Vertebral veins
- Posterior longitudinal ligament
- Vertebral artery
- Pedicle
- Annulus fibrosus
- Vertebral body
- Intervertebral cartilage (disk)
- Nucleus pulposus
- Anterior longitudinal ligament

Typical Vertebrae (Superior View)

- Cervical vertebra
- Thoracic vertebra
- Lumbar vertebra

Structural Features of an Intervertebral Disk (Schematic)

- Nucleus pulposus
- Annulus fibrosus

Note alternating obliquity of collagen fibrils.

The nucleus pulposus is the central gelatinous cushioning part of the intervertebral disk enclosed in several layers of cartilaginous laminae. The nucleus pulposus becomes dehydrated with age.

Function of Intervertebral Disks

- Normal
- Weight
- Body
- Disk
- Annulus fibrosus
- Nucleus pulposus

The disk, which contains nucleus pulposus, functions to protect the vertebrae from pressure.

Pathology

Osteoporosis

Osteoporosis develops when the body loses bone more quickly than it can make new bone. As a result, bones become less dense at the core and lose thickness at the surface. This increases the bones' susceptibility to fracture.

When osteoporosis involves the lumbar region, the vertebral bodies become markedly biconcave and the disks are ballooned.

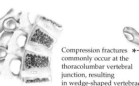

Compression fractures * commonly occur at the thoracolumbar vertebral junction, resulting in wedge-shaped vertebrae.

* Fractures of laminae, pedicles, or transverse processes of the vertebrae are common.

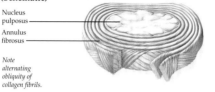

A B C

A. Hyperkyphosis
An excessive rounding of the thoracic vertebral column (humpback or hunchback)

B. Scoliosis
A curvature of the spine, often with twisting of the spinal column

C. Hyperlordosis
A forward/anterior curvature of the cervical and lumbar (lower back) regions of the spine. In the lumbar region, it is also called "swayback."

Causes of Pain in the Back or Extremities

Shown below are other causes of pain that the examining physician should consider in making the diagnosis.

Lower Spine (Lateral View)

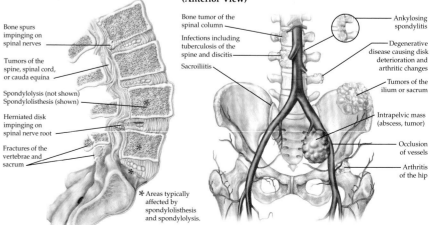

- Bone spurs impinging on spinal nerves
- Tumors of the spine, spinal cord, or cauda equina
- Spondylolysis (not shown) Spondylolisthesis (shown)
- Herniated disk impinging on spinal nerve root
- Fractures of the vertebrae and sacrum

Lower Spine and Pelvic Region (Anterior View)

- Bone tumor of the spinal column
- Infections including tuberculosis of the spine and discitis
- Sacroiliitis
- Ankylosing spondylitis
- Degenerative disease causing disk deterioration and arthritic changes
- Tumors of the ilium or sacrum
- Intrapelvic mass (abscess, tumor)
- Occlusion of vessels
- Arthritis of the hip

* Areas typically affected by spondylolisthesis and spondylolysis.

ANATOMY AND INJURIES OF THE SPINE

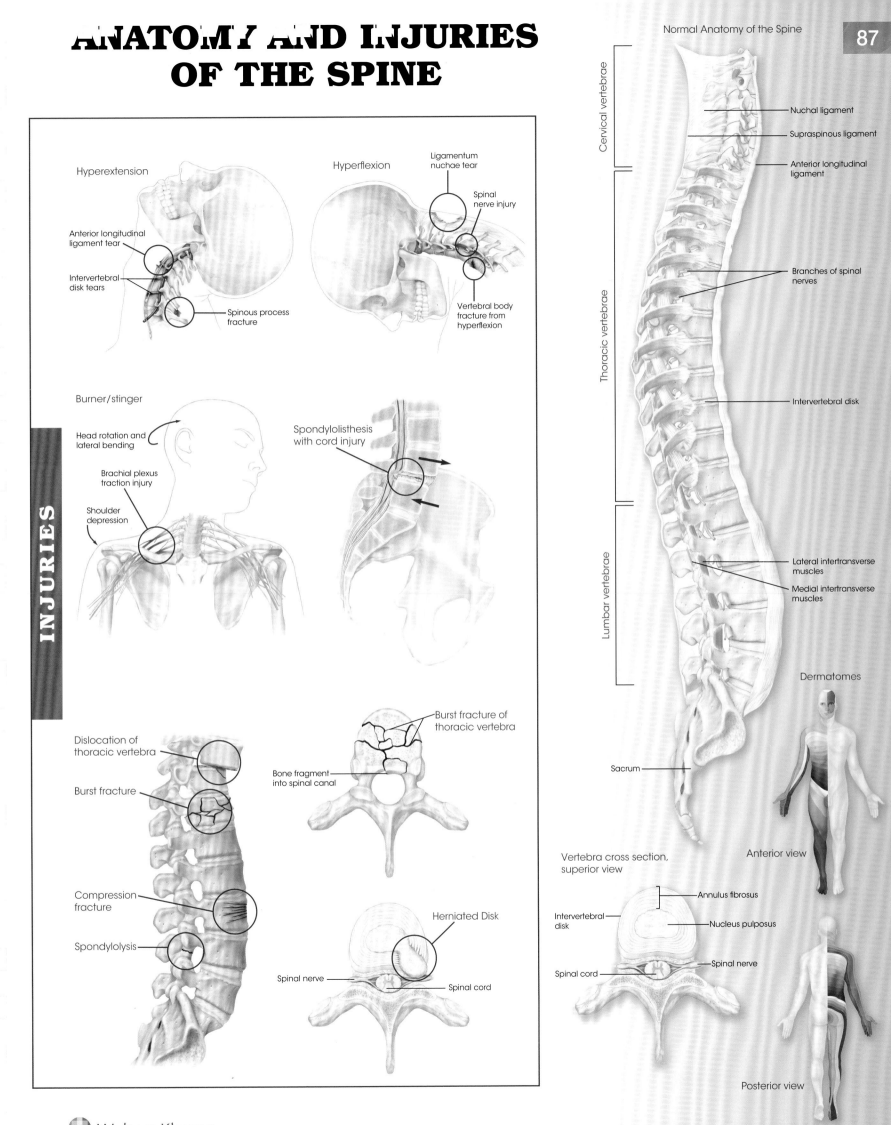

INJURIES

Hyperextension

Anterior longitudinal ligament tear

Intervertebral disk tears

Spinous process fracture

Hyperflexion

Ligamentum nuchae tear

Spinal nerve injury

Vertebral body fracture from hyperflexion

Burner/stinger

Head rotation and lateral bending

Brachial plexus traction injury

Shoulder depression

Spondylolisthesis with cord injury

Dislocation of thoracic vertebra

Burst fracture

Compression fracture

Spondylolysis

Burst fracture of thoracic vertebra

Bone fragment into spinal canal

Herniated Disk

Spinal nerve

Spinal cord

Normal Anatomy of the Spine

Cervical vertebrae

Nuchal ligament

Supraspinous ligament

Anterior longitudinal ligament

Thoracic vertebrae

Branches of spinal nerves

Intervertebral disk

Lumbar vertebrae

Lateral intertransverse muscles

Medial intertransverse muscles

Sacrum

Dermatomes

Anterior view

Posterior view

Vertebra cross section, superior view

Annulus fibrosus

Intervertebral disk

Nucleus pulposus

Spinal cord

Spinal nerve

The Effects of Osteoporosis

Osteoporosis often is called a silent disease because it causes no symptoms except after fractures have occurred. Effects of osteoporosis include the following:

- Low back pain
- Loss of height over time, accompanied by a stooped posture
- Fractures that occur after a fall or a nonmajor injury

Vertebrae Showing the Effects of Osteoporosis

Bone Comparison

This is what the inside of a healthy bone looks like compared to a bone with osteoporosis.

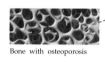

Healthy bone

Bone with osteoporosis

Vertebral body
Intervertebral disc

What Is Osteoporosis?

Osteoporosis develops when the body loses bone more quickly than it can make it. As a result, bones become less dense at the core and lose thickness at the surface. This increases the bones' susceptibility to fracture.

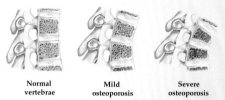

Normal vertebrae

Mild osteoporosis

Severe osteoporosis

Risk Factors

With aging, everyone has some bone loss. Certain people are likely to have even greater bone loss. Here are some factors that create a higher risk.

- Female (women are at a higher risk for osteoporosis than men are).
- Advancing age (over 50 years old).
- Family history of osteoporosis.
- Inactive lifestyle.
- Thin or small body size.
- Low-calcium diet.
- Vitamin D deficiency.
- Went through menopause at an early age.
- Smoking.
- Frequent alcohol use.
- Other medical conditions, such as chronic kidney failure, intestinal disease, and overactive thyroid.
- Certain medications, such as glucocorticoids (which caused to control diseases such as arthritis and asthma), some antiseizure drugs, certain sleeping pills, some hormones used to treat endometriosis, and some cancer drugs.
- Race—Caucasians and Asians have a higher risk of developing osteoporosis.

Common Sites of Osteoporosis

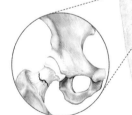

Fractures in the lower spine result from a decrease in the strength of the vertebral bodies. They can occur even without trauma. Deformities of the spine may occur due to a collapse of these injured vertebrae.

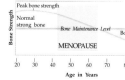

Fractures of the hip may be caused by a fall or other relatively minor accidents. A femoral prosthesis can be used to repair a broken hip.

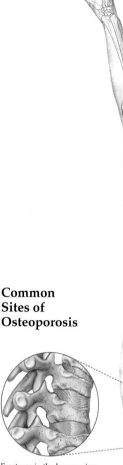

Prevention and Treatment

Strategies to reduce the chances of developing osteoporosis include the following:

- Good eating and exercise habits, ideally from early in life. Building strong bones at a young age will lessen the affect of the natural bone loss that begins to occur around age 30.
- Adequate intake of calcium-rich foods.
- Regular exercise, including weight-bearing activities, which put stress on the bones.
- Not smoking.
- Limiting alcohol use.
- Consulting with a physician to find out if you should have a bone mineral density (BMD) test.

How Much Calcium Do I Need?
Children 800 mg (4-8 years)
Teenagers 1,300 mg (9-18 years)
Adults 1,000 mg (19-50)
Adults 1,200 mg (51 or older)
Women 1,200 mg (pregnant or nursing)
Women 1,200-1,500 mg (postmenopausal)

Drug therapy can be used to prevent and to treat osteoporosis. The following drugs have been approved by the U.S. Food and Drug Administration to preserve or increase bone mass and maintain bone quality to reduce the risk of fractures:

- Estrogen replacement therapy (ERT)*
- Hormone replacement therapy (HRT)*
- Biosphosphonates
- Selective estrogen receptor modulators (SERMs)
- Hormones to regulate calcium and bone metabolism

Other methods to prevent and treat osteoporosis are being studied. Consult with your doctor to determine the best plan of treatment.
* Because of the non–bone-related effects of these drugs, their long-term use in managing osteoporosis must be carefully considered.

How Do I Know If I Have Low Bone Mass?

Bone density is a term that describes how solid your bones are. In order to determine your bone density and fracture risk for osteoporosis, a BMD test must be done. In general, the lower your bone density, the higher your risk for fracture. There are several different machines that measure bone density. All are painless, noninvasive, and safe. In many testing centers you don't even have to change into an examining robe.

Ask your doctor about this test if you think you at a risk for osteoporosis, if you are a woman around the age of menopause, or if you are a man or woman over age 65.

What's Your T-score?

Your T-score	What It Means
Above –1.0	Bone mass is about normal.
–1.0	Bone mass is about 10% below normal.
–1.5	Bone mass is about 15% below normal.
–2.0	Bone mass is about 20% below normal.
You are considered osteoporotic if your T-score is –2.5 or less.	

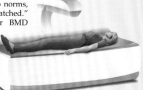

Your BMD is compared to two norms, "young normal" and "age-matched." Your T-score compares your BMD to the peak bone density of a 30-year-old healthy adult. Your fracture risk increases when your BMD falls below "young normal" levels.

Women's Bone Strength Changes With Age

Estrogen is a female hormone that helps keep bones strong. As a woman experiences menopause, the resulting decline of estrogen leads to the weakening of bones.

Peak bone strength
Normal strong bone
Bone Maintenance Level
Bone becomes weak
MENOPAUSE
Bone Strength
Age in Years
20 30 40 50 60 70 80 90

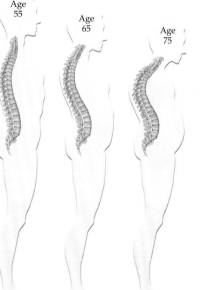

Age 55
Age 65
Age 75

Progressive Spinal Deformity in Osteoporosis

Osteoporosis weakens the bones, which can lead to fractures of the vertebrae. The vertebral fractures lead to loss of height and to kyphosis (humpback). Although vertebral fractures may be painful, the majority occur without any symptoms. Individuals may be aware only of deformity and progressive loss of height.

Fractures of the wrist often result from a fall on an outstretched hand.

ANATOMY AND INJURIES OF THE HEAD AND NECK

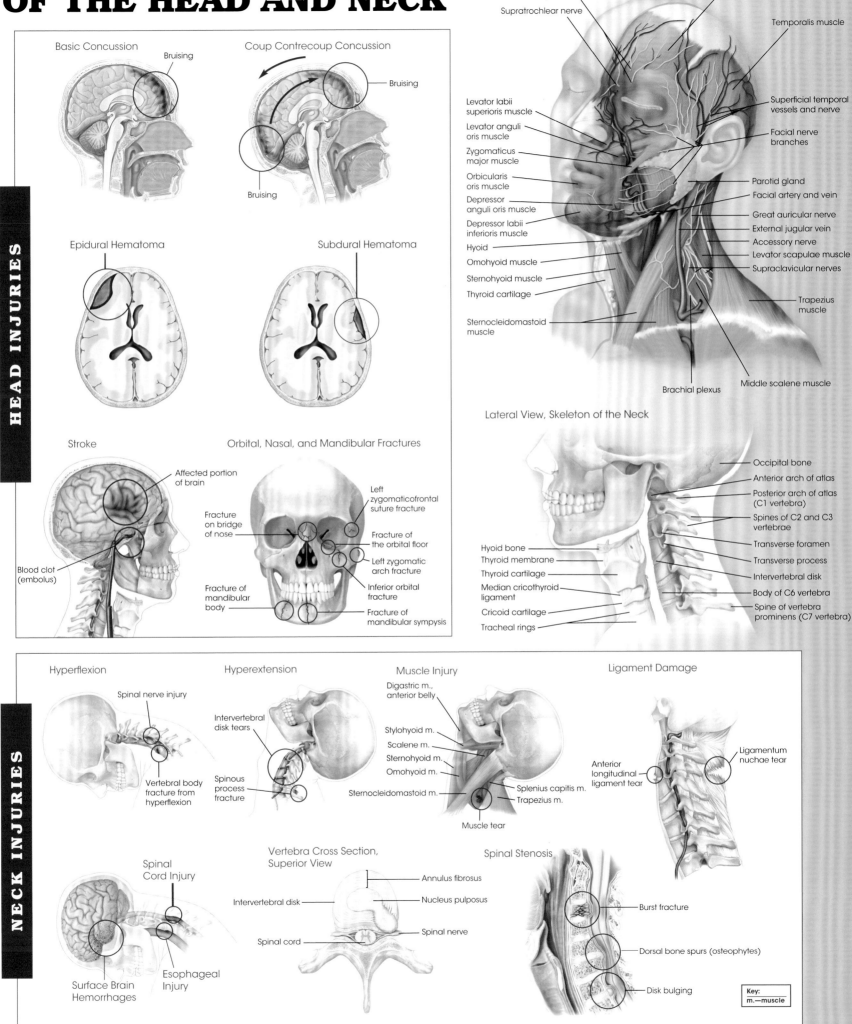

HEAD INJURIES

Basic Concussion
Bruising

Coup Contrecoup Concussion
Bruising
Bruising

Epidural Hematoma

Subdural Hematoma

Stroke
Affected portion of brain
Blood clot (embolus)

Orbital, Nasal, and Mandibular Fractures
Fracture on bridge of nose
Left zygomaticofrontal suture fracture
Fracture of the orbital floor
Left zygomatic arch fracture
Inferior orbital fracture
Fracture of mandibular body
Fracture of mandibular sympysis

Supraorbital nerve
Supratrochlear nerve
Frontalis muscle
Temporalis muscle
Superficial temporal vessels and nerve
Facial nerve branches
Levator labii superioris muscle
Levator anguli oris muscle
Zygomaticus major muscle
Orbicularis oris muscle
Depressor anguli oris muscle
Depressor labii inferioris muscle
Hyoid
Omohyoid muscle
Sternohyoid muscle
Thyroid cartilage
Sternocleidomastoid muscle
Parotid gland
Facial artery and vein
Great auricular nerve
External jugular vein
Accessory nerve
Levator scapulae muscle
Supraclavicular nerves
Trapezius muscle
Brachial plexus
Middle scalene muscle

Lateral View, Skeleton of the Neck
Hyoid bone
Thyroid membrane
Thyroid cartilage
Median cricothyroid ligament
Cricoid cartilage
Tracheal rings
Occipital bone
Anterior arch of atlas
Posterior arch of atlas (C1 vertebra)
Spines of C2 and C3 vertebrae
Transverse foramen
Transverse process
Intervertebral disk
Body of C6 vertebra
Spine of vertebra prominens (C7 vertebra)

NECK INJURIES

Hyperflexion
Spinal nerve injury
Vertebral body fracture from hyperflexion

Hyperextension
Intervertebral disk tears
Spinous process fracture

Muscle Injury
Digastric m., anterior belly
Stylohyoid m.
Scalene m.
Sternohyoid m.
Omohyoid m.
Sternocleidomastoid m.
Splenius capitis m.
Trapezius m.
Muscle tear

Ligament Damage
Anterior longitudinal ligament tear
Ligamentum nuchae tear

Spinal Cord Injury
Surface Brain Hemorrhages
Esophageal Injury

Vertebra Cross Section, Superior View
Intervertebral disk
Annulus fibrosus
Nucleus pulposus
Spinal nerve
Spinal cord

Spinal Stenosis
Burst fracture
Dorsal bone spurs (osteophytes)
Disk bulging

Key: m.—muscle

WHIPLASH INJURIES OF THE HEAD AND NECK

Whiplash injury of the head and neck is caused by a sudden exaggerated thrust of the head backward, forward, and sometimes sideways. Abnormal forces are applied to muscles, ligaments, nerves, bones, intervertebral disks, blood vessels, and eyes as the head moves beyond normal physiological limits. There may be no visible bruises or abrasions from this type of injury, yet victims report classic symptoms. These symptoms result from injuries to vertebrae and to soft tissues of the head and neck.

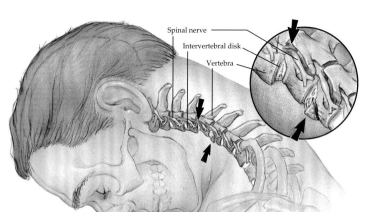

Spinal nerve
Intervertebral disk
Vertebra

Hyperflexion
The head is propelled in a forward and downward motion in hyperflexion. A wedge-shaped deformity of the bone may be created if the anterior portions of the vertebrae are crushed. Intervertebral disks may be damaged. The disks may bulge or rupture, irritating spinal nerves.

Hyperextension
The head is forced backward in hyperextension. Pieces of bone may be pulled from cervical vertebrae by a tear of the anterior longitudinal ligament. Spinous processes of the vertebrae may be fractured. Intervertebral disks may be compressed posteriorly and torn anteriorly. Vertebral arteries may be stretched, pinched, or torn, causing reduced blood flow to the brain. Nerves of the cervical sympathetic chain may also be injured.

Intervertebral disk
Vertebral artery
Cervical sympathetic chain
Spinous process

Spinal Ligaments
Vertebrae are held in place by a complex arrangement of ligaments. Some of the ligaments are barely a centimeter long, and all are only a few millimeters thick. In a whiplash injury, ligaments may be badly stretched, partially torn, or completely ruptured as shown in the image below.

Intervertebral disk
Anterior longitudinal ligament
Vertebra
Interspinous ligament
Posterior longitudinal ligament

Muscle Injury
Whiplash can cause injuries of neck muscles, ranging from minor strains and microhemorrhages to severe tears. Commonly affected muscles include the sternocleidomastoid muscle, scalene muscles, splenius capitis muscle, and longus colli muscle.

Scalene muscles
Splenius capitis muscle
Sternocleidomastoid muscle

Ligament Damage
The anterior longitudinal ligament, running vertically along the anterior surface of the vertebrae, may be injured during hyperextension. The posterior longitudinal ligament, running on the posterior surface of the vertebral bodies, may be injured in hyperflexion. The broad ligamentum nuchae may also be stretched or torn.

Ligamentum nuchae
Interspinous ligament
Posterior longitudinal ligament
Anterior longitudinal ligament

Spinal Cord Injury
When tears occur in ligaments that surround the vertebrae, the vertebrae may slip out of normal alignment and the spinal cord may be injured. An injured spinal cord can cause paralysis and even death. Whiplash may also jar the brain, producing minute hemorrhages on its surface. The esophagus may even be injured as it scrapes against sharp edges of arthritic bone or is pinched between vertebrae.

Spinal cord
Esophagus
Brain (Cerebral cortex)
Eyeball

REPRODUCTIVE DISEASES & DISORDERS

- Benign Breast Disease
- Common Gynecological Disorders
- Infertility
- Understanding Erectile Dysfunction
- The Prostate
- Sexually Transmitted Infections (STIs)
- Diseases of the Urinary Tract

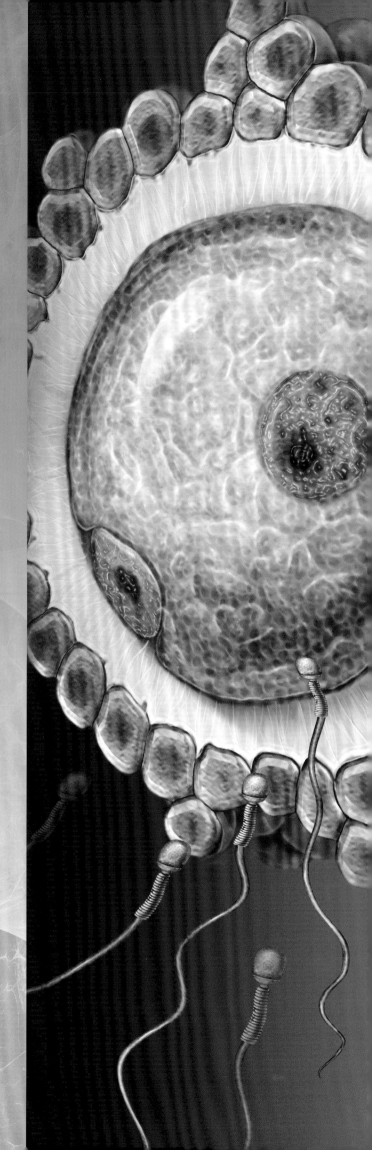

What is Benign Breast Disease?

Certain types of noncancerous conditions found in the breast are called **benign breast disease**. The most common types of benign breast disease are **benign breast tumors, breast inflammation and infection**, and **fibrocystic changes**. Normal hormonal changes probably are to blame for the growth of most benign breast changes.

There are two main types of breast tissue, **glandular** and **stromal**. The milk-producing lobules and their ducts are found in the glandular tissue. The stromal tissue is made up of fatty tissue and ligaments that support the breast.

Breast Self-Examination

A breast self-examination (BSE) should be done at the same time every month. The best time to do a BSE is several days after your period ends. If you no longer menstruate (have periods), pick a certain day such as the first day of every month. Regular BSEs teach you how your breasts normally feel so you can more readily detect any changes.

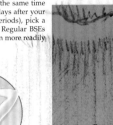

A. Stand in front of a mirror. Check each breast for anything unusual, such as dimpling, puckering, or scaliness of the skin. Check for discharge from the nipples. With your hands clasped behind your head, look for any change in the shape or contour of your breasts.

B. Press your hands firmly on your hips. Bend slightly toward the mirror as you pull your shoulders and elbows forward. Gently, squeeze each nipple and look for discharge.

C. Raise one arm. Use the pads of the fingers of your other hand to check each breast. Make sure also to check the underarm up to the collarbone and all of the way over the shoulder. Feel for any unusual lump or mass under the skin. Some women find this step easier to perform when standing in the shower using soap and water.

D. Repeat step C while lying on your back. Place one arm over your head and a pillow or rolled-up towel under the same shoulder to raise the breast tissue and make it easier to check.

Circles   Edges   Lines

Feel the tissue by pressing your fingers in small, overlapping areas. Be sure to cover the entire breast. Take your time, and follow a definite pattern such as **circles**, **edges**, or **lines**.

Symptoms

Health care providers often first find benign breast lumps during a clinical breast examination or mammogram. BSEs also are helpful in finding lumps. Symptoms of benign breast disease can include the following:

- Pain
- Tenderness
- Nipple pain or retraction
- Redness or scaliness of the breast skin or nipple
- Lump or swelling
- Skin irritation
- Tenderness (turning inward)
- A discharge other than milk

If you experience any of these symptoms, call your health care provider.

Treatment

Treatment for benign breast disease may include medications, changes in diet, or minor surgical procedures. Treatment will be determined based on:

- The patient's overall health and medical history
- Extent of the disease
- The patient's tolerance for specific medications, procedures, or therapies
- Outlook for the course of the disease
- The patient's opinion or preference

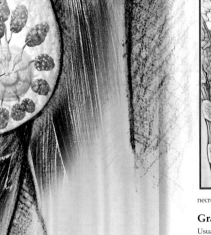

Pectoralis major muscle

Stromal tissue: Fat

Glandular tissue: Gland lobule

Glandular tissue: Lactiferous duct

Nipple

Glandular tissue: Ampulla

Areola

External abdominal oblique muscle

Diagnostic Procedures for a Detected Breast Abnormality

1) Medical History and Physical Examination

A health care provider performs a complete physical examination to locate the lump. He/she will note its texture, size, and relationship to the skin and chest muscles.

2) Nipple Discharge Evaluation

If there is nipple discharge, some of the fluid may be collected and examined. Most nipple discharge is benign.

3) Imaging Tests
- **Diagnostic mammography** is an x-ray examination of the breast that can show masses and tiny mineral deposits in the breast tissue.
- **Ultrasound** uses high-frequency sound waves to outline the breasts.

4) Biopsy

A biopsy is the removal and microscopic examination of a piece of tissue. Types of biopsies include the following:
- **Fine needle aspiration** uses a thin needle to remove fluid from a cyst or tissue from a mass.
- **Core needle biopsy** uses a somewhat larger needle with a special cutting edge. It removes a small sample of tissue.
- A **surgical biopsy** either removes the entire mass and a small area of surrounding tissue or removes only a small part of the mass.

Fibrocystic Breast Disease

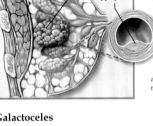

Fibrocystic breast disease

Glandular tissue: Gland lobules

Cyst

Adenosis

Epithelial hyperplasia

The term **fibrocystic breast disease** describes a variety of benign changes of the breast. It also is called fibrocystic change, cyclic disease, chronic cystic mastitis, or mammary dysplasia. There are several types of solitary breast lumps that can be classified as fibrocystic breast disease. These include **cysts, galactoceles, adenosis**, and **epithelial hyperplasia**.

Cysts

Cysts (fluid-filled sacs) found in the breast, often get bigger and become tender just before a menstrual period. They range in size from lumps that are too small to be felt to 1-2 inches in diameter. Cysts usually appear as movable, smooth, rounded lumps.

Galactoceles

Galactoceles look like cysts but instead they are filled with milk. They can occur in women who are pregnant or breast-feeding. Usually they appear as smooth, movable lumps, but on occasion, they can be hard or unmovable.

Adenosis

The excessive growth of lobule tissue is called adenosis. Since it can easily be mistaken for cancer, a biopsy is usually required. Women with adenosis do have a slight chance of getting breast cancer.

Epithelial Hyperplasia

An increase in the number of normal cells that line either the ducts or the lobules of the breast is called epithelial hyperplasia. Women with this condition have a greater chance of getting breast cancer.

Benign Breast Tumors

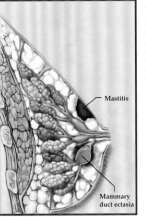

Fibroadenoma

Glandular tissue: Gland lobules

Intraductal papilloma

Glandular tissue: Lactiferous ducts

Nipple

Glandular tissue: Ampulla

Fat necrosis

Fibroadenomas

Fibroadenomas are common benign breast tumors. They range in size from microscopic to several inches in diameter. Often fibroadenomas stop growing or even shrink on their own without treatment.

Intraductal Papilloma

Intraductal papillomas are small, benign growths that most often develop in the large milk duct (lactiferous duct) near the nipple. They often cause bloody discharge.

Fat Necrosis

Fat necrosis is a benign condition in which fat cells die, usually after injury to the breast. Many times, scar tissue forms at the site of injury. Areas of fat necrosis sometimes form a saclike collection of greasy fluid called an oil cyst.

Granular Cell Tumors

Usually found in the mouth or skin, granular cell tumors are sometimes found in the breast. They are movable, firm lumps and measure between 1/2 and 1 inch in diameter. At first, they can be mistaken for breast cancer.

Phyllodes Tumors

A phyllodes (or phylloides) tumor is a rare type of breast tumor. It forms in the connective tissue of the breast. Usually benign, on rare occasions it can be cancerous and can spread.

Breast Infection and Inflammation

Mastitis

Any infection or inflammation of the breast is called mastitis. Most commonly, it affects women who are breast-feeding. If the skin around the nipple cracks, bacteria can enter the breast, leading to infection. If not treated early enough, a collection of pus (abscess) can result and may need to be drained. Signs of mastitis usually include redness, heat, and pain in the breast.

Mastitis

Mammary Duct Ectasia

When the ducts leading to the nipple become swollen and then fill with fluid, infection and inflammation can result. This is called mammary duct ectasia. If it is not treated, scar tissue can form, which may pull the nipple inward. Mammary duct ectasia can be painful and produces a thick, sticky discharge.

Mammary duct ectasia

Common GYNECOLOGICAL DISORDERS

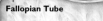

Fallopian Tube
Fundus of Uterus
Ovarian Ligament
Cavity of Uterus
Fimbia
Ovary
Ovum (egg) Released (ovulation)
Uterus:
Endometrium
Myometrium
Perimetrium
Cervical canal
Cervix
Vagina

NORMAL MENSTRUAL CYCLE

Monthly, from puberty through menopause, the menstrual cycle occurs in response to normal hormonal variations. The endometrial lining of the uterus thickens in preparation for the implantation of a fertilized egg. If pregnancy does not occur, the lining of the uterus is shed, resulting in a menstrual period. A normal menstrual cycle is 21-35 days.

ABNORMAL MENSTRUAL CYCLE

Abnormal vaginal bleeding is a flow of blood from the vagina that occurs either at the wrong time during a cycle or in inappropriate amounts brought on by various factors. Any history of abnormal vaginal bleeding warrants a visit to your doctor.

LACK OF MENSTRUAL BLEEDING
—Absence of menstruation (amenorrhea) may be due to anovulation, low estrogen levels, or a physical abnormality of the uterus. Causes include the following:

Asherman Syndrome

Bandlike adhesions

Asherman syndrome is the presence of bandlike adhesions that cross the lining of the uterus. This condition usually occurs after a surgical procedure such as dilatation and curettage (D&C).

Prolactinoma

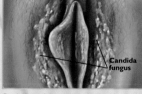

Pituitary gland

A prolactinoma is a benign (noncancerous) tumor of the pituitary gland that causes excess secretion of the prolactin hormone.

IRREGULAR BLEEDING
—Menstrual bleeding that is not regular or predictable is classified as irregular. Irregular bleeding tends to be anovulatory (ovulation does not occur) because the normal cyclic hormonal changes are inconsistent interfering with ovulation. Women may experience lack of menstruation or unpredictable bleeding. Causes include the following:

Polycystic Ovary Syndrome

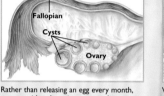

Fallopian
Cysts
Ovary

Rather than releasing an egg every month, women with polycystic ovary syndrome (PCOS) have ovarian follicles that develop into small cysts and remain in the ovary.

Eating Disorders and Extreme

Eating disorders or long, strenuous exercise programs may cause anovulatory cycles. These women may experience absence of menstruation or irregular menstrual cycles and may also be at risk for osteoporosis.

Medications

Many medications, including certain psychiatric and antiseizure drugs, can cause anovulation and irregular bleeding. Hormones found in oral contraceptives or hormone therapy can cause abnormal bleeding as a side effect.

Vaginal and Uterine Atrophy (With Menopause)

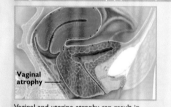

Vaginal atrophy

Vaginal and uterine atrophy can result in vaginal bleeding. Similarly, postmenopausal bleeding can be associated with endometrial hyperplasia and uterine cancer.

Hormonal Imbalances

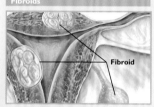

Thyroid gland

Abnormal activity of the thyroid gland (hyper- or hypothyroidism) can affect ovulation. Hyperprolactinemia (abnormally high level of the hormone prolactin) can also block ovulation.

REGULAR HEAVY BLEEDING
—Menstrual bleeding that is regular (monthly and predictable) and heavy or regular with bleeding in between periods (spotting) may be due to conditions that distort the uterine cavity or the body of the uterus. These conditions include benign tumors and growths. If bleeding is regular, it is likely that cyclic hormonal changes are also regular and that ovulation is occurring. Causes include the following:

Fibroids

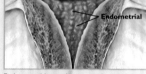

Fibroid

Fibroids are benign tumors of the muscle and connective tissue that develop within or are attached to the wall of the uterus; these may also cause painful periods.

Polyps

Polyps

Polyps are benign growths of the endometrium that can cause irregular bleeding and spotting.

Cervical Lesions

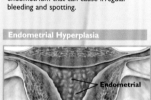

Cervix
Lesions

Cervical lesions are caused by the human papillomavirus (HPV). If left untreated, they may progress to cervical cancer.

Endometrial Hyperplasia

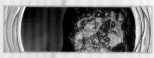

Endometrial

Endometrial hyperplasia is an abnormal overgrowth of the uterine lining (endometrium).

von Willebrand Disease

von Willebrand disease is an inherited bleeding disorder that may cause excessive bleeding during menstruation and/or surgery.

ABNORMAL VAGINAL DISCHARGE
—Normal vaginal discharge is a clear white or off-white. The amounts are different for each individual and may change over time. Abnormal vaginal discharge has an unpleasant smell and can cause itching. The following conditions are associated with abnormal vaginal discharge:

Candidiasis (Yeast Infection)

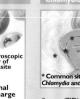

Candida fungus

Candidiasis of the vagina occurs when there is an overgrowth of the fungus called *Candida*. The discharge may resemble cottage cheese or may be watery, often has no smell, and usually causes vaginal itching.

Bacterial Vaginitis

Cervix
Milky discharge

The most common vaginal infection occurring in women of reproductive age, bacterial vaginitis occurs when there is an overgrowth of bacteria. There is usually a thin, milky discharge with a fishy odor that may be more noticeable after sexual intercourse.

Trichomoniasis Vaginitis

Cervix
Microscopic view of parasite
Vaginal discharge

Trichomonas is a parasite that is generally spread through sexual contact. This infection may be asymptomatic (presenting no symptoms) but is generally associated with vaginal discharge, odor, and burning with urination.

Chlamydia and Gonorrhea

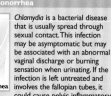

* Common sites for *Chlamydia* and Gonorrhea

Chlamydia is a bacterial disease that is usually spread through sexual contact. This infection may be asymptomatic but may be associated with an abnormal vaginal discharge or burning sensation when urinating. If the infection is left untreated and involves the fallopian tubes, it could cause pelvic inflammatory disease (PID) and infertility.

Gonorrhea is a sexually transmitted infectious disease caused by a bacterium that can infect the genital tract, the mouth, and the rectum. It is usually spread through sexual contact. Early symptoms can include bleeding during intercourse, painful/burning urination, and/or yellow or bloody vaginal discharge.

GYNECOLOGICAL/PELVIC PAIN
—Pain related to the pelvic and gynecological organs is a common symptom for many women. Pain can be caused by a variety of conditions. When experiencing pain, it is important to try to characterize the type of pain (crampy, sharp, etc.), the duration, and its relation to your menstrual cycle. This will help your health care provider to determine the cause of the pain.

Ovarian Cysts

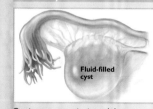

Fluid-filled cyst

Ovarian cysts range in size and the symptoms that they produce. Symptoms can range from asymptomatic, to dull ache/pressure, to pain. Some women may experience pain during intercourse.

Pelvic Inflammatory Disease and Pelvic Adhesions

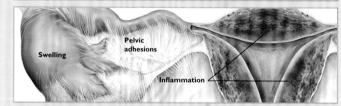

Pelvic adhesions
Swelling
Inflammation

PID is a general term that refers to infection of the uterus, fallopian tubes, and other reproductive organs. Pelvic adhesions can occur following surgery or a pelvic infection. Depending upon their location, they can be the cause of pelvic pain.

Endometriosis

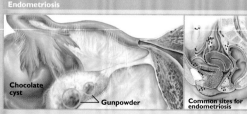

Chocolate cyst
Gunpowder
Common sites for endometriosis

Endometriosis occurs when the endometrium (the lining of the uterus) grows outside of the uterus. Pain symptoms can occur before and during periods and during or after intercourse.

Adenomyosis

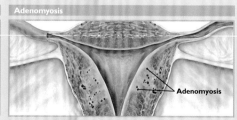

Adenomyosis

Adenomyosis occurs when endometrial cells grow within the wall of the uterus. This can cause heavy and painful menstrual cycles.

© 2008 Wolters Kluwer Published by Anatomical Chart Company, Skokie, IL.

INFERTILITY

Ovum (Egg)

Nucleus
Nucleolus
Ooplasm
Polar body
Zona pellucida
Corona radiata

What Is Infertility?

Infertility is commonly defined as 1 year of unprotected intercourse without conception.

Spermatozoon (Sperm)

Mitochondrial sheath Acrosome
Tail Middle Head

Semen Analysis

The first step in diagnosing male infertility is a semen analysis. This test checks for sperm motility (movement), sperm morphology (shape and structure), and sperm count.

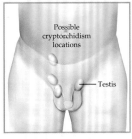

Possible cryptorchidism locations
Testis

Cryptorchidism

Cryptorchidism is the failure of one or both testes to descend into the scrotum. In this congenital disorder, the testes remain in the abdomen or inguinal canal or at the external inguinal ring. Although this condition may be bilateral, it more commonly affects the right testis. True undescended testes remain along the path of normal descent.

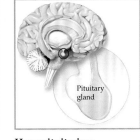

Pituitary gland

Hypopituitarism

The pituitary gland in the brain produces follicle-stimulating hormone (FSH) and luteinizing hormone (LH). Both of these hormones act on the testes and are necessary for normal sperm production. A deficiency in the production of these hormones may cause abnormal sperm production.

Female Internal Genital Organs

Early cell division of zygote
Two-cell stage
Four-cell stage
Eight-cell stage
Morula
Fertilization
Ovum
Implanted blastocyst
Ovarian ligament
Fallopian tube Infundibulum
Ectopic pregnancy
Corpus luteum
Uterus
Body of cervix
Mucous plug
Cervix (external os)
Vagina
Ovary Fimbria

Fertilization and Implantation

During monthly ovulation, an ovum is released from the ovary into the fallopian tube, where it travels toward the uterus. If sperm are ejaculated during sexual intercourse, they move through the fallopian tube, where they meet the ovum.

If a sperm penetrates the ovum, fertilization occurs, and the ovum becomes a zygote. The zygote continues to travel toward the uterus, dividing many times until it becomes a blastocyst. There it implants in the uterine lining and, in a normal pregnancy, continues to develop over the next 9 months.

Blocked Fallopian Tubes

The egg is fertilized by the sperm within the fallopian tube and then travels into the uterine cavity, where it may become implanted. If the fallopian tubes are blocked, the fertilized egg cannot enter the uterus. Sometimes, a fertilized egg implants within the fallopian tube, causing an ectopic (outside the uterus) pregnancy.

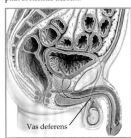

Vas deferens

Obstruction

Obstruction or absence of the vas deferens is a rare cause of infertility. The vas deferens carries the sperm from the testis through to the penis. If this structure is blocked or absent, sperm may be prevented from reaching the ejaculatory duct.

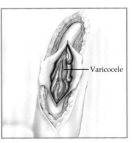

Varicocele

Varicocele

Varicocele is a mass of dilated and tortuous varicose veins in the spermatic cord. Blood pools in the plexus of veins rather than flowing into the venous system. Inadequate blood flow through the testis may affect sperm production and may lead to testicular atrophy.

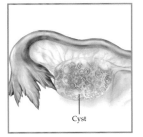

Cyst

Polycystic Ovarian Syndrome

Polycystic ovarian syndrome (PCOS) is associated with infrequent and irregular ovulation and multiple, small ovarian cysts. Some women with PCOS may also be overweight, may have increased acne and hair growth, and are at risk for developing diabetes and uterine lining abnormalities.

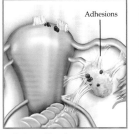

Adhesions

Pelvic Adhesions

The fallopian tube must be able to move freely in order to engulf the ovum (egg) after release from the ovary. Pelvic adhesions from previous infection, surgery, or endometriosis can interfere with the fallopian tube's mobility. The scar tissue can also affect the ovaries.

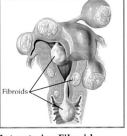

Adhesions
Fibroids

Intrauterine Fibroids

Fibroids are benign tumors of the uterus. Large submucosal fibroids can protrude into the uterine cavity and interfere with proper implantation of a fertilized egg. Fibroids can also block the opening of the fallopian tubes into the uterus and prevent a fertilized egg from entering the uterine cavity.

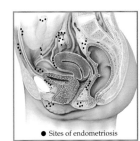

● Sites of endometriosis

Endometriosis

Endometriosis occurs when the tissue that normally lines the uterus grows outside it and in other areas of the body. It can cause scar tissue, pain, and infertility. In some cases the infertility may be attributed to the scar tissue, but there may also be an immunologic component.

Common Causes of Infertility

MALE

Abnormal sperm factors:
If there is an abnormality in the semen analysis, further referral to a urologist may be needed. The World Health Organization (WHO) has published rough guidelines for normal semen analysis values.

Pretesticular factors:
• Hypopituitarism—not enough pituitary hormones
• Hyperprolactinemia—too much prolactin hormone
• Hypothalamic dysfunction

Testicular factors:
• Certain drugs—can depress sperm quantity and quality
• Chemotherapy/radiation—may affect sperm count
• Testicular dysgenesis—failure of testes to form properly
• Cryptorchidism—failure of the testes to descend into the scrotum

Posttesticular factors:
• Obstruction or absence of the vas deferens.
• Varicocele—dilated and tortuous veins in the spermatic cord.
• Retrograde ejaculation—sperm are deposited into the bladder following ejaculation. This can occur as a result of diabetes or neurologic disease, or occasionally following removal of the prostate gland.
• Coital dysfunction—inability to ejaculate.

Infertility Percentage Chart

The pie chart depicts the approximate distribution of the common causes of infertility among couples.

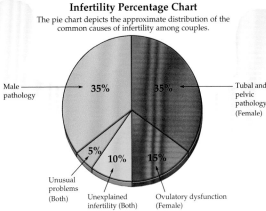

Male pathology — 35%
Tubal and pelvic pathology (Female) — 35%
Unusual problems (Both) — 5%
Unexplained infertility (Both) — 10%
Ovulatory dysfunction (Female) — 15%

FEMALE

Ovulatory dysfunction factors:
The woman fails to ovulate or ovulates irregularly. Causes include the following:
• Polycystic ovarian syndrome
• Age > 35 (increases the chance of decreased ovulation)
• Hyperprolactinemia—too much prolactin hormone
• Excessive exercise or dieting
• Drug or alcohol abuse
• Obesity

Tubal and pelvic pathology factors:
Problems with fallopian tubes and ovaries, including the following:
• Pelvic adhesions—scar tissue affecting the fallopian tubes and ovaries
• Hydrosalpinx—fluid in the fallopian tubes
• Blocked fallopian tubes
• Endometriosis

Unusual problems, anatomic abnormalities, thyroid disease factors:
• Cervical factors like abnormal cervical mucus or prior cervical surgery
• Intrauterine fibroids or congenital abnormalities
• Immunologic antibody-mediated sperm damage
• Hyper- or hypothyroidism
• Intrauterine adhesions

Unexplained infertility factors: Sometimes fertility test results are normal. Although there is probably a cause, it cannot be diagnosed with routine tests.

What Is Erectile Dysfunction?

Erectile dysfunction (*impotence*) is the persistent inability to obtain and maintain an erection sufficient for intercourse. Some men may experience complete erectile dysfunction, while others may achieve partial or brief erections. It is estimated that as many as 52% of men in the United States are affected. Erectile dysfunction affects all age groups but increases in frequency with age.

What Causes Erectile Dysfunction?

A variety of medical conditions, the use of certain medicines, and psychological problems may cause erectile dysfunction.

- **Blood vessel (*vascular*) disease**
Problems with the blood vessels that carry blood to the penis can reduce blood flow enough to impede erection. **Atherosclerosis** (*hardening of the arteries*) is the most common cause. **Cardiovascular disease, hypertension** (*high blood pressure*), and hypercholesterolemia (*high blood cholesterol*) can worsen the condition.

- **Diabetes**
Diabetes is a common cause of erectile dysfunction because diabetes can cause changes in blood flow through narrowing of the arteries or damage to nerve endings in the penis.

- **Neurologic disease**
Brain, spinal cord, or **nerve injuries** (*especially to the nerves leaving the spinal cord, called the cauda equina*), as well as neurological diseases such as Alzheimer disease, **stroke**, multiple sclerosis, and Parkinson disease can lead to erectile dysfunction.

- **Hormone imbalance**
Hormone imbalance, such as insufficient testosterone, causes only a small percentage of cases of erectile dysfunction. Testosterone is not directly involved in the vascular and neurologic events associated with penile erection.

- **Pelvic surgery, trauma, or radiation**
Surgery, trauma, or radiation to the prostate, bladder, rectum, or colon can cause damage to the nerves or blood vessels in the surrounding area. Damage to pelvic nerves or arteries can result in erectile dysfunction.

- **Psychological problems**
Depression, anxiety, stress, low self-esteem, and other mental conditions may lead to erectile dysfunction.

- **Alcohol and drugs**
Alcoholism and drug abuse are associated with erectile dysfunction, as is the use of certain **prescription drugs**. Medicines used to treat high blood pressure, heart disease, depression, psychosis, and heartburn are among the most common medicines that interfere with the ability to have an erection.

- **Chronic tobacco use**
Smoking has been shown to affect the arteries in the penis, thus reducing blood flow necessary to maintain an erection.

How Is Erectile Dysfunction Treated?

The treatment depends on the cause of the erectile dysfunction. Behavior changes such as eliminating alcohol and drug abuse, cessation of smoking, and reducing stress may improve erectile function.

Treatments include the following:

- **Oral medication**
Oral medication works directly on the blood vessels, causing the arteries to the penis to expand. It will cause an erection only when the man is sexually aroused.
Side effects: headaches, facial flushing, backache, upset stomach, bluish tinge to vision

- **Intraurethral pellets**
The patient uses an applicator to insert a small pellet of medication into the opening at the end of the penis (*the urethra*). The medication causes blood vessels to relax, so the penis fills with blood and becomes erect.
Side effects: pain, burning sensation

- **Vacuum therapy**
A cylinder is placed over the penis. By withdrawing air, a vacuum is created, mechanically enhancing the flow of blood into the penis. A rubber ring is placed at the base of the erect penis to trap the blood and maintain the erection.
Side effects: bruising, pain, diminished ejaculation

- **Penile injections**
The patient uses a small needle to inject a powerful muscle relaxant into the base of the penis. The relaxation of muscle tissue allows blood to flow into the erectile tissues in the penis, creating an erection.
Side effects: pain, scarring, bleeding, and, rarely, prolonged erection

- **Penile implants**
This requires a surgical intervention. Two inflatable balloons are implanted in the penis, as well as a pump into the scrotum and a reservoir near the bladder. When the pump is inflated, fluid from the reservoir flows into the inflatable balloons, creating an erection.
Side effects: infection, pain, or malfunction

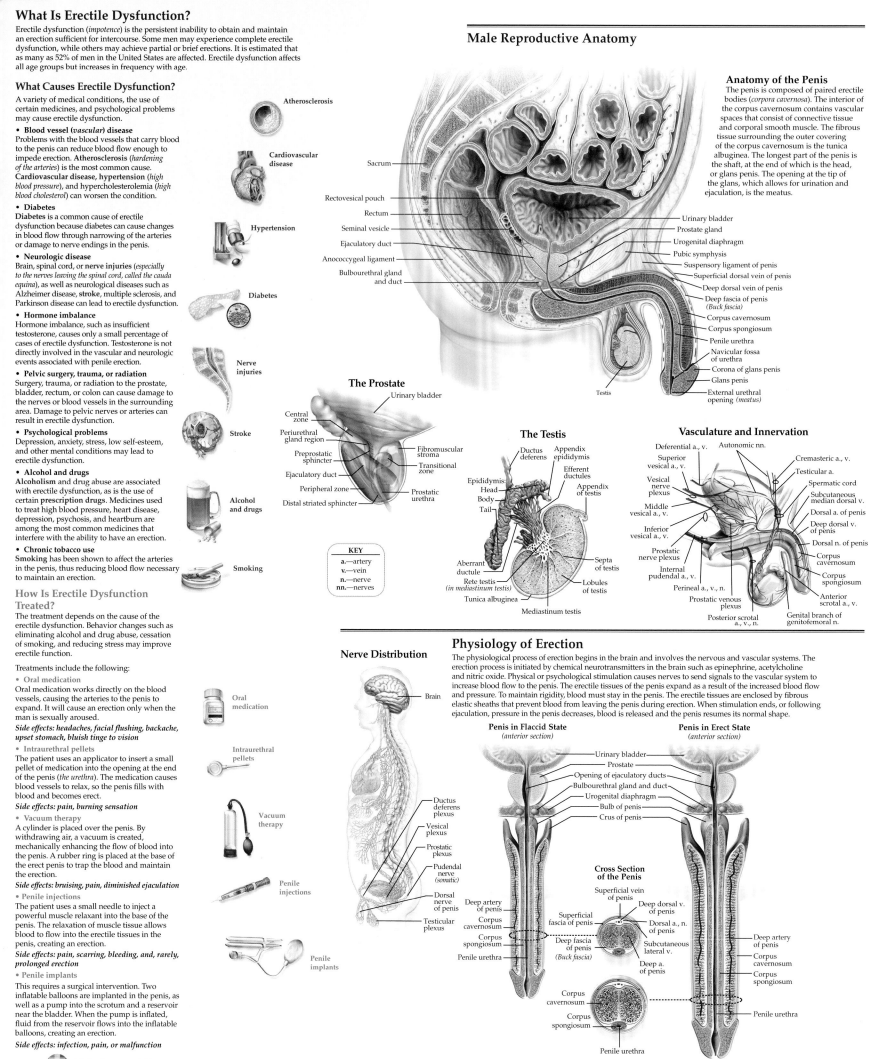

Atherosclerosis

Cardiovascular disease

Hypertension

Diabetes

Nerve injuries

Stroke

Alcohol and drugs

Smoking

Oral medication

Intraurethral pellets

Vacuum therapy

Penile injections

Penile implants

Male Reproductive Anatomy

Anatomy of the Penis
The penis is composed of paired erectile bodies (*corpora cavernosa*). The interior of the corpus cavernosum contains vascular spaces that consist of connective tissue and corporal smooth muscle. The fibrous tissue surrounding the outer covering of the corpus cavernosum is the tunica albuginea. The longest part of the penis is the shaft, at the end of which is the head, or glans penis. The opening at the tip of the glans, which allows for urination and ejaculation, is the meatus.

Sacrum
Rectovesical pouch
Rectum
Seminal vesicle
Ejaculatory duct
Anococcygeal ligament
Bulbourethral gland and duct

Urinary bladder
Prostate gland
Urogenital diaphragm
Pubic symphysis
Suspensory ligament of penis
Superficial dorsal vein of penis
Deep dorsal vein of penis
Deep fascia of penis (*Buck fascia*)
Corpus cavernosum
Corpus spongiosum
Penile urethra
Navicular fossa of urethra
Corona of glans penis
Glans penis
External urethral opening (*meatus*)
Testis

The Prostate

Urinary bladder
Central zone
Periurethral gland region
Preprostatic sphincter
Ejaculatory duct
Peripheral zone
Distal striated sphincter
Fibromuscular stroma
Transitional zone
Prostatic urethra

The Testis

Ductus deferens
Appendix epididymis
Efferent ductules
Appendix of testis
Epididymis:
Head
Body
Tail
Septa of testis
Aberrant ductule
Rete testis (*in mediastinum testis*)
Lobules of testis
Tunica albuginea
Mediastinum testis

Vasculature and Innervation

Deferential a., v.
Autonomic nn.
Superior vesical a., v.
Cremasteric a., v.
Testicular a.
Vesical nerve plexus
Spermatic cord
Subcutaneous median dorsal v.
Middle vesical a., v.
Dorsal a. of penis
Deep dorsal v. of penis
Inferior vesical a., v.
Dorsal n. of penis
Prostatic nerve plexus
Corpus cavernosum
Internal pudendal a., v.
Corpus spongiosum
Perineal a., v., n.
Anterior scrotal a., v.
Prostatic venous plexus
Posterior scrotal a., v., n.
Genital branch of genitofemoral n.

KEY
a.—artery
v.—vein
n.—nerve
nn.—nerves

Nerve Distribution

Brain
Ductus deferens plexus
Vesical plexus
Prostatic plexus
Pudendal nerve (*somatic*)
Dorsal nerve of penis
Testicular plexus

Physiology of Erection

The physiological process of erection begins in the brain and involves the nervous and vascular systems. The erection process is initiated by chemical neurotransmitters in the brain such as epinephrine, acetylcholine and nitric oxide. Physical or psychological stimulation causes nerves to send signals to the vascular system to increase blood flow to the penis. The erectile tissues of the penis expand as a result of the increased blood flow and pressure. To maintain rigidity, blood must stay in the penis. The erectile tissues are enclosed by fibrous elastic sheaths that prevent blood from leaving the penis during erection. When stimulation ends, or following ejaculation, pressure in the penis decreases, blood is released and the penis resumes its normal shape.

Penis in Flaccid State (*anterior section*)
Penis in Erect State (*anterior section*)

Urinary bladder
Prostate
Opening of ejaculatory ducts
Bulbourethral gland and duct
Urogenital diaphragm
Bulb of penis
Crus of penis

Cross Section of the Penis

Superficial vein of penis
Deep dorsal v. of penis
Superficial fascia of penis
Dorsal a., n. of penis
Deep fascia of penis (*Buck fascia*)
Subcutaneous lateral v.
Deep a. of penis
Deep artery of penis
Corpus cavernosum
Corpus spongiosum
Penile urethra

Deep artery of penis
Corpus cavernosum
Corpus spongiosum
Penile urethra
Corpus cavernosum
Corpus spongiosum
Penile urethra

THE PROSTATE

Hormonal Influence on the Prostate

The prostate functions continuously, producing fluid that empties into the urethra. Hormones from the **pituitary gland** direct the **adrenal glands** and the **testes** to send chemical signals to the **prostate** to promote fluid production.

- Pituitary
- Adrenal gland
- Kidney
- Ureter
- Urinary bladder
- Prostate
- Testis

What Is the Prostate?

The prostate is a gland consisting of fibrous, muscular, and glandular tissue surrounding the urethra below the urinary bladder. Its function is to secrete prostatic fluid as a medium for semen, helping it to reach the female reproductive tract. Within the prostate, the urethra is joined by two ejaculatory ducts. During sexual activity, the prostate acts as a valve between the urinary and reproductive tracts. This enables semen to ejaculate without mixing with urine. Prostatic fluid is delivered by the contraction of muscles around gland tissue. Nerve and hormonal influences control the secretory and muscular functions of the prostate.

Normal Prostate (sagittal section)

- Ureteral orifice
- Trigone
- Bladder wall
- Urinary bladder
- Seminal vesicles
- Internal urethral sphincter
- Ejaculatory ducts
- Prostatic capsule
- Anterior rectal wall
- Prostatic urethra
- Prostatic utricle
- External urethral sphincter
- Bulbourethral gland
- Membranous urethra
- Pubic symphysis
- Internal urethral sphincter
- Prostatovesicular junction
- Prostate gland
- Deep dorsal vein of the penis

Posterior View (dissected)

- Fibromuscular wall of bladder
- Ductus deferens
- Ureter
- Ampulla of ductus deferens
- Seminal vesicles
- Levator ani m.
- Prostatic utricle
- Peritoneal covering over bladder dome
- Retropubic space
- Membranous urethra

Anterior View With Exposed Prostatic Urethra

- Interureteric fold
- Orifice of ureter
- Trigone
- Muscular wall of bladder
- Urethra in bladder neck
- Base
- Venous plexus
- Openings of urethral gland
- Prostatic utricle
- Prostatic sinus
- Apex
- Prostatic urethra
- Orifice of ejaculatory duct
- Urethral crest
- Membranous urethra

Superior View (transverse section)

- Ejaculatory ducts
- Prostatic utricle
- Prostate glandular tissue lobes
- Prostatic urethra

Vasculature and Innervation

- Umbilical a.
- Ureter
- Ductus deferens
- Pelvic plexus
- Urinary bladder
- Vesical plexus
- Superior vesical a., v.
- Middle vesical a., v.
- Pubic symphysis
- Inferior vesical a., v.
- Prostatic nerve plexus
- Deep dorsal vein of the penis
- Urogenital diaphragm
- Prostate gland

Zones of the Prostate

Prostatic urethra

- A—Central zone
- B—Fibromuscular zone
- C—Transitional zone
- D—Peripheral zone
- E—Periurethral gland region

Ejaculatory duct

Glands of the Prostate

The prostate is mainly filled with secretory glands. These glands are made of many ducts with grape-shaped-saccule ends or "acini." Secretory cells lining the ducts are stimulated by hormones to expel prostatic fluid. During sexual activity, muscle contracts and expels the fluid. The basal cell, also found lining the ducts of the prostate, may be responsible for most types of prostatic hyperplasia as a result of uncontrolled prostatic tissue growth.

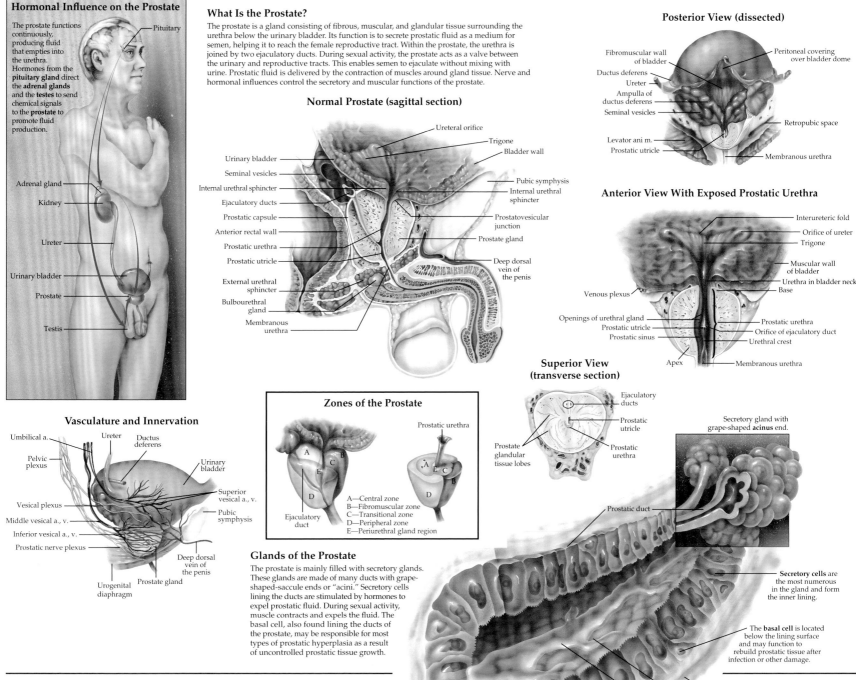

Secretory gland with grape-shaped **acinus** end.

- Prostatic duct
- **Secretory cells** are the most numerous in the gland and form the inner lining.
- The **basal cell** is located below the lining surface and may function to rebuild prostatic tissue after infection or other damage.
- Fibromuscular stroma
- Ductal lumen
- Prostatic fluid

Benign Prostatic Hyperplasia

Benign prostatic hyperplasia (BPH) is the most common type of tumor in mature men. It is a benign growth, which means it may enlarge but will not spread to other locations in the body. The tumor can cause discomfort and may grow to completely close the bladder neck, preventing urination. This condition occurs because the tumor usually grows in the transitional zone and periurethral gland region located at the prostate base near the bladder neck.

Early BPH:

Narrowing of the prostatic urethra causing difficulty in starting, maintaining, and stopping urination

- Prostatic urethra

Prostatitis

Prostatitis is an uncomfortable condition in which the prostate becomes inflamed and swollen due to an infection. Prostatitis can make urinating painful.

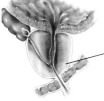

- Prostatitis (inflamed prostate tissues)

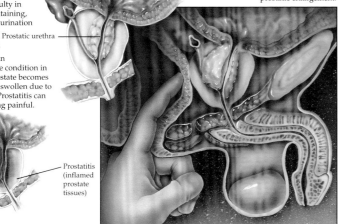

A **digital rectal examination** is very useful in detecting early signs of prostatic enlargement.

Prostate Cancer

Prostate carcinoma is the most common malignant tumor in men. Unlike BPH, prostate cancer not only enlarges but also metastasizes (spreads) to other parts of the body. This disease is complicated by the simple transfer of cancer cells directly to other parts of the body through a local plexus of veins.

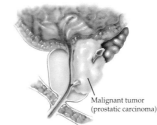

- Malignant tumor (prostatic carcinoma)

Pathway for Plexiform Venous Arborizations

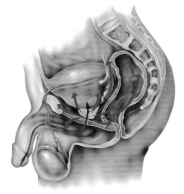

SEXUALLY TRANSMITTED INFECTIONS (STIs)

What Are Sexually Transmitted Infections?

Sexually transmitted infections (STIs) are diseases you can get by having sex with someone who has an infection. There are more than 20 types of STIs, which can be spread during vaginal, oral, and anal sexual contact. STIs can be painful, and may have serious consequences (including death) if not treated. **Bacterial** STIs like gonorrhea and chlamydia are relatively easy to cure if treated early, but **viral** STIs, like genital herpes and the human immunodeficiency virus (HIV), cannot be cured. Other STIs such as trichomoniasis are caused by **protozoa** (single-celled organisms), and **parasites** are responsible for pubic lice and scabies.

Complications

Without treatment, STIs can lead to serious health problems—especially in women. In addition, STIs increase the risk of acquiring and transmitting HIV, the virus that causes AIDS. Some complications of STIs and the organs affected are listed below:

A **Brain and Nervous System**—Headaches, brain damage, meningitis (inflamed lining of the brain), stroke, neurological disorders (nervous system problems), psychiatric illness, spinal damage

B **Eyes**—Conjunctivitis, blindness

C **Mouth and Throat**—Thrush (infection of the oral tissues), pharyngitis (inflamed throat)

D **Lungs**—*Pneumocystis carinii* (form of pneumonia common in people with reduced immunity)

E **Heart and Blood Vessels**—Aortic stenosis (narrowing of artery and/or valve of the heart), inflammation of the aorta, aneurysm (bulging) of the aorta, Kaposi's sarcoma (AIDS-related cancer affecting certain lymphatic vessels)

F **Skin**—Rashes, itching, blisters, ulcers

G **Intestines**—Dysentery (inflammation of the intestine, with abdominal pain and frequent, watery stools)

H **Urinary System**—Cystitis (inflammation of the bladder), urinary tract infections, urethritis (inflammation of urethra)

I **Bones and Joints**—Arthritis, bone aches

Reproductive system complications include the following:

Male Prostatitis (inflammation of the prostate gland), sterility, impotence, epididymitis (inflammation of the epididymis), urethral stricture

Female Pelvic scarring, genital damage, cervical cancer, infertility, vulvovaginitis (inflammation of vulva and vagina), ectopic (tubal) pregnancy

Signs and Symptoms

The table below lists some of the most common symptoms of STIs. It is important to remember that many women and men who have an STI often do not experience any symptoms at all. If you are experiencing any of the symptoms listed below or if you believe you have an STI, talk to your health care provider as soon as possible.

Possible STIs

Symptoms	Chancroid	Chlamydia	Gonorrhea	Hepatitis B	Genital herpes	HIV/AIDS	Genital warts	PID	Pubic lice	Scabies	Syphilis	Trichomoniasis
Unusual vaginal discharge		✓	✓					✓				✓
Unusual vaginal bleeding		✓	✓					✓				
Fever	✓	✓	✓	✓	✓	✓		✓				
Fatigue				✓		✓						
Sores or blisters					✓						✓	
Penile discharge		✓	✓									✓
Burning or pain when urinating		✓	✓		✓							✓
Lower abdominal pain		✓	✓					✓				
Persistent vaginal yeast infections						✓						
Swollen and/or painful testicles	✓	✓	✓									
Bumps on or around genitals					✓		✓		✓		✓	
Yellowing of eyes or skin				✓								
Rash			✓		✓	✓			✓	✓	✓	
Itching in genital area									✓	✓		✓
Itching on body				✓						✓		
Hair loss											✓	
Rectal pain or discharge		✓	✓									
Swollen glands in the groin	✓				✓							✓
Loss of appetite				✓		✓						
Flu-like symptoms				✓		✓						
Enlarged lymph nodes				✓		✓					✓	

Genital Warts

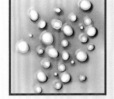

Genital warts are painless growths found on or around the genital and anal areas. They are caused by the human papillomavirus (HPV). Despite treatment, genital warts cannot be cured and often recur. In women, infection with certain strains of HPV can increase the risk of developing cervical cancer.

Genital Herpes

Genital herpes is a viral infection that causes painful sores on and around the genitals or anal area. It is easily spread, and the disease tends to recur, especially in the first few years after initial infection. There is no cure, but there are medications that can help relieve symptoms.

Chancroid

Soft, ragged edges / Pus

Chancroid (shan-kroid) is a bacterial infection that causes painful ulcers on the genitals. The chancroid ulcer can be difficult to distinguish from ulcers that are caused by genital herpes and syphilis. Symptoms usually appear within a week of exposure.

Syphilis

Hard, raised edges

Syphilis is a bacterial infection that can damage organs over time if untreated. The first symptom of syphilis is an ulcer called a **chancre** (shan-ker). Left untreated, about one-third of cases will go onto the later, more damaging, stages.

Trichomoniasis

One of the most common STIs, trichomoniasis (trick-oh-moh-nye-uh-sis) is a genital-tract infection caused by a protozoan (single-celled organism). This STI is usually transmitted through sexual intercourse, but a woman can also transmit the infection to her baby during childbirth.

HIV/AIDS

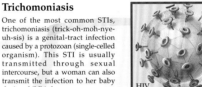

HIV (AIDS virus)

HIV (human immunodeficiency virus) infects and gradually destroys cells in the immune system. HIV severely weakens the body's response to infections and cancers. Eventually, AIDS (acquired immunodeficiency syndrome) is diagnosed. With AIDS, a variety of infections can overtake the body and eventually cause death.

Pelvic Inflammatory Disease (PID)

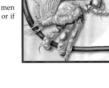

Pus / Adhesions

PID is a term used to describe an infection of the uterus, fallopian tubes, or ovaries. It is the most common, serious infection among young women. PID infection can cause scarring of the tissue inside the fallopian tubes, which can damage the tubes or block them completely. If untreated, PID can result in infertility, ectopic pregnancy, miscarriage, or chronic pain.

Hepatitis B

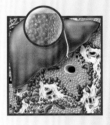

The liver disease hepatitis B is caused by a virus carried in the blood, saliva, semen, and other body fluids of an infected person. It is spread through sexual contact and can be spread from a mother to her baby during childbirth or during breast-feeding. Recovery usually happens within 6 months, but in rare cases hepatitis B can lead to liver damage and an increased risk of liver cancer.

Pubic Lice

Pubic lice are tiny parasites that live in pubic hair and survive by feeding on human blood. They are most often spread by sexual activity, but in rare cases they can be spread through contact with infested clothing or bedding. It is unusual for pubic lice to cause any serious health problems, but the itching they cause can be very uncomfortable.

Scabies

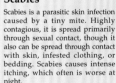

Scabies is a parasitic skin infection caused by a tiny mite. Highly contagious, it is spread primarily through sexual contact, though it also can be spread through contact with skin, infested clothing, or bedding. Scabies causes intense itching, which often is worse at night.

Chlamydia

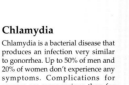

Female Reproductive Anatomy

Chlamydia is a bacterial disease that produces an infection very similar to gonorrhea. Up to 50% of men and 20% of women don't experience any symptoms. Complications for women are more serious than for men. In women chlamydia can cause irreversible damage, such as pelvic inflammatory disease and infertility.

★ = sites of infection for both chlamydia and gonorrhea

Gonorrhea

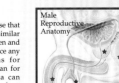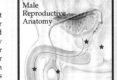

Male Reproductive Anatomy

Gonorrhea is a curable STI that can infect the genital tract, the mouth, and the rectum. It is usually spread through sexual contact, but an infected woman can pass the disease to her baby during delivery. Often there are no symptoms. Untreated, it can cause sterility in both sexes.

★ = sites of infection for both chlamydia and gonorrhea

Prevention and Treatment

The only way to eliminate the risk of acquiring an STI is to avoid sex *completely*. But there are several measures you can take to *reduce* your risk and to avoid transmitting STIs:

- Avoid sex with multiple partners.
- Use a condom.
- Get a hepatitis B immunization (shot).
- Become familiar with the symptoms of STIs.
- Know your sexual partner's sexual history.

- Have regular checkups for STIs, even if you have no symptoms.
- Seek medical help immediately if any suspicious symptoms develop.

- If infected, tell any past or present partner(s) so that they may get treated.
- Avoid all sexual activity while being treated for an STI.

Most STIs are easily treated. The earlier a person seeks treatment, the less likely the disease will cause permanent physical damage, be spread to others, or be passed on from a mother to her newborn baby.

8492 ISBN# 1-58779-849-2 (Paper) ISBN# 1-58779-850-6 (Laminated)

© 2004 Wolters Kluwer

Anatomical Chart Company, Skokie, IL. Medical illustrations by Liana Bauman, MAMS, in consultation with Michèle Till, MD.

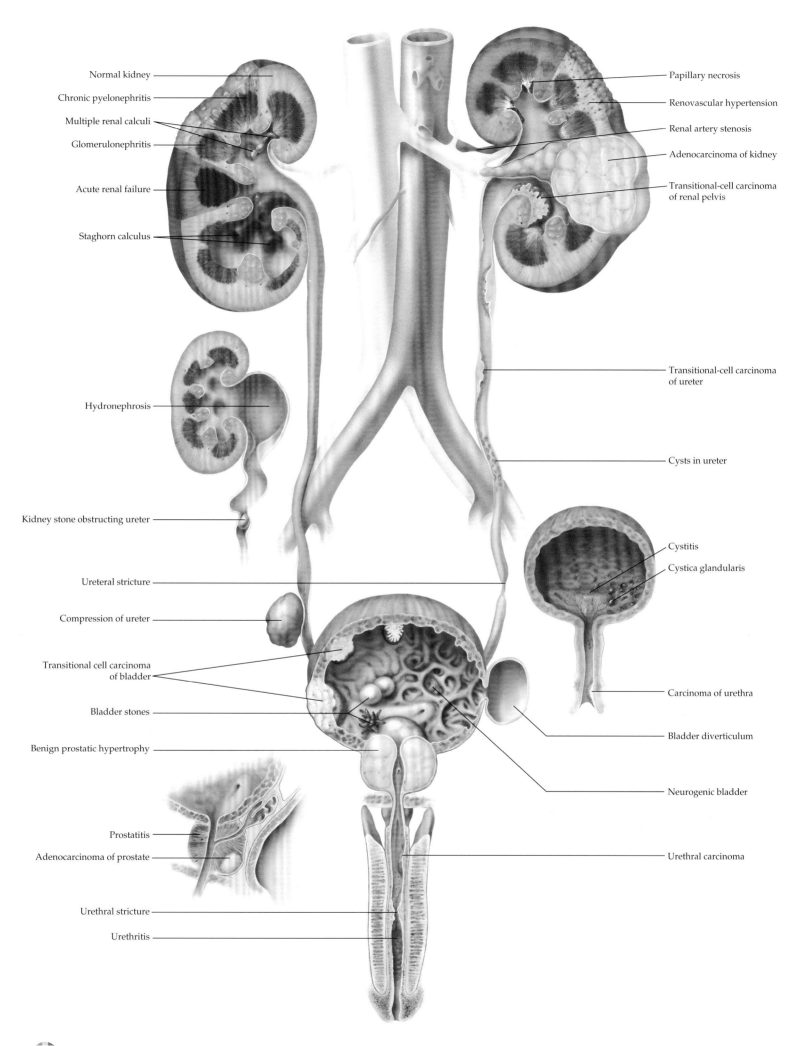

Normal kidney

Chronic pyelonephritis

Multiple renal calculi

Glomerulonephritis

Acute renal failure

Staghorn calculus

Hydronephrosis

Kidney stone obstructing ureter

Ureteral stricture

Compression of ureter

Transitional cell carcinoma of bladder

Bladder stones

Benign prostatic hypertrophy

Prostatitis

Adenocarcinoma of prostate

Urethral stricture

Urethritis

Papillary necrosis

Renovascular hypertension

Renal artery stenosis

Adenocarcinoma of kidney

Transitional-cell carcinoma of renal pelvis

Transitional-cell carcinoma of ureter

Cysts in ureter

Cystitis

Cystica glandularis

Carcinoma of urethra

Bladder diverticulum

Neurogenic bladder

Urethral carcinoma

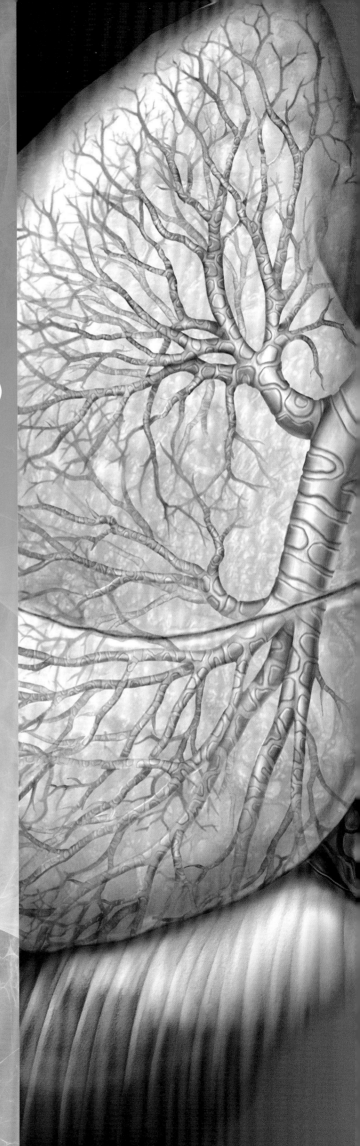

RESPIRATORY DISEASES & DISORDERS

- **Understanding Allergies**
- **Understanding Asthma**
- **Chronic Obstructive Pulmonary Disease (COPD)**
- **Diseases of the Lung**

UNDERSTANDING ALLERGIES

What Is an Allergy?

An allergy is an overreaction or hypersensitivity of the body's immune system to normally harmless substances, called allergens. An allergic reaction occurs when the body's immune system responds to an allergen as if the substance were disease causing. Subsequent exposures to this substance can result in physical symptoms that range from mild to life threatening.

Who Gets Allergies?

The tendency to develop allergies is thought to be inherited, because they commonly develop in those who have a family history of allergies. It is possible for anyone to develop allergies at any age. Environmental factors can make our immune systems overly sensitive. This could then trigger allergies in people with no family history or hasten the onset in those with a family history.

What Are Common Allergens?

Allergens can enter the body in a number of different ways, including inhaling, eating/drinking, injection (as with bee venom), and contact with the skin or eyes. Common allergens include pollen, mold, animal hair or dander, dust mites, certain medications (eg, penicillin), and certain foods (eg, peanuts, eggs, milk, wheat, and seafood).

Anaphylaxis: An Allergic Emergency

Anaphylaxis is a life-threatening reaction. The onset of this reaction may occur within seconds or minutes of exposure. Symptoms may include a red rash over most of the body. Skin becomes warm to the touch, intense tightening and swelling of the airways make breathing difficult, and there is a drop in blood pressure. Breathing can stop, and the body may slip into shock. If medication is not administered quickly, heart failure and death can result within minutes in the most severe reactions. Allergens in insect venom and medications such as antibiotics are more likely to cause anaphylaxis than are any other allergens. Anaphylaxis is not a common reaction and can be controlled with prompt medication and the help of a physician.

Managing Allergies

The first step in managing allergies is to identify the type of reaction you are having, whether it is watery eyes, sneezing, or difficulty breathing. Second, try to identify the trigger or the situation that led to the symptoms. Ask yourself a few questions:

- *Where did the reaction occur?*
- *Inside or outside?*
- *Were you eating or drinking?*
- *Were there any animals or insects near you?*
- *Were you wearing any new clothing?*
- *Did you use a new soap or detergent?*

A physician can perform skin or blood allergy tests with a variety of common allergens. Once the allergen has been identified, manage your allergies by following some tips:

- *Avoid allergens when possible.*
- *Avoid tobacco smoke and other irritants.*
- *Use medication as prescribed.*
- *See a doctor regularly.*
- *Stay healthy.*

Seafood

Drugs

Mold

Peanuts

Pollen

Dander

Dust mites

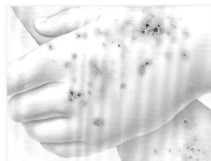

Hay Fever (Allergic Rhinitis)

Commonly caused by exposure to ragweed and some tree pollens. It affects the eyes and nose. It causes sneezing; runny nose; watery, itchy eyes; irritated, itchy throat; and sometimes, a stuffy, blocked nose.

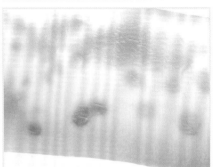

Sinusitis

An inflammation, or swelling, of the tissue lining the sinuses. Symptoms may include facial pain/pressure, a "stuffy head" (congestion), nasal stuffiness, nasal discharge, and loss of sense of smell.

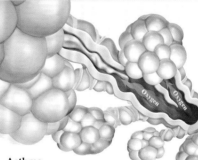

Eczema (Atopic Dermatitis)

A group of medical conditions that cause the skin to become inflamed or irritated. It causes itchy, red rashes of the skin characterized by lesions, scaling, and flaking.

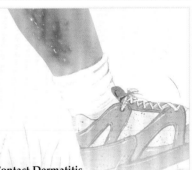

Hives (Urticaria)

An outbreak of swollen, pale red bumps or patches (wheals) on the skin, as a result of the body's adverse reaction to certain allergens, or for unknown reasons.

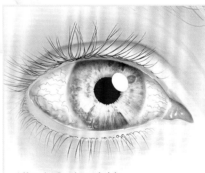

Asthma

Affects the respiratory system, causing coughing, wheezing, and chest tightness after exposure to an allergen. Common allergens that worsen asthma include plant pollens and dust mites.

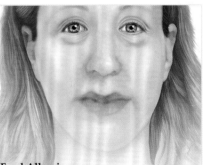

Contact Dermatitis

An inflammation of the skin caused by direct contact with an irritating or allergy-causing substance (such as poison ivy or latex gloves). It causes redness, itching, swelling, or rashes on the skin.

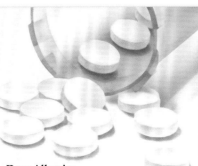

Allergic Conjunctivitis

An inflammation of the conjunctiva, the tissue that lines the eyeball and inside of the eyelid, associated with allergies. The eye becomes red, itchy, and watery.

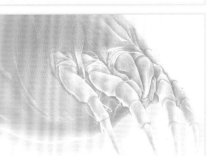

Food Allergies

Symptoms include swelling of lips, throat, face, and tongue; upset stomach; vomiting; abdominal cramps; hives; and skin rashes. Food allergies may be life threatening.

Drug Allergies

Certain medicines can trigger allergic reactions ranging from mild rashes to life-threatening symptoms, which can affect any tissue or organ in the body.

Household Allergies

Dust mites are microscopic organisms that feed on live and shed skin tissue. Mites are commonly found on pillows, mattresses, and upholstered furniture. Mite feces are responsible for a majority of the year-round types of allergies, and are a major cause of asthma.

© 2005 Wolters Kluwer

Published by Anatomical Chart Company, Skokie, IL. Medical illustrations by Lik Kwong, MFA, in consultation with David Lipson, MD.

UNDERSTANDING ASTHMA

Carbon dioxide exhaled

Oxygen inhaled

What Happens in an Asthma Attack?

What Is Asthma?
Asthma is a chronic disease of the lungs in which inflammation causes the airways to narrow, making breathing more difficult.

What Causes Asthma?
Although the actual cause of asthma is not known, many studies have shown that it may be due to a combination of factors. We do know that asthma is not contagious like the flu. We also know that people have a higher risk of developing asthma if a family member has had an asthma attack or if they live with people who smoke.

How Is Asthma Diagnosed?
There is no single or definitive test for asthma. It is diagnosed based on a review of the patient's medical history and those of his or her family. There are many tests your doctor may use to get more information about your condition. These include pulmonary function tests, allergy tests, blood tests, and chest and sinus x-rays.

A Smooth muscle tightens the airways.

Smooth muscle

Alveoli

B Sides of airways have become inflamed and swollen, making it harder for oxygen to get to alveoli.

Oxygen

C Excess mucus has formed inside the airways.

Sides of airways are thin to allow more space for oxygen to get to alveoli.

Oxygen

Bronchiole During an Asthma Attack

Healthy Bronchiole

How Do the Lungs Work?
When you breathe, you draw in (inhale) fresh air and oxygen into your lungs and expel (exhale) stale air and carbon dioxide from your lungs.

1. The incoming air goes through a network of airways (bronchial tubes) that reach the lungs.
2. As the air moves through the lungs, the bronchial tubes become progressively smaller, like branches of a tree.
3. At the end of the smallest tubes are alveolar sacs, the site of gas exchange between the lungs and the circulatory system.
4. Oxygen enters the alveolar sacs, where it passes to the bloodstream and is then used by the body.
5. Carbon dioxide (waste product) from the bloodstream enters the alveolar sacs to be carried out of the lungs.

Monitoring Your Asthma by Zone

Green Zone	Yellow Zone	Red Zone
No asthma symptoms. Able to do usual activities and sleep without coughing, wheezing, or breathing difficulty.	There may be coughing, wheezing, and mild shortness of breath. Sleep and usual activities may be disturbed. May be more tired than usual.	Symptoms may include frequent, severe cough; severe shortness of breath; wheezing; trouble talking while walking; rapid breathing.
Action: Keep controlling/preventing your asthma symptoms. Continue to take your asthma medicines exactly as prescribed by your health care specialist, even if you have no symptoms and feel fine.	**Action:** Keep controlling your asthma symptoms and add your prescribed quick-relief medicine. Call to discuss the situation with your doctor or health care specialist.	**Action:** Go to an emergency room.

Symptoms of Asthma
Symptoms of asthma often vary from time to time in an individual. The severity of an asthma attack can increase rapidly, so it is important to treat your symptoms.

Adult Symptoms
• Wheezing
• Chest tightness
• Coughing
• Difficulty breathing
• Shortness of breath

Childhood Symptoms
• Coughing at night or during sleep
• Diminished responsiveness
• Constant rattly cough
• Frequent chest colds
• Rapid breathing
• Weak cry
• Grunt when nursing or have difficulty feeding
• Chest might feel "funny"
• Unexplained irritability

Common Asthma Triggers
The airways in an asthmatic person are extremely sensitive to certain factors known as triggers. When stimulated by these triggers, the airways overreact with abnormal inflammation that leads to swelling, increased mucus secretion, and muscle contraction of the air passages. Examples of asthma triggers include the following:

• Pollution: cigarette smoke,* smog, strong odors from painting or cooking, scented products
• Allergens: animal dander, dust mites, cockroaches, pollen, mold
• Cold air or changes in weather
• Illness and infections
• Exercise
• Medications such as pain relievers
• Sulfites or other additives in food and beverages
• GERD (gastroesophageal reflux disease)

The proteins on dust mites are among the allergens that may trigger an asthma attack.

People can have trouble with one or more triggers. Your doctor can help you identify your asthma triggers and ways to avoid them.

*The risk of asthma is increased in children who are regularly exposed to cigarette smoke.

Management of Asthma
Asthma is a chronic disease that can be controlled to allow normal daily activities. By controlling your asthma every day, you can prevent serious symptoms and take part in all activities. If your asthma is not well controlled, you are likely to have symptoms that can make you miss school or work and keep you from doing other things you enjoy. Although there is no cure, here are some important prevention strategies:
• Recognize attacks early.
• Take medication as directed.
• Avoid tobacco smoke.
• Identify and avoid triggers.
• Talk with your doctor to find ways to improve your health.
• Get the influenza vaccination (flu shot) every year and a pneumococcal vaccination (pneumonia shot) every 5 years.

Wolters Kluwer Anatomical Chart Co., Skokie, IL. Medical illustrations by Dawn Scheuerman, MAMS, in consultation with David A. Lipson, MD.

Chronic Obstructive Pulmonary Disease (COPD)

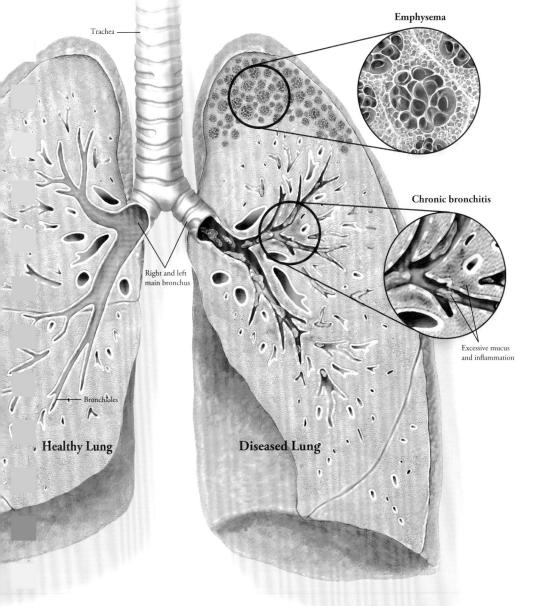

Trachea

Right and left main bronchus

Bronchioles

Healthy Lung

Diseased Lung

Emphysema

Chronic bronchitis

Excessive mucus and inflammation

COPD is a term used to describe chronic airflow obstruction that is mainly associated with emphysema and chronic bronchitis.

In normal healthy breathing, air moves in and out of the lungs to meet the demands of the body; this is impaired in COPD. Patients with COPD may develop a chronic cough and shortness of breath. Symptoms may be minimal early in the disease, but tend to worsen with time.

COPD is a major global health problem that causes significant disability. It is the fourth leading cause of death in the United States, and its global prevalence continues to rise.

Emphysema

When you inhale, air travels down your windpipe (trachea) and into your lungs through branching tubes (bronchi). These tubes continue to divide, like the branches of a tree, into smaller tubes that end in tiny air sacs (alveoli). The air sacs have very thin walls full of tiny blood vessels (capillaries). Emphysema causes inflammation within the small airways and the fragile walls of the air sacs. This inflammation can destroy some of the wall's elasticity and cause small airways to collapse when you exhale; stale air is trapped in your lungs, leaving you to work harder to get adequate oxygen in and carbon dioxide out. Destruction of the air sacs prevents oxygen from getting into the bloodstream and creates holes in the lung. This contributes to breathlessness.

Chronic Bronchitis

Prolonged inhalation of irritants, such as cigarette smoke, inflames the airways. Chronic bronchitis is characterized by ongoing persistent inflammation, cough, and excessive production of mucus that blocks the airways.

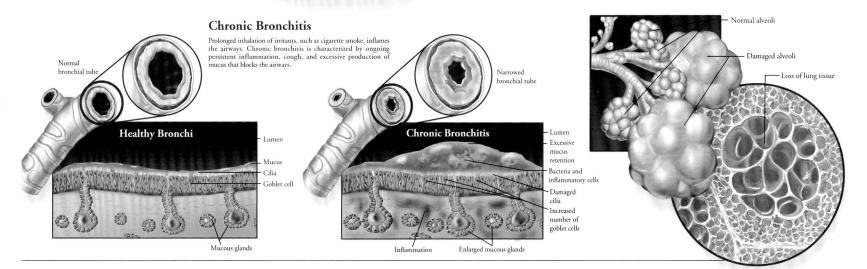

Normal bronchial tube

Healthy Bronchi

Lumen

Mucus

Cilia

Goblet cell

Mucous glands

Narrowed bronchial tube

Chronic Bronchitis

Lumen

Excessive mucus retention

Bacteria and inflammatory cells

Damaged cilia

Increased number of goblet cells

Inflammation

Enlarged mucous glands

Normal alveoli

Damaged alveoli

Loss of lung tissue

Signs and Symptoms

Subtle at first, these problems worsen with age and as the disease progresses. Patients may have the following:

- Persistent cough
- Increased mucus production
- Shortness of breath, even on minimal exertion
- Frequent respiratory infections
- Wheezing
- Oxygen deficiency in the blood
- Abnormal pulmonary function

At an advanced stage, chronic bronchitis and emphysema may be associated with chest deformities, heart enlargement, depression and anxiety, severe respiratory failure, overwhelming deconditioning and disability, and death.

Diagnosis

Chest Imaging—Chest x-rays or CAT (computerized axial tomography) scans display lung tissue and chest structures. They may help to rule out other conditions such as pneumonia and lung cancer.

Pulmonary Function Test—Spirometry is the most common lung function test to measure lung capacity and airway obstruction.

Arterial Blood Gas Analysis—Measures the amount of oxygen and carbon dioxide in the blood.

Sputum Analysis—Detects respiratory infections.

Risk Factors

Smoking—Cigarette smoking is by far the most important risk factor for COPD. Smoking increases inflammation in the lung; some inflammatory changes may partially reverse if the person stops smoking. However, the risk of disease increases with an increased rate of smoking. Pipe smokers, cigar smokers, and those exposed to large amounts of secondhand smoke are also at risk.

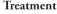

Air Pollution—Occupational or long-term exposure to ozone, chemical fumes, vapors, and dust can irritate and inflame your lungs, especially if you also smoke.

Recurrent or Chronic Respiratory Infections—Frequent viral and bacterial infections may increase the risk of developing COPD. Long-standing asthma, especially if poorly controlled, may also increase the risk.

Genetics—A genetic disorder known as alpha-1 antitrypsin deficiency may predispose a person to the development of COPD. Researchers suspect that other genetic factors may also make certain smokers more susceptible to the disease.

Prevention

Unlike some diseases, the vast majority of COPD cases are linked directly to cigarette smoking. The best way to prevent COPD is by not starting to smoke or by quitting smoking. Avoid places where other people smoke; secondhand smoke exposure can cause disease and premature death in children and adults who do not smoke. Secondhand smoke contains hundreds of chemicals known to be toxic or cancer causing.

Avoid exposure to chemical fumes and dust. If you work with specific lung irritants, talk to your supervisor about the best ways to protect yourself.

Treatment

Treatment objectives for COPD include relieving symptoms such as breathlessness and cough, slowing the decline in lung function, decreasing the risk of exacerbation, and improving quality of life.

Smoking Cessation—Stopping all smoking is the most essential step in any treatment plan for smokers with COPD. There are many treatment options and organizations that can provide you with additional support.

Bronchodilators and Inhaled Steroids—There are several different types of bronchodilators that can help relax the muscles around the airways to improve airflow and help cough and secretion clearance. Inhaled steroids can reduce airway inflammation. Combinations of bronchodilators and steroids can reduce the rate of decline of lung function and reduce the risk of exacerbation. Other long-acting bronchodilators may improve quality of life and reduce exacerbation risk also. Various medications may be prescribed to help maximize symptom control.

Oxygen Therapy—For patients who require it, supplemental oxygen can lessen breathlessness with exertion and prolong survival. Oxygen concentrators can be provided for home use, and portable oxygen may be used outside the home to aid activities.

Antibiotics and Vaccinations—Antibiotics help treat bacterial infections that can aggravate COPD symptoms. Pneumococcal vaccination and annual influenza vaccinations are important in preventing complications.

Pulmonary Rehabilitation—This is a comprehensive program to improve quality of life, strength, conditioning, and sense of well-being. Pulmonary rehabilitation may improve activities of daily living.

Surgical Treatments—Select patients with advanced disease may be candidates for lung reduction surgery or lung transplantation.

Control Your Breathing—Your physician or respiratory therapist can offer breathing and relaxation techniques to help you breathe more easily and efficiently. Effective coughing, postural drainage, and chest physiotherapy can help mobilize secretions.

DISEASES OF THE LUNG

Influenza (Flu)

The flu is a contagious viral infection of the nose, throat, and lungs. The flu leaves the body susceptible to other lung diseases if not properly treated.

Signs and Symptoms:

- Runny or stuffy nose
- Sore throat
- Headache
- Nasal congestion
- Muscle aches
- High fever
- Cough

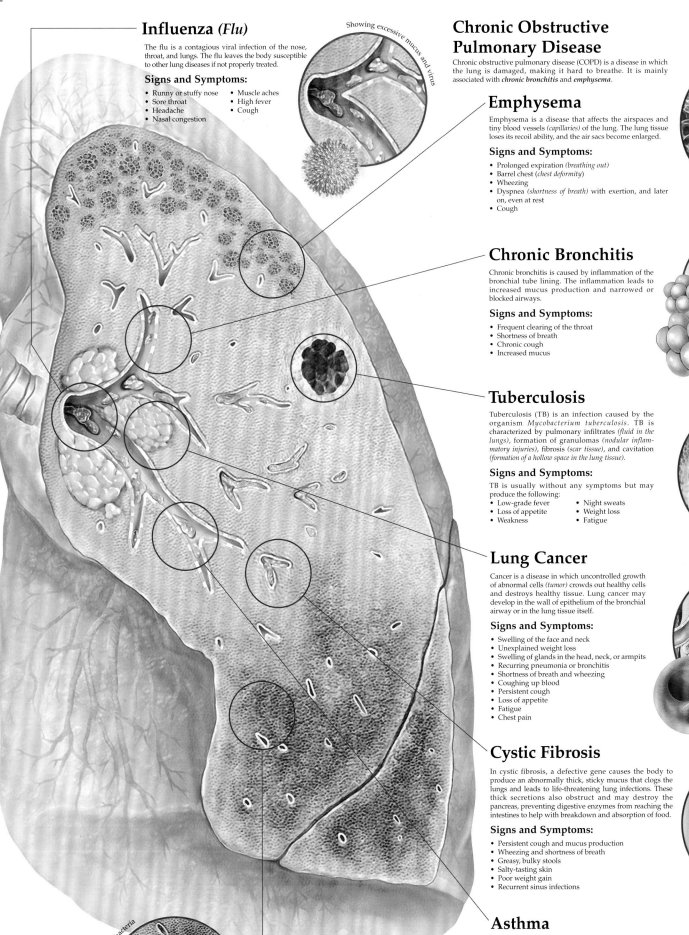

Showing excessive mucus and virus

Chronic Obstructive Pulmonary Disease

Chronic obstructive pulmonary disease (COPD) is a disease in which the lung is damaged, making it hard to breathe. It is mainly associated with *chronic bronchitis* and *emphysema*.

Emphysema

Emphysema is a disease that affects the airspaces and tiny blood vessels *(capillaries)* of the lung. The lung tissue loses its recoil ability, and the air sacs become enlarged.

Signs and Symptoms:

- Prolonged expiration *(breathing out)*
- Barrel chest *(chest deformity)*
- Wheezing
- Dyspnea *(shortness of breath)* with exertion, and later on, even at rest
- Cough

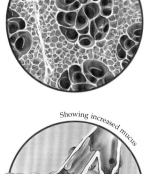

Showing enlarged air sacs

Chronic Bronchitis

Chronic bronchitis is caused by inflammation of the bronchial tube lining. The inflammation leads to increased mucus production and narrowed or blocked airways.

Signs and Symptoms:

- Frequent clearing of the throat
- Shortness of breath
- Chronic cough
- Increased mucus

Showing increased mucus

Tuberculosis

Tuberculosis (TB) is an infection caused by the organism *Mycobacterium tuberculosis*. TB is characterized by pulmonary infiltrates *(fluid in the lungs)*, formation of granulomas *(nodular inflammatory injuries)*, fibrosis *(scar tissue)*, and cavitation *(formation of a hollow space in the lung tissue)*.

Signs and Symptoms:

TB is usually without any symptoms but may produce the following:

- Low-grade fever
- Loss of appetite
- Weakness
- Night sweats
- Weight loss
- Fatigue

Showing cavity in lung tissue

Lung Cancer

Cancer is a disease in which uncontrolled growth of abnormal cells *(tumor)* crowds out healthy cells and destroys healthy tissue. Lung cancer may develop in the wall of epithelium of the bronchial airway or in the lung tissue itself.

Signs and Symptoms:

- Swelling of the face and neck
- Unexplained weight loss
- Swelling of glands in the head, neck, or armpits
- Recurring pneumonia or bronchitis
- Shortness of breath and wheezing
- Coughing up blood
- Persistent cough
- Loss of appetite
- Fatigue
- Chest pain

Showing tumor and bronchoscopic view

Cystic Fibrosis

In cystic fibrosis, a defective gene causes the body to produce an abnormally thick, sticky mucus that clogs the lungs and leads to life-threatening lung infections. These thick secretions also obstruct and may destroy the pancreas, preventing digestive enzymes from reaching the intestines to help with breakdown and absorption of food.

Signs and Symptoms:

- Persistent cough and mucus production
- Wheezing and shortness of breath
- Greasy, bulky stools
- Salty-tasting skin
- Poor weight gain
- Recurrent sinus infections

Showing thick, sticky mucus

Asthma

Asthma is a disease in which the bronchial airways of the lungs become narrow. An asthma episode is the body's reaction to an irritating substance or allergen that has been inhaled. During an asthma episode, the walls of the airways in the lungs become narrowed, thick, and swollen with sticky mucus, making breathing difficult.

Signs and Symptoms:

- Tightness in the neck and/or chest area
- Wheezing or coughing, especially at night or after exercise
- Difficulty breathing
- Symptoms may worsen during an upper respiratory or sinus infection

Showing narrowed airway and increased mucus

Pneumonia

Pneumonia is an infection in which the air sacs in the lungs become filled with pus or other fluids. This can impair oxygen delivery through the lungs to other tissue and can cause cells to function improperly.

Signs and Symptoms:

- Sputum *(phlegm)* production
- Chest pain on inspiration *(breathing in)*
- Shaking chills
- Cough
- Fever

Showing inflammation and bacteria

  Wolters Kluwer Anatomical Chart Company, Skokie, IL. Medical illustrations by Lik Kwong, MFA, in consultation with David Lipson, MD.

HEALTHY LIFESTYLE ISSUES

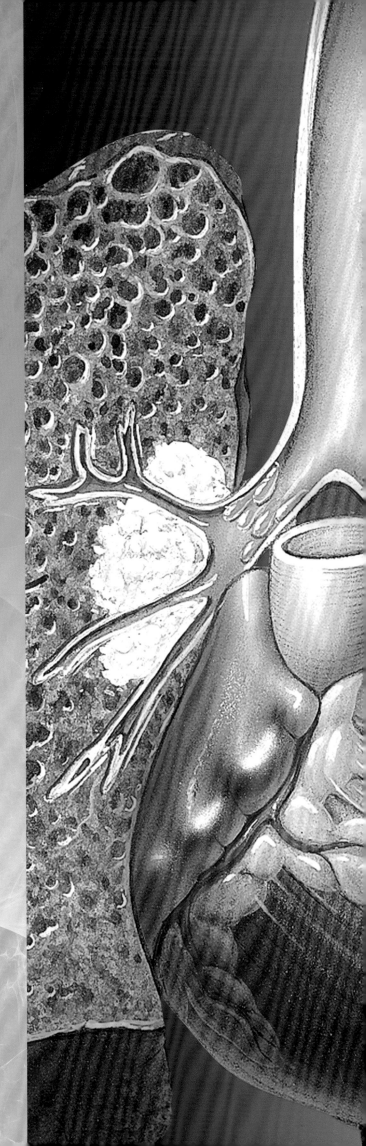

Understanding
Menopause

Menopause is defined as the date after 12 consistent months without periods. It occurs when the production of the hormones estrogen and progesterone significantly declines. The average age at which menopause occurs in the United States is now 51. Menopause is a natural aging process. However, it can also occur due to premature ovarian failure (decreased ovarian hormone production in women under age 40) or surgical removal of the ovaries. Menopause is the start of a menstrual-free lifestyle and no need for birth control.

Perimenopause is the transition into menopause. It can begin as early as a few months to several years prior to menopause and ends with menopause. During this stage, women experience menstrual irregularities (changes in cycle lengths or missed periods) and symptoms of menopause.

What Are the Changes I Might Expect?

While some women may only experience the irregularity and eventual ending of menstrual periods, other women may experience a variety of physical and mental/emotional changes.

The most common signs and symptoms of menopause are no periods for 12 months, hot flashes/night sweats, sleep difficulties, and vaginal dryness.

Some changes you may experience:

Hair Growth
- Thinning of scalp hair
- Darkening/thickening of body hair, such as facial hair

Breasts and Body Changes
- Less firm breasts
- Weight gain

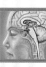
Emotional and Mental Symptoms
- Mood changes/disturbances
- Irritability
- Decreased sex drive
- Lack of concentration/forgetfulness
- Depression
- Nervousness

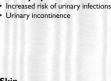
Urinary System
- Increased risk of urinary infections
- Urinary incontinence

Heart and Circulatory System
- Increased risk of heart disease, high blood pressure, and high cholesterol

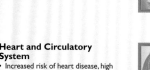
Reproductive System
- Amenorrhea (no more periods)
- Painful intercourse caused by vaginal thinning and dryness
- Increased risk of vaginal infections
- Decreased size of fibroids (noncancerous tumors)
- Decreased symptoms of endometriosis (uterus lining grows outside of the uterus) in women who had it prior to menopause

Skin
- Hot flashes—redness and/or sweating on the face, neck, and chest
- Sleep disturbances and night sweats (hot flashes occurring at night)
- Thinning of skin, loss of elasticity
- Sensitivity to sun exposure

Bone
- Increased risk of osteoporosis (loss of bone mass)

Medications

Other medications for specific symptoms are available; these include medicines for hot flashes, urinary incontinence, and maintenance of bone strength.

Hormone Therapy
Taking hormone therapy (HT) may be a complicated decision for many women; there may be both potential risks and significant benefits to HT. It is important to explore individual risks and benefits with your health care provider before starting HT.

Benefits of Hormone Therapy Include the Following:
- Decreased hot flashes
- Decreased vaginal dryness and irritation
- Slowed bone loss and decreased risk of fractures
- Improved sleep/decreased mood swings
- Decreased risk of colorectal cancer (with estrogen plus progestin therapy)

Risks of Hormone Therapy Include the Following:
- Blood clots
- Heart attack
- Stroke
- Breast cancer
- Gallbladder disease
- Endometrial cancer (with estrogen alone)

Complementary and Alternative Medicine (CAM)
Talk to your health care provider before starting CAM; some may be beneficial and safe (black cohosh), while others may be ineffective and even dangerous (ginseng, red clover, vitamin E). Current studies do not provide conclusive evidence, and more research is being conducted to determined its safety and effectiveness.

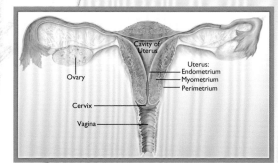

Cavity of Uterus

Uterus:
- Endometrium
- Myometrium
- Perimetrium

Ovary

Cervix

Vagina

The Role of Hormones

The changes experienced during menopause are the body's reaction to the decrease in estrogen and progesterone (hormones produced by the ovaries).

Estrogen
- Declining estrogen production causes inconsistent ovulation and irregular periods.
- Decreased estrogen is also associated with increased risk of heart disease and bone loss.

Progesterone
- Declining progesterone levels may lead to irregular periods and "spotting."

Staying Healthy After Menopause
Women should take advantage of preventive options such as the following:
- Avoid the triggers that can cause hot flashes including:
  - Hot environments
  - Hot or spicy foods
  - Alcohol
  - Caffeine
  - Stress
- Don't smoke.
- Use a water-based vaginal lubricant or moisturizer. Stay sexually active.
- Exercise regularly. Include weight-bearing exercise (such as walking, jogging, or dancing) at least 3 days a week; this may slow down bone loss and improve overall health.
- Get adequate sleep—avoid exercise and alcohol before sleeping.
- Eat a healthy diet that is high in fiber and calcium and low in fat and cholesterol.

In addition to eating right, exercising, getting enough sleep, and avoiding toxins like tobacco and excessive alcohol, it is important to continue regular visits to your health care provider for the following examinations and tests:

Examination	Frequency
Pelvic examination and Pap smear	Every 2-3 years after 3 consecutive negative annual tests
Breasts examination	Self breast examinations once a month and at annual visits
Mammogram	Once every 1-2 years for women aged 40-49; every year for women aged 50+
Blood work to check thyroid function (TSH test)	Every 5 years
Blood work to check lipid profile (cholesterol and triglyceride levels)	Every 5 years
Fasting glucose (blood sugar) test	Every 3 years
Blood pressure check	At every checkup/exam (at least annually)
Fecal occult blood test (FOBT)—to check for hidden blood in the stool	Annually (may vary based on an individual's risk factors)
Colonoscopy	Every 5 years (may vary based on an individual's risk factors)
Bone scan, such as a DEXA (dual-energy x-ray absorptiometry scan)	Every 2 years (may vary based on an individual's risk factors)
Skin cancer check	Self skin checks and with annual physical exams (may vary based on an individual's risk factors)

Dangers of Alcohol

The form of alcohol we drink is ethyl alcohol. It is made from sugar, starch, and other carbohydrates by the process of fermentation with yeast.

Nervous System

Alcohol can damage many body tissues including the brain and nerves. Excessive intake of alcohol can cause temporary memory loss (blackouts), loss of consciousness, or coma. Heavier drinkers may suffer with more persistent short-term memory loss and are at an increased risk of stroke. Chronic alcoholics may develop double vision, loss of balance, and profound memory loss. The alcoholic who suddenly stops drinking may experience withdrawal symptoms, which can include shakiness, anxiety, hallucinations, and seizures. Permanent damage from alcoholism can include pain and loss of sensation in the arms and legs and loss of intelligence.

Neuron

Liver cell

Alcohol passing into liver cell

Excess alcohol continues to circulate

Hepatic sinusoid in liver tissue

Alcohol passing through sinusoid wall

Stomach wall absorbing alcohol

Alcohol Absorption

Alcohol is absorbed through the walls of the stomach and small intestine; it is carried by the blood vessels to the liver to be metabolized. Here, alcohol in the blood flows through the sinusoids, passes through the sinusoid walls, and enters the liver cells. The liver can only process about 1 oz of alcohol per hour, which is roughly equal to a standard drink; any excess amount will continue to circulate throughout the entire body until the liver is able to process more.

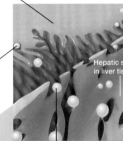

Esophageal cancer

Esophageal varices

Gastritis

Gastric ulcer

Duodenal ulcer

Stomach cancer

Pancreatitis

The Digestive System

Alcohol can damage many of the organs of the digestive system. Irritation of the stomach lining, gastritis, can lead to vomiting or even bleeding from small tears in the stomach. Chronic irritation can result in gastric and duodenal ulcers. Alcoholics may also develop acute and chronic pancreatitis. Alcoholics with cirrhosis frequently develop esophageal varices, which are dilated veins in the esophagus; these may rupture and bleed profusely. A number of cancers are linked to heavy alcohol consumption and are a major cause of death among alcoholics; these include cancers of the larynx, esophagus, stomach, and liver. Alcoholics who smoke are at a particularly high risk for developing these cancers.

Excessive drinking can lead to alcohol abuse and dependence, the disease of alcoholism. Some individuals may be genetically predisposed to alcoholism. Consequences of the misuse of alcohol include destroyed relationships, loss of job, poor health, and death.

However, moderate alcohol consumption may have health benefits, particularly in preventing cardiovascular disease. Moderate drinking is defined as two drinks (or less) a day for males under 65 years of age and one drink (or less) per day for males over the age of 65 years and females.

Complications

Alcohol passing through placental barrier

Maternal blood

Fetal blood vessels

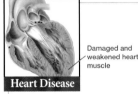

Heart Disease

Damaged and weakened heart muscle

Short-term effects from a drink may include an increased pulse rate and dilation of blood vessels. Chronic alcohol use can cause serious damage such as high blood pressure and cardiomyopathy, a damaged and weakened heart muscle. Heavy drinkers are also at risk for an abnormal heart rhythm.

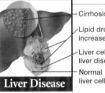

Liver Disease

Cirrhosis

Lipid droplets increased

Liver cell in fatty liver disease

Normal liver cell

The liver is frequently affected in chronic alcohol abuse. Consequences may include fatty liver disease (an accumulation of fat droplets inside liver cells), alcohol-induced hepatitis, and cirrhosis. In cirrhosis, liver cells die and scar tissue irreversibly changes the normal architecture of the liver tissue.

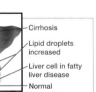

Reproduction

Excessive alcohol consumption may cause impotence and damage to sperm in men. For women, alcohol use may cause interruptions in menstruation and damage to eggs. Alcohol may also cause serious problems for the developing fetus that can affect its entire life. The baby can be born with fetal alcohol syndrome, be underweight, grow slower, and have birth defects, as well as have a smaller brain and a lower IQ, or mental retardation. Alcohol may be passed to a baby through breast milk as well.

Intoxication: The blood alcohol concentration (the amount of alcohol in the blood) roughly correlates with the level of mental and physical impairment (intoxication). The level of alcohol measured in breath tests closely parallels the blood alcohol concentration. Given the same amount of alcohol, levels from person to person can vary depending on body weight, body fat, recent meals, tolerance, and how quickly the alcohol was consumed. Women and older individuals tend to be more sensitive to the effects of alcohol. Once alcohol is in your blood, the only effective cure for intoxication is time. The legal limit for driving in all U.S. states is 80 mg/dL or 0.08%.

The intoxicating effects of alcohol may increase the likelihood of being injured or dying a premature accidental death. Many auto accidents, suicides, and murders are alcohol related.

Intoxicating Effects
(Nonalcoholics)

More than 25 mg/dL or 0.025% (blood alcohol concentration)	More than 100 mg/dL or 0.1% (blood alcohol concentration)	If alcohol levels continue to rise...
• Mild intoxication • Altered mood • Impaired thinking • Incoordination	• Decreased inhibition • Euphoria followed by depression • Hostility • Slurred speech • Double vision	• Stupor • Coma

Chronic Bronchitis

A persistent cough is the major symptom of chronic bronchitis. In the large airways, the size and number of mucus-secreting glands are increased. In the small airways, there are increased secretions, impaired handling of secretions, and inflammation that can impair or obstruct airflow.

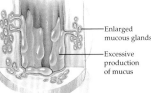

Enlarged mucous glands

Excessive production of mucus

Tobacco smoke is a highly dangerous substance that contains more than 200 known poisons. Every time a smoker lights up, he or she is being injured to some degree by inhaling these poisons. A two-pack-a-day smoker shortens his or her life expectancy by 8 years, and even light smokers shorten their life expectancy by 4 years. To date, lung cancer is one of the leading causes of death in men, yet incidence is increasing among women often resulting in death at an earlier age than men.

Stroke

Smoking is a major cause of arteriosclerosis, or hardening of the arteries. In turn, arteriosclerosis is a chief cause of stroke. Strokes occur when one of the arteries of the brain ruptures, forms a blood clot, or bleeds into the brain. Once brain tissue is destroyed, it cannot be repaired.

Blood clot

Increased amount of secretion obstructing small airways

Brain

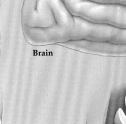

Emphysema

With emphysema, the lungs irreversibly lose their ability to take up oxygen, causing great breathing difficulty. Lung tissue loses its elasticity, air sacs tear, and stale air becomes trapped, eventually causing death from lack of oxygen.

Dilation and destruction of bronchiole walls

Tongue

Mouth and Throat Cancer

Cancer-causing chemicals from tobacco products increase the risk of cancer of the lip, cheek, tongue, and larynx (voice box). The removal of these cancers can be disfiguring and can result in loss of the larynx.

Cancer of the tongue

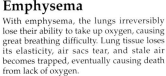

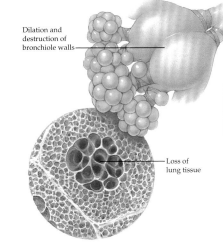

Loss of lung tissue

Smoker's Lung

Healthy Lung

Heart Disease

Arteriosclerosis is responsible for most heart attacks. Plaque, deposits of cholesterol, collecting in the coronary arteries narrows the vessels until eventually the oxygen supply to the heart is stopped. Smoking accelerates this process.

Plaque in coronary artery wall

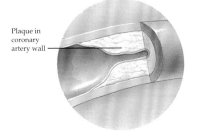

Heart

Lung Cancer

Tobacco smoke is the most common cause of lung cancer. One in 10 heavy smokers will get lung cancer, and in most cases it will be fatal. It is the leading cause of death by cancer because it is difficult to detect, and it is likely to spread early to the liver, brain, and bones.

Stomach

Gastric Ulcer

Smoking increases the production of gastric juices, raising the acidity level and eroding the lining of the stomach. Painful ulcers result from these eroded areas and increase the risk for hemorrhage and perforation of the stomach lining.

Ulcer in lining of stomach

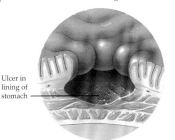

Metastasis to hilar lymph nodes

Tumor projecting into bronchi

Metastasis to carinal lymph nodes

Bladder Cancer

Chemicals from tobacco are absorbed into the bloodstream and leave the body through the urine. These cancer-causing chemicals are always in contact with the bladder, increasing the risk for bladder cancer.

Maternal blood supply

Placenta

Maternal blood containing chemicals mixes with fetal blood supply

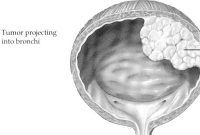

Fetal blood vessels

Tumor projecting into bronchi

Bronchoscopic View

Tumor

Fetal Risk

Carbon monoxide in smoke reduces the oxygen level in the fetus' (unborn child's) blood, while nicotine restricts the blood flow from the mother to the fetus. Smoking is thought to retard the growth of the fetus, resulting in low birth weight. Smoking also increases the risk of premature birth and infant death.

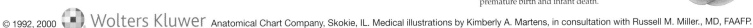

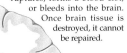

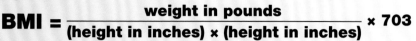
BMI and Waist Circumference

Body Mass Index

The BMI (body mass index) is a way to interpret the risk of weight for your height. The higher the BMI, the higher the risk.

English Formula

$$BMI = \frac{\text{weight in pounds}}{(\text{height in inches}) \times (\text{height in inches})} \times 703$$

Metric Formula

$$BMI = \frac{\text{weight in kilograms}}{(\text{height in meters}) \times (\text{height in meters})}$$

BMI does have some limitations:
- It may overestimate body fat in athletes or people with muscular build.
- It may underestimate body fat in older person and others who have lost muscle mass.
- There may be differences in what constitutes healthy and unhealthy BMIs among different ethnic groups, such as people of Asian descent.

Waist Circumference

The waist circumference measurement is useful in assessing risk for adults who are normal or overweight according to the BMI table. It is a good indicator of abdominal fat.

People with high-risk waistlines are at higher risk for developing other diseases such as diabetes, hypertension (high blood pressure), dyslipidemia (abnormal blood fats such as high LDL cholesterol, high triglycerides and/or low HDL cholesterol), and cardiovascular disease.

High-Risk Waistline

For Men: Over 40 inches (102 cm)
For Women: Over 35 inches (88 cm)

If a patient has a normal or overweight BMI and has a high-risk waistline, he or she is considered one (1) risk category above that defined by the BMI. Please note that there may be differences in what constitutes a higher risk waistline among different ethnic groups.

How to measure: The measurement for waist circumference is at the ILIAC CREST.

Classification	BMI
Underweight	Below 18.5
Normal	18.5-24.9
Overweight	25.0-29.9
Obese Class I	30.0-34.9
Obese Class II	35.0-39.9
Obese Class III (Extreme Obesity)	40.0+

Body Mass Index (BMI) Table

To determine your BMI, look down the left column to find your height and then look across that row and find the weight that is nearest your own. Now look to the top of the column to find the number that is your BMI.

BMI	Normal						Overweight					Obese										Extreme Obesity															
---	19	20	21	22	23	24	25	26	27	28	29	30	31	32	33	34	35	36	37	38	39	40	41	42	43	44	45	46	47	48	49	50	51	52	53	54
Height (feet & inches)													Body Weight (pounds)																							
4'10" (58")	91	96	100	105	110	115	119	124	129	134	138	143	148	153	158	162	167	172	177	181	186	191	196	201	205	210	215	220	224	229	234	239	244	248	253	258
4'11" (59")	94	99	104	109	114	119	124	128	133	138	143	148	153	158	163	168	173	178	183	188	193	198	203	208	212	217	222	227	232	237	242	247	252	257	262	267
5'0" (60")	97	102	107	112	118	123	128	133	138	143	148	153	158	163	168	174	179	184	189	194	199	204	209	215	220	225	230	235	240	245	250	255	261	266	271	276
5'1" (61")	100	106	111	116	122	127	132	137	143	148	153	158	164	169	174	180	185	190	195	201	206	211	217	222	227	232	238	243	248	254	259	264	269	275	280	285
5'2" (62")	104	109	115	120	126	131	136	142	147	153	158	164	169	175	180	186	191	196	202	207	213	218	224	229	235	240	246	251	256	262	267	273	278	284	289	295
5'3" (63")	107	113	118	124	130	135	141	146	152	158	163	169	175	180	186	191	197	203	208	214	220	225	231	237	242	248	254	259	265	270	278	282	287	293	299	304
5'4" (64")	110	116	122	128	134	140	145	151	157	163	169	174	180	186	192	197	204	209	215	221	227	232	238	244	250	256	262	267	273	279	285	291	296	302	308	314
5'5" (65")	114	120	126	132	138	144	150	156	162	168	174	180	186	192	198	204	210	216	222	228	234	240	246	252	258	264	270	276	282	288	294	300	306	312	318	324
5'6" (66")	118	124	130	136	142	148	155	161	167	173	179	186	192	198	204	210	216	223	229	235	241	247	253	260	266	272	278	284	291	297	303	309	315	322	328	334
5'7" (67")	121	127	134	140	146	153	159	166	172	178	185	191	198	204	211	217	223	230	236	242	249	255	261	268	274	280	287	293	299	306	312	319	325	331	338	344
5'8" (68")	125	131	138	144	151	158	164	171	177	184	190	197	203	210	216	223	230	236	243	249	256	262	269	276	282	289	295	302	308	315	322	328	335	341	348	354
5'9" (69")	128	135	142	149	155	162	169	176	182	189	196	203	209	216	223	230	236	243	250	257	263	270	277	284	291	297	304	311	318	324	331	338	345	351	358	365
5'10" (70")	132	139	146	153	160	167	174	181	188	195	202	209	216	222	229	236	243	250	257	264	271	278	285	292	299	306	313	320	327	334	341	348	355	362	369	376
5'11" (71")	136	143	150	157	165	172	179	186	193	200	208	215	222	229	236	243	250	257	265	272	279	286	293	301	308	315	322	329	338	343	351	358	365	372	379	386
6'0" (72")	140	147	154	162	169	177	184	191	199	206	213	221	228	235	242	250	258	265	272	279	287	294	302	309	316	324	331	338	346	353	361	368	375	383	390	397
6'1" (73")	144	151	159	166	174	182	189	197	204	212	219	227	235	242	250	257	265	272	280	288	295	302	310	318	325	333	340	348	355	363	371	378	386	393	401	408
6'2" (74")	148	155	163	171	179	186	194	202	210	218	225	233	241	249	256	264	272	280	287	295	303	311	319	326	334	342	350	358	365	373	381	389	396	404	412	420
6'3" (75")	152	160	168	176	184	192	200	208	216	224	232	240	248	256	264	272	279	287	295	303	311	319	327	335	343	351	359	367	375	383	391	399	407	415	423	431
6'4" (76")	156	164	172	180	189	197	205	213	221	230	238	246	254	263	271	279	287	295	304	312	320	328	336	344	353	361	369	377	385	394	402	410	418	426	435	443

Source: National Heart, Lung, and Blood Institute.

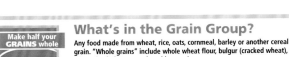

Your food and physical activity choices each day affect your health—how you feel today, tomorrow, and in the future.

By making small changes each day, you can create a lifetime of health.

The COLORS of Health

Fruits and vegetables are great sources of many vitamins and minerals that may help protect you from chronic diseases.

To get a healthy variety, think color. Eating fruits and vegetables of different colors gives your body a wide range of valuable nutrients, like fiber, folate, potassium, and vitamins A and C. Some examples include green spinach, orange sweet potatoes, black beans, yellow corn, purple plums, red watermelon, and white onions. For more variety, try new fruits and vegetables regularly.

Tips for Healthy Eating

Enjoy your food, but eat less and avoid oversized portions.

Foods to Increase

- Increase vegetable and fruit intake.
- Eat a variety of vegetables, especially dark-green and red and orange vegetables and beans and peas.
- Consume at least half of all grains as whole grains.
- Increase intakes of fat-free or low-fat milk and milk products, such as milk, yogurt, cheese, or fortified soy beverages.
- Choose a variety of protein foods, which include seafood, lean meat and poultry, eggs, beans and peas, soy products, and unsalted nuts and seeds.
- Increase the amount and variety of seafood consumed by choosing seafood in place of some meat and poultry.
- Replace protein foods that are higher in solid fats with choices that are lower in solid fats and calories and/or are sources of oils.
- Use oils to replace solid fats where possible.
- Choose foods that provide more potassium, dietary fiber, calcium, and vitamin D, which are nutrients of concern in American diets. These foods include vegetables, fruits, whole grains, milk and milk products.

Foods to Reduce

- Cut back on salt and sodium; learn to enjoy the natural taste of foods.
- Reduce daily sodium (salt) intake to <2,300 milligrams (mg) and further reduce intake to 1,500 mg among persons who are 51 and older.
- Cut back on sweet treats. Skip the soda.
- Cut back on solid fats, saturated fats, and/or trans fats. Solid fats are found in whole milk, cheese, higher-fat meats, and other foods such as butter, lard, chicken skin, and shortening. Some oils such as palm, palm kernel, and coconut are also higher in saturated fats.
- Keep dietary cholesterol to <300 milligrams a day. Reduce dietary cholesterol by cutting back on animal sources of food, such as beef, poultry, and eggs. If an item is high in saturated fat, it's probably also high in cholesterol.
- Drink water instead of sugary drinks.

GRAINS

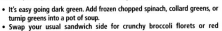
Make half your GRAINS whole

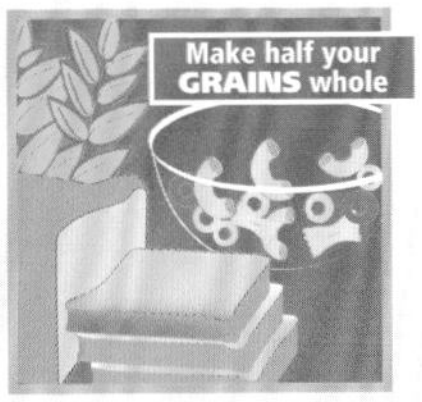

What's in the Grain Group?

Any food made from wheat, rice, oats, cornmeal, barley or another cereal grain. "Whole grains" include whole wheat flour, bulgur (cracked wheat), oatmeal, whole cornmeal, and brown rice.

- Get a whole grain head start with oatmeal or whole grain cereal.
- Use whole grains in mixed dishes such as barley in vegetable soup or stews, bulgur in casseroles, or brown rice in stir fries.
- Change it up. Make your sandwich on 100% whole wheat or oatmeal bread. Snack on popcorn or whole grain crackers. Examples of refined grain products are white flour, degermed cornmeal, white bread, and white rice.

Daily Recommendation: Most people consume enough grains, but few are whole grains. At least 1/2 of all grains eaten should be whole grains. The amount you eat depends on your age, sex, and level of physical activity.

VEGETABLES

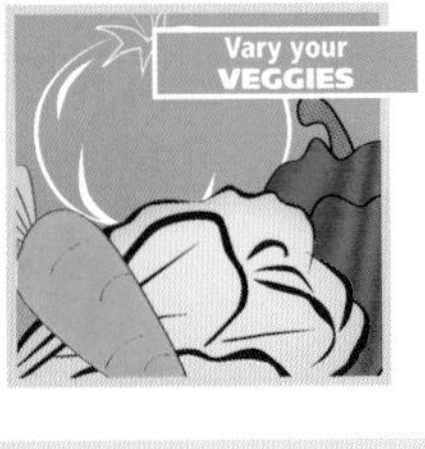

Vary your VEGGIES

What's in the Vegetable Group?

Any vegetable or 100% vegetable juice. Vegetables may be raw or cooked; fresh, frozen, canned or dried/dehydrated.

- It's easy going dark green. Add frozen chopped spinach, collard greens, or turnip greens into a pot of soup.
- Swap your usual sandwich side for crunchy broccoli florets or red pepper strips.
- Microwave a sweet potato for a delicious side dish.

Daily Recommendation: The amount of vegetables you need to eat depends on your age, sex, and level of physical activity. Total daily amounts range from 1 to 3 cups.*

FRUIT

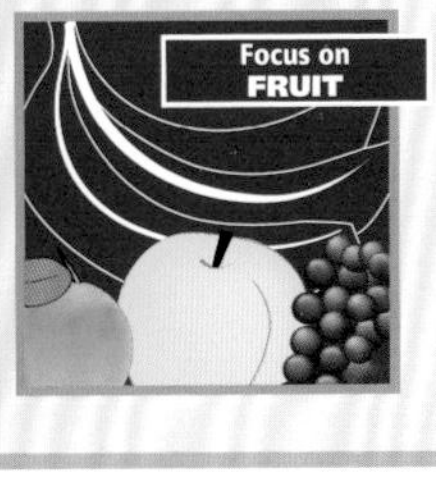

Focus on FRUIT

What's in the Fruit Group?

Any fruit or 100% fruit juice. Fruits may be fresh, canned, frozen, or dried; and may be whole, cut up, pureed, raw, or cooked.

- Bag some fruit for your morning commute. Toss in an apple to munch with lunch and some raisins to satisfy you at snack time.
- Buy fresh fruits in season when they taste best and cost less.
- Never be fruitless! Stock up on peaches, pears, and apricots canned in fruit juice or frozen so they're always on hand.

Daily Recommendation: The amount of fruit you need to eat depends on age, sex, and level of physical activity. Recommended daily amounts range from 1 to 2 cups per day.*

DAIRY

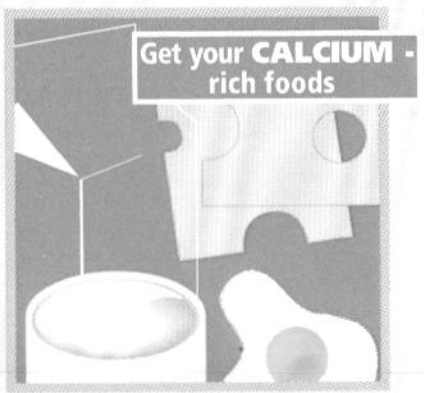

Get your CALCIUM-rich foods

What's in the Dairy Group?

All fluid milk products and many foods made from milk. Examples include cheese and yogurt. Make your milk group choices fat free or low fat.

- Use fat-free or low-fat milk instead of water when you make oatmeal, hot cereals, or condensed cream soups, such as cream of tomato.
- Snack on low-fat or fat-free yogurt. Try it as a dip for fruits and veggies and a topper for baked potatoes.
- Order your latte or hot chocolate with fat-free (skim) milk.

Daily Recommendation: Most milk group choices should be fat free or low fat. The amount of food from the dairy group you need to eat depends on age, sex, and level of physical activity. Recommended daily amounts range from 2 to 3 cups.*

Special Tip: Although cream cheese, cream and butter are made from milk, they don't count in the Milk group because they contain little or no calcium. Instead, if you eat these foods, count them as "extra" calories from solid fats.

PROTEIN

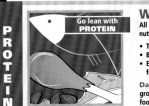
Go lean with PROTEIN

What's in the Protein Group?

All foods made from beef, pork, poultry, fish, dry beans or peas, eggs, nuts, and seeds. Make your meat and poultry choices lean or low-fat.

- Trim visible fat from meat, and remove skin from poultry.
- Broil, grill, roast, or poach meat, poultry, or fish instead of frying.
- Enjoy pinto or kidney beans on a salad or a hearty split pea or lentil soup for extra protein.

Daily Recommendation: Most people eat enough food from this group but need to make leaner and more varied selections of these foods. The amount of food from the protein foods group you need to eat depends on age, sex, and level of physical activity. Daily protein requirements range from 2 to 6 ounces per day.*

These amounts are appropriate for individuals who get <30 minutes per day of moderate physical activity, beyond normal daily activities. Those who are more physically active may be able to consume more while staying within calorie needs.

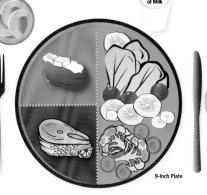

Here's a trick to make sure your meals include appropriate portions of key food groups:

As you plan a meal, keep in mind that fruits or vegetables should cover half your dinner plate, and lean protein and whole grains should each take a quarter of the plate.

8 oz. Glass of Milk

9-Inch Plate

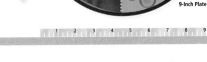

OILS/FATS

Limit your OILS/FATS

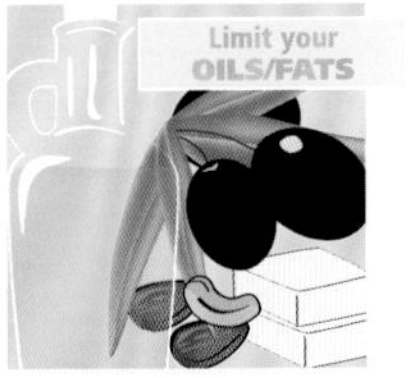

Oils—Know Your Fats: Oils are fats that are liquid at room temperature such as canola, corn, and olive oils. Mayonnaise and certain salad dressings are made with oils. Nuts, olives, avocados, and some fish such as salmon are naturally rich in oils.

- Use some vegetable oil instead of butter for cooking and baking.
- Toss salad with salad oil and flavored vinegar.
- Try thin slices of avocado on a sandwich, or sprinkle some nuts on a salad.

Some common oils are canola oil, corn oil, cottonseed oil, olive oil, safflower oil, soybean oil, and sunflower oil.

Solid fats are fats that are solid at room temperature, like butter and shortening. Solid fats come from many animal foods and can be made from vegetable oils through a process called hydrogenation.

Some common solid fats are butter, beef fat (tallow, suet), chicken fat, pork fat (lard), stick margarine, and shortening.

Daily Recommendation: Most people consume enough oil in the foods they eat, such as nuts, fish, cooking oil, and salad dressings. A person's allowance for oils depends on age, sex, and level of physical activity but should be kept to a minimum.

How to Read a Nutrition Label

1 Serving Size: Compare the serving size listed on the label with your own portion and then multiply each nutrient accordingly. For example, if a serving of cereal is 1 cup and you've poured yourself 2 cups, you must double all the nutrient values on the label (eg, 2 g of fat/serving becomes 4 g).

Be aware that the amount of food contained in what looks like a single-serving package, like a small bag of chips, may be more than one serving.

2 Calories: More than half of Americans are overweight or obese. Therefore, consumers are advised to watch their calorie intake. According to the Food and Drug Administration, 40 calories per serving is low, 100 calories is moderate, and 400 calories or more is high.

3 Nutrients: Eating too much saturated and trans fat, dietary cholesterol, and sodium is linked to heart disease, some cancers, and obesity. These nutrients should be limited as much as possible.

**4 Many American adults do not get their daily requirement of fiber, vitamins A and C, calcium, and iron. Lacking these nutrients can contribute to diseases such as certain cancers, osteoporosis, and anemia. Consumers should make sure their intake of these vitamins and minerals is adequate.

5 Footnote: The Daily Values (DV) that were determined by public health and nutrition experts are listed in the footnote section of the nutrition label. DV, or recommended intakes for certain nutrients, are based on a 2,000-calorie diet. Be aware of the following statement, which precedes the DV information: "Percent Daily Values are based on a 2,000 calorie diet. Your Daily Values may be higher or lower depending on your calorie needs."

6 % Daily Value: The percent DV is shown in the right-hand column of the nutrition label. Keep in mind that the DV is based on the serving amount. If a larger portion is consumed, multiply the DV percent accordingly. Use the guidelines when interpreting the DV percentages: 5% DV or less is low; 20% DV or more is high.

Note:
Trans fat does not have a DV because this type of fat should be avoided as much as possible.

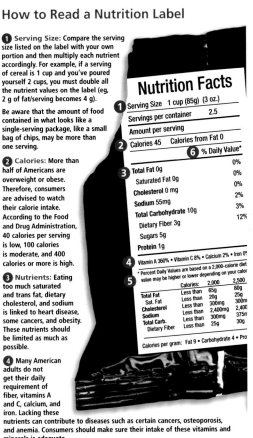

Nutrition Facts

1 Serving Size 1 cup (85g) (3 oz.)
Servings per container 2.5
Amount per serving

2 Calories 45   Calories from Fat 0

6 % Daily Value*

	% Daily Value*
3 Total Fat 0g	0%
Saturated Fat 0g	0%
Cholesterol 0 mg	0%
Sodium 55mg	2%
Total Carbohydrate 10g	3%
Dietary Fiber 3g	12%
Sugars 5g	
Protein 1g	

4 Vitamin A 360% • Vitamin C 8% • Calcium 2% • Iron 0%

*Percent Daily Values are based on a 2,000-calorie diet. Your Daily Values may be higher or lower depending on your calorie needs:

	Calories:	2,000	2,500
Total Fat	Less than	65g	80g
Sat. Fat	Less than	20g	25g
Cholesterol	Less than	300mg	300mg
Sodium	Less than	2,400mg	2,400mg
Total Carb.	Less than	300mg	375mg
Dietary Fiber	Less than	25g	30g

Calories per gram: Fat 9 • Carbohydrate 4 • Protein 4

© 1993, 1999, 2003, 2005, 2011 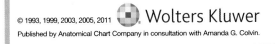 Wolters Kluwer

Published by Anatomical Chart Company in consultation with Amanda G. Colvin.

MyPyramid.gov
STEPS TO A HEALTHIER YOU

How to Use the Food Pyramid

MyPyramid was developed to be consistent with USDA dietary guidelines. The color-coded vertical slices of the pyramid correspond with each of the six food groups. Fruits, vegetables, and grains, the wider sections of the pyramid, are the recommended staples of a balanced diet.

A personalized feature of this pyramid is an online interactive tool that calculates an adult's suggested daily calorie needs (based on height, weight, and activity level). Additionally, the climbing figure across the side of the pyramid underscores the importance of daily physical activity for weight control.

Variety and proportionality of all food groups are also emphasized in MyPyramid (www.mypyramid.gov).

Healthy Diet Plan

If you are concerned about your diet, no particular food plan is magical and no particular food must be either included or avoided. Your diet should consist of foods that you like or can learn to like, that are available to you, and that are within your means. The most effective diet programs for weight loss and maintenance are based on physical activity and reasonable serving sizes, with less frequent consumption of foods high in fat and refined sugars.

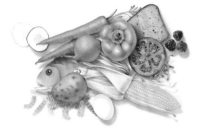

Physiological Hazards That Accompany Low-Carbohydrate Diets

- **Heart Failure**
  Carbohydrates maintain sodium and fluid balance. A carbohydrate deficiency promotes loss of sodium and water, which can adversely affect blood pressure and cardiac function if not corrected.

- **High Blood Cholesterol**
  Low-carbohydrate diets can raise blood cholesterol because in these diets, fruits, vegetables, breads, and cereals are replaced by meat and dairy products, which are rich in fat and protein. High fat and protein intakes, especially from meat and dairy products, raise LDL and total cholesterol.

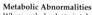
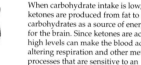

- **Metabolic Abnormalities**
  When carbohydrate intake is low, ketones are produced from fat to replace carbohydrates as a source of energy for the brain. Since ketones are acids, high levels can make the blood acidic, altering respiration and other metabolic processes that are sensitive to an increase or decrease in acidity.

The Risk in Low-Carbohydrate Diets

Low-carbohydrate diets, especially if undertaken without medical supervision, can be dangerous. Low-carbohydrate diets are designed to cause rapid weight loss by promoting an undesirably high concentration of ketone bodies (a by-product of fat metabolism). The sales pitch is that you'll never feel hungry and that you'll lose weight faster than you would on any "ordinary diet"; however, these claims are misleading. Fast weight loss means loss of water and lean tissue, which are rapidly regained when people begin eating their usual diets again. The amount of body fat lost will be the same as with a conventional low-calorie diet. Fat loss is always equal to the difference between energy consumed in food and energy expended in activity.

Overweight Problems

As the amount of body fat increases, especially around the abdomen, so does the risk of:

- Respiratory disease
- Obstructive sleep apnea
- Complications during surgery
- Gallbladder disease
- Stroke
- Non–insulin-dependent (type 2) diabetes
- Some forms of cancer, especially breast and colon
- Coronary heart disease
- Hypertension

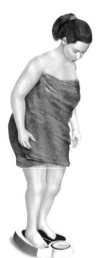

Strategies for Diet Planning:

- Adopt a realistic long-term plan.
- Individualize your diet, include foods that you like, and indulge yourself once in a while.
  - Include foods from all five food groups.
  - Eat foods that contain a lot of nutrients.
  - Stress the Dos and not the Don'ts in your diet and your way of living.
  - Eat on a regular schedule at least 3 times a day. Don't skip meals.

Suggestions and Tips for Physical Activity:

- Walk at least 10-20 minutes daily.
- Take the stairs instead of the elevator.
- Sports (basketball, baseball, tennis...).
- Dance classes.
- Aerobics classes.
- Incorporate exercise into your normal routine.
- Concentrate on strengthening your muscles as well as your heart and lungs.

What Is Your Body Mass Index?

Your body mass index (**BMI**) is your weight in kilograms divided by the square of your height in meters. It is used to indicate whether or not you are overweight or underweight.

How to Calculate Your Body Mass Index:

1. Convert your weight in pounds (lb) to kilograms (kg) by dividing your weight in pounds by 2.2 kg.
2. Convert your height in inches (in.) to meters (m) by multiplying your height in inches by 0.0254 m.
3. Take your height in meters and square it by multiplying it by itself.
4. Divide your weight in kilograms by your height in meters squared (your calculated height from step 3).

Example: Mark weighs 150 lb and is 5 ft, 10 in. tall (70 in.).

1. 150 lb ÷ by 2.2 kg = 68.18 kg
2. 70 in. × 0.0254 m = 1.778 m
3. 1.778 m × 1.778 m = 3.161 m^2
4. 68.18 kg ÷ 3.161 m^2 = 21.56

Mark's BMI is 21.56

Acceptable Weight for Height Based on Body Mass Index

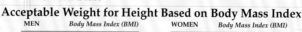
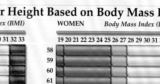

MEN	*Body Mass Index (BMI)*	WOMEN	*Body Mass Index (BMI)*

Color key for weight: = under = average = marginal = over = severely over

Source: Compiled from Body Mass Index Table from Hamilton, Whitney, and Sizer. 1991. *Nutrition Concepts and Controversies.* New York: West and Body Mass Index from 1998 Centers for Disease Control and Prevention.

Excess Fat Distribution

Apple Shaped: Excess fat is distributed around the abdomen. Common in men, in postmenopausal women, and with aging. Associated with increased risk of Type 2 diabetes.

Pear Shaped: Excess fat is distributed around the hips and buttocks. Common in women. Associated with increased risk of osteoarthritis.

Understanding Calories

Calories are a standard measurement of heat energy. Technically, 1 calorie is 1 kilocalorie, which is the amount of heat required to raise the temperature of 1 kg of water by 1°C.

A person's energy needs are determined by the amount of lean tissue or muscle and by the level of activity. A small, elderly, sedentary woman may need only about 1,200 calories to meet her energy needs each day, while a tall, young, physically active man may need as many as 4,000 calories daily.

How to Calculate Your Total Daily Energy (Calorie) Needs

1. Convert your weight from pounds (lb) to kilograms (kg) by dividing your weight in pounds by 2.2 lb/kg.
2. Multiply your weight in kilograms by 30 kcal/kg if you are a man and 25 kcal/kg if you are a woman.

Example

1. 150 lb ÷ by 2.2 lb/kg = 68.18 kg
2. 68.18 kg × 30 kcal/kg = 2,045 kcal

Result: A 150 lb man needs approximately 2,045 kcal (calories) a day to maintain his weight.

Energy Demands of Activities

Activity	Body Weight (lb)				
	110	125	150	175	200
	CALORIES PER MINUTE				
Aerobics	6.8	7.8	9.3	10.9	12.4
Basketball (vigorous)	10.7	12.1	14.6	17.0	19.4
Bicycling *13 miles per hour*	5.0	5.6	6.8	7.9	9.0
Cross-country skiing *8 miles per hour*	11.4	13.0	15.6	18.2	20.8
Golf (carrying clubs)	5.0	5.6	6.8	7.9	9.0
Rowing (vigorous)	10.7	12.1	14.6	17.0	19.4
Running *5 miles per hour*	6.7	7.6	9.2	10.7	12.2
Soccer	10.7	2.1	14.6	17.0	19.4
Studying	1.2	1.4	1.7	1.9	2.2
Swimming *20 yards per minute*	3.5	4.0	4.8	5.6	6.4
Walking (brisk pace) *3.5 miles per hour*	3.9	4.4	5.2	6.1	7.0

Source: Compiled from Hamilton, Whitney, and Sizer. 1991. *Nutrition Concepts and Controversies.* New York: West.

Underweight Problems

When body weight decreases to 15%-20% below desirable weight (BMI < 18.5), the amount of energy being consumed is not sufficient to support the function of vital organs. Lean tissue is being broken down and utilized for energy to make up the deficit. The results are as follows:

- Low body temperature
- Abnormal electrical activity in the brain
- Altered blood lipids
- Dry skin
- Impaired immune response
- Loss of digestive function
- Abnormal hormone levels
- Malnutrition
- Anemia

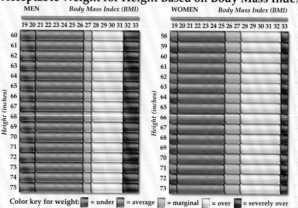

Risks of Obesity

What Is Obesity?

- Obesity has become a major public health problem, with both genetic and environmental causes.
- The term **obesity** is defined as weight that is higher than what is considered healthy for a given height.
- The percentage of body tissue that is body fat varies according to gender and age. People are considered obese if their weight is 20% or more above their ideal weight range.
- Morbid obesity is when a person is 50% or more above their ideal weight range.
- Obesity is a long-term disease that increases the risk of developing other serious health problems, including high blood pressure, high blood cholesterol, type 2 diabetes, heart disease, and stroke.

Causes of Obesity

- Genetic, behavioral, and hormonal factors can affect weight. The main cause of obesity is energy imbalance—when more energy (calories) is taken in from food than is used through physical activity.
- Other factors that can contribute to a person's weight are age, gender, genetics, environmental factors, psychological factors, illness, and medication.

Obesity and Children

- The prevalence of child obesity is increasing rapidly worldwide. In the United States alone, 1 out of 5 children is overweight.
- When compared to children with a healthy weight, overweight children are more likely to have an increased risk of heart disease, high blood pressure, and type 2 diabetes.
- Children who are obese are also more likely to grow up to be obese adults.
- As with adults, lack of exercise, unhealthy eating habits, genetics, and lifestyle can all influence a child's weight.
- Doctors or health care professionals are the best people to help determine if your child is overweight. By considering your child's age and growth patterns, they can decide if the child's weight is healthy.

How Is Body Fat Measured?

There are two ways in which body fat is measured.

- Waist circumference is a common measurement used to assess abdominal (stomach) fat. People with excess fat that is situated mostly around the abdomen are at risk for many of the serious conditions associated with obesity. A high-risk waistline is one that is 35 in. or greater in women and 40 in. or greater in men.
- BMI is a measure of weight in relation to a person's height. For most people, BMI has a strong relationship to weight.

To calculate your BMI, use the following equations:

English Formula

$$BMI = \left(\frac{\text{weight in pounds}}{(\text{height in inches}) \times (\text{height in inches})}\right) \times 703$$

Metric Formula

$$BMI = \left(\frac{\text{weight in kilograms}}{(\text{height in meters}) \times (\text{height in meters})}\right)$$

Treatment for Adult Obesity

- Obesity is a chronic disease, and it needs long-term management. The usual focus is to reduce the risk for developing health problems and to lose the excess weight.
- If you are obese, it is best to consult a health care professional to help determine how much weight you should lose and what kind of weight loss program is appropriate.
- A good plan is to gradually reduce your weight. Weight loss of 1-2 pounds per week is a safe and healthy strategy. A successful treatment plan can include one or more of the following options: diet, physical activity, behavioral therapy, counseling, drug therapy, and surgery.

Diet

- For weight loss, a low calorie, well-balanced diet that is low in fat is recommended. Dietary therapy involves reducing the number of calories that are eaten and learning how to select portion sizes, which types of food to buy, and how to read nutrition labels. Speak with a health care professional to determine your ideal calorie intake.

Physical Activity

- Daily moderate physical activity for a total of 150-250 minutes per week (or 30 minutes per day) is important for weight loss, maintenance of weight loss, and general good health. Physical activity doesn't only involve exercise. It also includes everyday activities such as walking up stairs or yard work.

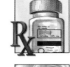

Counseling

- Sometimes, social problems (alcohol or drugs) or psychological problems (depression or anxiety) play an important part in weight gain. Individual or group counseling is an important treatment if psychological or social problems lead to overeating.

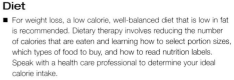

Drug Therapy

- If prescribed, drug treatment should be used in combination with a healthy diet and physical activity. Patients should have regular visits with their health care professional to monitor their progress and any side effects the medication may have.

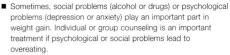

Surgery

- Surgery should be considered only for patients with morbid obesity who have not been able to lose weight with other treatment options and who are at high risk for developing other life-threatening health problems. The goal of these types of surgeries is to modify the gastrointestinal tract to reduce the amount of food that can be eaten.

Behavioral Therapy

- A successful weight loss plan involves changing eating and physical activity habits to new patterns that will promote successful weight loss and weight control.
- Behavioral therapy can include strategies such as keeping a food diary to help recognize eating habits, identifying high-risk situations (having high-calorie foods in the house) and then consciously avoiding them, and changing unrealistic beliefs related to a patient's body image. A support network, such as family, friends, or a support group, is beneficial as well.

Health Risks Associated with Obesity

If you are obese, you have a greater risk of developing serious health problems. If you lose weight, the risk is reduced. The following is a list of diseases and disorders that can develop as a result of obesity.

A Brain
Psychological disorders (low self-esteem, depression), stroke

B Esophagus
Gastroesophageal reflux disease (GERD), heartburn

C Arteries
High blood pressure, arteriosclerosis (atherosclerosis, arteriolar sclerosis), high blood cholesterol

D Lungs
Asthma, sleep apnea (interrupted breathing while sleeping)

E Heart
Coronary heart disease, heart attack

F Gallbladder
Gallstones, cancer, inflammation of the gallbladder, gallbladder disease

G Pancreas
Insulin resistance, type 2 diabetes, hyperinsulinemia

H Kidneys
Cancer, uric acid nephrolithiasis (stones in the kidneys)

I Colon
Cancer

J Bladder
Cancer, bladder control problems (stress incontinence)

K Bones
Gout (type of arthritis that deposits uric acid within the joints), osteoarthritis (degeneration of cartilage and bone in the joints)

Other possible health consequences of obesity include endometrial, breast, and prostate cancer; poor female reproductive health (menstrual irregularities, infertility, irregular ovulation, complications of pregnancy); and premature death.

For adults, BMI can also be found by using the table below. To use the BMI table, first find your weight at the bottom of the graph. Go straight up from that point until you reach the line that matches your height. Then look to see what weight group you fall in.

Healthy weight: BMI from 18.5 to 25   **Overweight:** BMI from 25 to 30   **Obese:** BMI 30 or greater

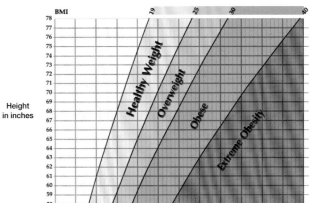

Height in inches / Weight in pounds

BMI does have some limitations. If a person is very muscular, BMI can overestimate the amount of body fat. It can also underestimate body fat if a person has lost muscle mass, as in the elderly. An actual diagnosis of obesity should be made by a health care professional.

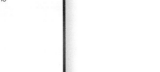

Understanding your weight

Body Weight Is Determined by Energy Balance

Obesity is excess body fat caused by long-term energy imbalance. Energy imbalance occurs when you consume more calories (energy intake through eating and drinking) than your body burns (energy expenditure through physical activity); this excess of energy intake is stored as fat in the body.

What Affects Your Energy Intake? (calories consumed)

The amount of calories consumed and absorbed by the body.

What Affects Your Energy Expenditure? (calories burned)

1. Metabolism—A process that produces the energy needed to run your body. The higher the metabolism, the more energy is burned.

Metabolism is affected by:

Muscle mass in the body—Muscle burns more calories than does fat, even when the body is resting. A variety of factors can influence the amount of muscle mass one has, including:

- **Age**—As people get older, they tend to lose muscle mass.
- **Gender**—Men usually have more muscle mass than do women.

Hormonal changes (menopause)—This can affect metabolism, but the effects are different for each person.

Genetics—The speed of metabolism can be inherited from your family.

Medications—Talk with your doctor about any prescription or over-the-counter drugs to find out more since some medications can increase or decrease metabolism.

Diet—Starvation, or abrupt calorie reduction, can cause significant drop in metabolism as the body tries to conserve energy to function.

Nicotine

Stress or emotional excitement

Body temperature due to fever or infection

Cold external temperature

2. Amount of physical activity—This includes any body movement throughout the day from walking through the grocery store, gardening, dancing, or any type of exercise.

3. Thermic effect of food—The energy required to digest, absorb, and metabolize food and drink.

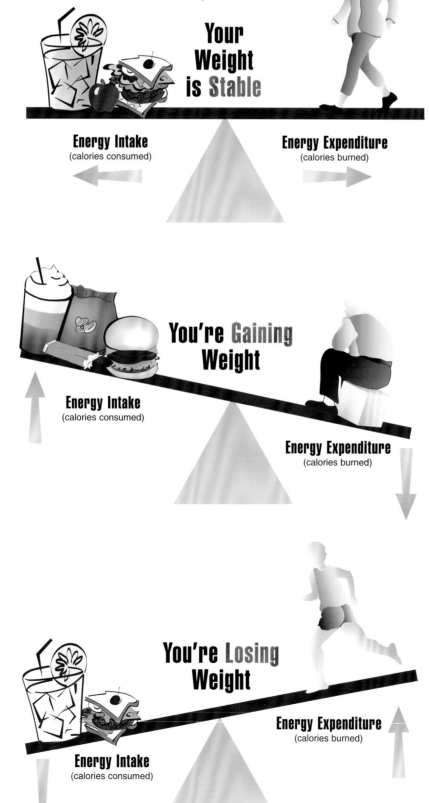

Your Weight is Stable

Energy Intake (calories consumed)

Energy Expenditure (calories burned)

You're Gaining Weight

Energy Intake (calories consumed)

Energy Expenditure (calories burned)

You're Losing Weight

Energy Intake (calories consumed)

Energy Expenditure (calories burned)

How to Lose Excess Weight

Set a reasonable goal for gradual weight loss—A realistic goal for weight loss is 5%-10% of your initial body weight in 6 months; this translates to about 1-2 lb of weight loss per week.

Improve your energy balance—Burn more calories through increased physical activity and metabolism than you consume through eating and drinking.

Focus on making small lifestyle changes—Over time these steps will add up to great results.

Track your diet and activity goals—Keep a diary or a log of all food intake and physical activity.

Talk to your doctor about other options—Medication or surgery may be a choice if you have not achieved sufficient weight loss through diet and exercise.

Ways to Help Improve Your Diet

Reduce 500-1000 calories—Decrease energy intake and increase energy expenditure each day by making better choices of food and drink and increasing your physical activity. Thirty-five hundred calories is equal to 1 lb; if you can reduce 500 calories every day from your diet and with physical activity, you will lose 1 lb in a week!

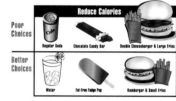

Recognize Your Eating Behaviors—One of the best ways to get a handle on eating behaviors is to keep a food dairy. Some common problems with eating patterns include the following:

- Eating large portions
- Mindless eating and grazing
- Not eating enough fruits and vegetables
- Skipping meals

Create a Supportive Environment

- **Request support**—Ask family members, friends, or coworkers to help/join you in your weight loss quest.
- **Replace unhealthy foods**—Keep healthy alternatives in your home and office.

Ways to Increase Your Physical Activity and Metabolism

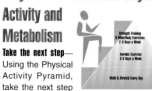

Take the next step—Using the Physical Activity Pyramid, take the next step up (from where you are) to increase the number of calories burned. Talk to your doctor about any medical limitations.

Look for ways throughout the day to be more active—Go on a walk break or take the stairs. Break your activities into 10-minute blocks, and try to add up to at least 30 minutes total per day. Track your activities every day with an activity log.

Add strength training—Use hand weights or resistance bands to increase muscle mass. This will increase metabolism and burn more calories.

CCS1020